3rd edition

review for
USMLE

**United States
Medical Licensing
Examination**

Step 1

National Medical Series

In the basic sciences

anatomy, 2nd edition
behavioral science, 2nd edition
biochemistry, 3rd edition
clinical epidemiology and
    biostatistics
genetics
hematology
histology and cell biology,
    2nd edition

human developmental anatomy
immunology, 2nd edition
introduction to clinical medicine
microbiology, 2nd edition
neuroanatomy
pathology, 3rd edition
pharmacology, 3rd edition
physiology, 2nd edition
radiographic anatomy

In the clinical sciences

medicine, 2nd edition
obstetrics and gynecology,
    3rd edition
pediatrics, 2nd edition
preventive medicine and
    public health, 2nd edition
psychiatry, 2nd edition
surgery, 2nd edition

In the exam series

review for USMLE Step 1,
    3rd edition
geriatrics

The National Medical Series for Independent Study

3rd edition

review for USMLE

United States Medical Licensing Examination

Step 1

John S. Lazo, Ph.D.

Chairman, Department of Pharmacology
Allegheny Foundation Professor of Pharmacology
University of Pittsburgh
  School of Medicine
Pittsburgh, Pennsylvania

Bruce R. Pitt, Ph.D.

Vice Chairman, Department of Pharmacology
Professor of Pharmacology
  and Anesthesiology
University of Pittsburgh
  School of Medicine
Pittsburgh, Pennsylvania

Joseph C. Glorioso, III, Ph.D.

Chairman, Department of Molecular
  Genetics and Biochemistry
William S. McEllroy Professor of
  Biochemistry
University of Pittsburgh
  School of Medicine
Pittsburgh, Pennsylvania

Harwal Publishing

Philadelphia • Baltimore • Hong Kong • London • Munich • Sydney • Tokyo

A Waverly Company

Harwal

Test I:

Figure 32–36, p 13, has been reprinted with permission from Harrison: *Principles of Internal Medicine,* 12th edition, New York, McGraw-Hill, 1991

Figure 50, p 18, has been reprinted with permission from Berne RM, Levy MN: *Human Physiology,* 3rd edition, St. Louis, CV Mosby, 1993

Figure 56, p 19, has been reprinted with permission from Murray J: *The Normal Lung,* Philadelphia, WB Saunders, 1976

Figure 59–60, p 20, has been reprinted with permission from Gilman AG, Rall TW, Nies AS, et al: Goodman and Gilman's: *The Pharmacologic Basis of Therapeutics,* 8th edition, Elmsford, NY, Pergamon Press, 1990

Figures 70–74 and 114–118, pp 23 and 33, have been reprinted with permission from Hoffman BF, and Cranefield PF: *Electrophysiology of the Heart,* New York, McGraw-Hill, 1960

Test III:

Figure 20–22, p 155, has been reprinted with permission from Robbins, SL: *Pathologic Basis of Disease,* 3rd edition, Philadelphia, WB Saunders, 1989

Figure 61–65, p 165, has been reprinted with permission from Bates DV, Macklem PT, Christie RV: *Respiratory Function in Disease,* 2nd edition, Philadelphia, WB Saunders, 1971

Figure 79–83, p 168, has been reprinted with permission from Wilson, Braunwald, Isselbacher: *Principles of Internal Medicine,* 12th edition, New York, McGraw-Hill, 1991

Test IV:

Figures 23, p 226, and 103, p 243, have been reprinted with permission from Guyton AC: *Textbook of Medical Physiology,* 8th edition, Philadelphia, WB Saunders, 1991

Figure 180–182, p 255, has been reprinted with permission from Sokolow M: *Clinical Cardiology,* 5th edition, East Norwalk, CT, Appleton & Lange, 1990

Library of Congress Cataloging-in Publication Data

Lazo, John S.
   Review for USMLE : United States medical licensing examination,
step 1 / John S. Lazo, Bruce R. Pitt, Joseph C. Glorioso III.—3rd ed.
    p. cm.—(The National medical series for independent study)
   ISBN 0-683-06265-4
   1. Medicine—Examinations, questions, etc. I. Pitt, Bruce R.
II. Glorioso, Joseph C. III. Title. IV. Title: Review for USMLE
step 1. V. Series.
   [DNLM: 1. Medicine—examination questions. W 18 L431ra 1994]
R834.5.L393 1994
610'.76—dc20
DNLM/DLC
for Library of Congress   93-41661
                                          CIP

ISBN 0-683-06265-4

10 9 8 7 6 5 4 3 2

Dedication

To Jacqui, Shayna, and Stacy

Contents

Preface

Much like the events that took place during the first quarter of this century, there are major changes currently occurring in the approach to medical education in the United States. There have been rapid advances in our understanding of the molecular basis of diseases; an enormous increase in the data that can be presented to medical students; and a consolidation of experimental methodologies in the basic sciences. As a result, there is now a general consensus that a greater emphasis should be placed on an integrated presentation of information during the first 2 years of medical school.

Few institutions provide students with a comprehensive examination that will test their grasp of the key concepts presented in their first 2 years of medical school. With the advent of the new USMLE Step 1 that de-emphasizes the traditional basic science disciplines and stresses the integrated approach, we believe it is especially important to provide students with a series of questions that will prepare them for this new format. Since the first edition, the *Review for USMLE Step 1* has undergone several iterations, reflecting the thoughtful comments of both students and faculty. In the most recent edition, we have substantially increased the patient-based questions that we hope will test your ability to integrate key basic science concepts with relevant clinical problems. We hope you will find this book useful, and we, as well as the publisher, welcome any comments you may have.

John S. Lazo
Bruce R. Pitt
Joseph C. Glorioso, III

Acknowledgments

The writing of this book could not have been accomplished without the assistance of many individuals in the Departments of Pharmacology, Molecular Genetics and Biochemistry, Human Genetics, Psychiatry, and Pathology who helped with the first two editions. We are particularly grateful to Mr. James White, MD/PhD student at the University of Pittsburgh School of Medicine, who authored many of the new questions in the third edition and without whose help this book would not have been published. Thanks are also extended to Dr. Jeff Towers and Dr. Laura Finn for supplying photomicrographs. Finally, this book could not have been succesfully published without the thoughtful and tireless assistance of Jane Velker and Donna Siegfried at Harwal Publishing.

Publisher's Note

In 1983, the National Board of Medical Examiners created a study committee to review the format of the National Board exam and to evaluate its effectiveness vis-à-vis the current state of medical education. The committee identified a number of deficiencies in format and made some sweeping recommendations on how to improve the exam. In 1986, following the recommendations of the committee, the National Board appointed Comprehensive Part I and Comprehensive Part II committees and charged them with the responsibility of creating new examinations. The results became the National Board Comprehensive Part I and Part II exams. The Part I exam was introduced in June 1991. As of 1992, this test is called the United States Medical Licensing Examination (USMLE) Step 1.

The comprehensive exam differs from the old exam in both intent and format. The intent is best described by *The Medical Board Examiner* (Winter 1990).

> (The new exam is) designed to be a broadly based, integrated examination for certification, rather than distinct achievement tests in individual basic science disciplines. Emphasis is on basic biomedical science concepts deemed important as part of the foundation for the current and future practice of medicine, including those related to the prevention of disease.

The format has been modified to reflect the objectives of the comprehensive exam. Concepts and information tested remain the same but are presented in a different framework. The new exam continues to use questions drawn from single disciplines but also includes questions designed to test whether the examinee understands and can apply concepts of basic biomedical science in an integrated, cross-discipline manner. Case studies, or vignettes, serve as clinical foundations for this approach.

The books in the National Medical Series (NMS) have always been exceptional sources of information for medical students. By using the narrative outline, the books facilitate learning a large amount of information in a short period of time. Whether they are used for course study, exam preparation, or Board review, the NMS books will continue to offer medical students a reliable low-cost way to excel.

This particular book on the NMS list is intended to be used along with the other NMS books and to help medical students:

- prepare for the USMLE Step 1 by reviewing all of the major content areas covered on the exam
- become acquainted and comfortable with the exam format
- determine areas where they may need further study through the use of the key concepts included at the beginning of each explanation

Use this book along with other material as you prepare for the exam. The authors and publisher have made every effort to ensure that all of the information in this book is accurate. Best of luck.

The Publisher

Taking a Test

One of the least attractive aspects of pursuing an education is the necessity of being examined on what has been learned. Instructors do not like to prepare tests, and students do not like to take them.

However, students are required to take many examinations during their learning careers, and little if any time is spent acquainting them with the positive aspects of tests and with systematic and successful methods for approaching them. Students perceive tests as punitive and sometimes feel that they are merely opportunities for the instructor to discover what the student has forgotten or has never learned. Students need to view tests as opportunities to display their knowledge and to use them as tools for developing prescriptions for further study and learning.

A brief history and discussion of the National Board of Medical Examiners (NBME) examinations [now the Unites States Medical Licensing Examination (USMLE)] are presented here, along with ideas concerning psychological preparation for the examinations. Also presented are general considerations and test-taking tips, as well as ways to use practice exams as educational tools. (The literature provided by the various examination boards contains detailed information concerning the construction and scoring of specific exams.)

Before the various NBME exams were developed, each state attempted to license physicians through its own procedures. Differences in the quality and testing procedures of the various state examinations resulted in the refusal of some states to recognize the licensure of physicians licensed in other states. This made it difficult for physicians to move freely from one state to another and produced an uneven quality of medical care in the United States.

To remedy this situation, the various state medical boards decided they would be better served if an outside agency prepared standard exams to be given in all states, allowing each state to meet its own needs and have a common standard by which to judge the educational preparation of individuals applying for licensure.

One misconception concerning these outside agencies is that they are licensing authorities. This is not the case; they are examination boards only. The individual states retain the power to grant and revoke licenses. The examination boards are charged with designing and scoring valid and reliable tests. They are primarily concerning with providing the states with feedback on how examinees have performed and with making suggestions about the interpretation and usefulness of scores. The states use this information as partial fulfillment of qualifications upon which they grant licenses.

Students should remember that these exams are administered nationwide and, although the general medical information is the same, educational methods and faculty areas of expertise differ from institution to institution. It is unrealistic to expect that students will know all the material presented in the exams; they may face questions on the exams in areas that were only

The author of this introduction, Michael J. O'Donnell, holds the positions of Assistant Professor of Psychiatry and Director of Biomedical Communications at the University of New Mexico School of Medicine, Albuquerque, New Mexico.

superficially covered in their classes. The testing authorities recognize this situation, and their scoring procedures take it into account.

The Exams

The first exam was given in 1916. It was a combination of written, oral, and laboratory tests, and it was administered over a 5-day period. Admission to the exam required proof of completion of medical education and 1 year of internship.

In 1922, the examination was changed to a new format and was divided into three parts. Part I, a 3-day essay exam, was given in the basic sciences after 2 years of medical school. Part II, a 2-day exam, was administered shortly before or after graduation, and Part III was taken at the end of the first postgraduate year. To pass both Parts I and II, a score equaling 75% of the total points available in each was required.

In 1954, after a 3-year extensive study, the NBME adopted the multiple-choice format. To pass, a statistically computed score of 75 was required, which allowed comparison of test results from year to year. In 1971, this method was changed to one that held the mean constant at a computed score of 500, with a predetermined deviation from the mean to ascertain a passing or failing score. The 1971 changes permitted more sophisticated analysis of test results and allowed schools to compare among individual students within their respective institutions as well as among students nationwide. Feedback to students regarding performance included the reporting of a passing or failing grade along with scores in each of the areas tested.

During the 1980s, the ever-changing field of medicine made it necessary for the NBME to examine once again its evaluation strategies. It was found necessary to develop questions in multidisciplinary areas such as gerontology, health promotion, immunology, and cell and molecular biology. In addition, it was decided that questions should test higher cognitive levels and reasoning skills.

To meet the new goals, many changes have been made in both the form and content of the examination. Changes include reduction in the number of questions to approximately 800 in Step 1 and Step 2 of the USMLE to allow students more time on each question, with total testing time reduced on Step 1 from 13 to 12 hours and on Step 2 from 12.5 to 12 hours. The basic science disciplines are no longer allotted the same number of questions, which permits flexible weighing of the exam areas. Reporting of scores to schools includes total scores for individuals and group mean scores for separate discipline areas. Only pass/fail designations and total scores are reported to examinees. There is no longer a provision for the reporting of individual subscores to either the examinees or medical schools. Finally, the question format used in the new exams is predominately multiple-choice, best-answer.

The New Format

New questions, designed specifically for Step 1, are constructed to test the student's grasp of the medical sciences in an integrated fashion—the questions are designed to be interdisciplinary. Many of these items are presented as vignettes, or case studies, followed by a series of multiple-choice, best-answer questions.

Whereas in the past the exams were scored on a normal curve, the new exam has a predetermined standard that must be met in order to pass. The exam no longer concentrates on the trivial; therefore, it has been concluded that there is a common base of information that all medical students should know in order to pass. In the past, the average student could expect to feel comfortable with only half the test and eventually would complete approximately 67% of the questions correctly, to achieve a mean score of 500. Although with the current method it is likely that the mean score will change and become higher, it is unlikely that the pass/fail rates will differ significantly from those in the past. During the first testing in 1991, there was not differential weighing of questions. However, in the future, the NBME will be researching methods of weighing questions based on both the time it takes to answer questions vis-à-vis their difficulty and the perceived importance of the information. In addition, the NBME is attempting to design a method of delivering feedback to the student that will have considerable importance in discovering weaknesses and pinpointing areas for further study if a retake is necessary.

Materials Needed for Test Preparation

In preparation for a test, many students collect far too much study material only to find that they simply do not have the time to go through all of it. They are defeated before they begin because either they leave areas unstudied, or they race through the material so quickly that they cannot benefit from the activity.

It is generally more efficient for the student to use materials already at hand: (1) class notes, (2) one good outline to cover or strengthen areas not locally stressed and to quickly review the whole topic, and (3) one good text as a reference for complex material that requires further explanation.

Also, many students attempt to memorize far too much information, rather than learning and understanding less material and then relying on that learned information to determine the answers to questions at the time of the examination. Relying too heavily on memorized material causes anxiety, and the more anxious students become during a test, the less learned knowledge they are likely to use.

Positive Attitude

A positive attitude and a realistic approach are essential to successful test taking. If the student concentrates on the negative aspects of tests or on the potential for failure, anxiety increases and performance decreases. A negative attitude generally develops if the student concentrates on "I must pass" rather than on "I can pass." "What if I fail?" becomes the major factor motivating the student to **run from failure rather than toward success**. This results from placing too much emphasis on scores rather than understanding that scores have only slight relevance to future professional performance.

The score received is only one aspect of test performance. Test performance also indicates the student's ability to use information during evaluation procedures and reveals how this ability might be used in the future. For example, when a patient enters the physician's office with a problem, the physician begins by asking questions, searching for clues, and seeking diagnostic information. Hypotheses are then developed, which will include several potential causes for the problem. Weighing the probabilities, the physician will begin to discard those hypotheses with the least likelihood of being correct. Good differential diagnosis involves the ability to deal with uncertainty, to reduce potential causes to the smallest number, and to use all learned information in arriving at a conclusion.

The same thought process can and should be used in testing situations. It might be termed **paper-and-pencil differential diagnosis**. In each question with five alternatives, of which one is correct, there are four alternatives that are incorrect. If deductive reasoning is used, as in solving a clinical problem, the choices can be viewed as having possibilities of being correct. The elimination of wrong choices increases the odds that a student will be able to recognize the correct choice. Even if the correct choice does not become evident, the probability of guessing correctly increases. Just as differential diagnosis in a clinical setting can result in a correct diagnosis, eliminating choices on a test can result in choosing the correct answer.

Answering questions based on what is incorrect is difficult for many students since they have had nearly 20 years' experience taking tests with the implied assertion that knowledge can be displayed only by knowing what is correct. It must be remembered, however, that students also can display knowledge by knowing something is wrong. **Students should begin to think in the present as they expect themselves to think in the future.**

Paper-and-Pencil Differential Diagnosis

The technique used to arrive at the answer to the following question is an example of the paper-and-pencil differential diagnosis approach.

A recently diagnosed case of hypothyroidism in a 45-year-old man may result in which of the following conditions?

(A) Thyrotoxicosis
(B) Cretinism
(C) Myxedema
(D) Graves' disease
(E) Hashimoto's thyroiditis

It is presumed that all of the choices presented in the question are plausible and partially correct. If the student begins by breaking the question into parts and trying to discover what the question is attempting to measure, it will be possible to answer the question correctly by using more than memorized charts concerning thyroid problems.

- The question may be testing if the student knows the difference between "hypo" and "hyper" conditions.
- The answer choices may include thyroid problems that are not "hypothyroid" problems.
- It is possible that one or more of the choices are "hypo" but are not "thyroid" problems; they are some other endocrine problems.
- "Recently diagnosed in a 45-year-old man" indicates that the correct answer is not a congenital childhood problem.
- "May result in" as opposed to "resulting from" suggests that the choices might include a problem that **causes** hypothyroidism rather than **results from** hypothyroidism, as stated.

By applying this kind of reasoning, the student can see that choice **A,** thyroid toxicosis, which is a disorder resulting from an overactive thyroid gland ("hyper") must be eliminated. Another piece of knowledge, that is, Graves' disease is thyroid toxicosis, eliminates choice **D.** Choice **B,** cretinism, is indeed hypothyroidism, but is a childhood disorder. Therefore, **B** is eliminated. Choice **E** is an inflammation of the thyroid gland—here the clue is the suffix "itis." The reasoning is that thyroiditis, being an inflammation, may **cause** a thyroid problem, perhaps even a hypothyroid problem, but there is no reason for the reverse to be true. Myxedema, choice **C,** is the only choice left and the obvious correct answer.

Preparing for Board Examinations

1. Study for yourself. Although some of the material may seem irrelevant, the more you learn now, the less you will have to learn later. Also, do not let the fear of the test rob you of an important part of your education. If you study to learn, the task is less distasteful than studying solely to pass a test.

2. Review all areas. You should not be selective by studying perceived weak areas and ignoring perceived strong areas. This is probably the last time you will have the time and the motivation to review **all** of the basic sciences.

3. Attempt to understand, not just memorize, the material. Ask yourself: To whom does the material apply? Where does it apply? When does it apply? Understanding the connections among these points allows for longer retention and aids in those situations when guessing strategies may be needed.

4. Try to **anticipate questions that might appear on the test**. Ask yourself how you might construct a question on a specific topic.

5. Give yourself a couple days rest before the test. Studying up to the last moment will increase your anxiety and potentially cause confusion.

Taking Board Examinations

1. In the case of the USMLE, be sure to **pace yourself** to use the time optimally. Each booklet is designed to take 2 hours. You should use all of your allotted time; if you finish too early, you probably did so by moving too quickly through the test.

2. Read each question and all the alternatives carefully before you begin to make decisions. Remember the questions contain clues, as do the answer choices. As a physician, you would not make a clinical decision without a complete examination of all the data; the same holds true for answering test questions.

3. Read the directions for each question set carefully. You would be amazed at how many students make mistakes in tests simply because they have not paid close attention to the directions.

4. It is not advisable to leave blanks with the intention of coming back to answer the questions later. Because of the way Board examinations are constructed, you probably will not pick up any new information that will help you when you come back, and the chances of getting numerically off on your answer sheet are greater than your chances of benefiting by skipping around. If you feel that you must come back to a question, mark the best choice and place a note in the margin. Generally speaking, it is best not to change answers once you have made a decision. Your intuitive reaction and first response are correct more often than changes made out of frustration or anxiety. **Never turn in an answer sheet with blanks.** Scores are based on the number that you get correct; you are not penalized for incorrect choices.

5. Do not try to answer the questions on a stimulus–response basis. It generally will not work. Use all of your learned knowledge.

6. Do not let anxiety destroy your confidence. If you have prepared conscientiously, you know enough to pass. Use all that you have learned.

7. Do not try to determine how well you are doing as you proceed. You will not be able to make an objective assessment, and your anxiety will increase.

8. Do not expect a feeling of mastery or anything close to what you are accustomed to. Remember, this is a nationally administered exam, not a mastery test.

9. Do not become frustrated or angry about what appear to be bad or difficult questions. You simply do not know the answers; you cannot know everything.

Specific Test-Taking Strategies

Read the entire question carefully, regardless of format. Test questions have multiple parts. Concentrate on picking out the pertinent key words that might help you begin to problem-solve. Words such as "always," "never," "mostly," "primarily," and so forth play significant roles. In all types of questions, distractors with terms such as "always" or "never" most often are incorrect. Adjectives and adverbs can completely change the meaning of questions—pay close attention to them. Also, medical prefixes and suffixes (e.g., "hypo-," "hyper-," "-ectomy," "-itis") are sometimes at the root of the question. The knowledge and application of grammar often are key to dissecting questions.

Multiple-Choice Questions

Read the question and the choices carefully to become familiar with the data provided. Remember, in multiple-choice questions there is one correct answer and four distractors, or incorrect answers. (Distractors are plausible and possibly correct or they would not be called distractors.) They are generally correct for part of the question but not for the entire question. Dissecting the question into parts aids in eliminating the distractors.

Many students think that they must always start at option A and make a decision before they move to B, thus forcing decisions that they are not ready to make. Your first decisions should be made on those choices you feel the most confident about.

Compare the choices to each part of the question. **To be wrong,** a choice needs to be **incorrect for only part** of the question. **To be correct,** it must be **totally** correct. If you believe a choice is partially incorrect, tentatively eliminate that choice. Make notes next to the choices regarding tentative decisions. One method is to place a minus sign next to the choices you are certain are incorrect and a plus sign next to those that potentially are correct. Finally, place a zero next to any choice you do not understand or need to come back to for further inspection. Do not feel that you must make final decisions until you have examined all choices carefully.

When you have eliminated as many choices as you can, decide which of those that remain has the highest probability of being correct. Remember to use paper-and-pencil differential diagnosis. Above all, be honest with yourself. If you do not know the answer, eliminate as many choices as possible and choose reasonably.

Vignette-Based Questions

Vignette-based questions are multiple-choice questions that use the same case, or grouped information, for setting the problem. The NBME has been researching question types that would test the student's grasp of the integrated medical basic sciences in a more cognitively complex fashion than can be accomplished with traditional testing formats. These questions allow the testing of information that is more medically relevant than memorized terminology.

It is important to realize that several questions, although grouped together and referring to one situation or vignette, are independent questions; that is, they are able to stand alone. Your inability to answer one question in a group should have no bearing on your ability to answer other questions in that group.

These are multiple-choice questions, and just as with single best-answer questions, you should use the paper-and-pencil differential diagnosis, as described earlier.

Single Best-Answer–Matching Sets

Single best-answer–matching sets consist of a list of words or statements followed by several numbered items or statements. Be sure to pay attention to whether the choices can be used more than once, only once, or not at all. Consider each choice individually and carefully. Begin with those with which you are the most familiar. It is important always to break the statements and words into parts, as with the other question formats. **If a choice is only partially correct, then it is incorrect.**

Guessing

Nothing takes the place of a firm knowledge base, but with little information to work with, even after playing paper-and-pencil differential diagnosis, you may find it necessary to guess at the correct answer. A few simple rules can help increase your guessing accuracy. Always guess consistently if you have no idea what is correct; that is, after eliminating all that you can, make the choice that agrees with your intuition or choose the option closest to the top of the list that has not been eliminated as a potential answer.

When guessing at questions that present with choices in numeric form, you will often find the choices listed in ascending or descending order. It is generally not wise to guess the first or last alternative, since these are usually extreme values and are most likely incorrect.

Using the USMLE to Learn

All too often, students do not take full advantage of practice exams. There is a tendency to complete the exam, score it, look up the correct answers to those questions missed, and then forget the entire thing.

In fact, great educational benefits can be derived if students would spend more time using practice tests as learning tools. As mentioned previously, incorrect choices in test questions are plausible and partially correct or they would not fulfill their purpose as distractors. This means that it is just as beneficial to look up the incorrect choices as the correct choices to discover specifically why they are incorrect. In this way, it is possible to learn better test-taking skills as the subtlety of question construction is uncovered.

In addition, it is advisable to go back and attempt to restructure each question to see if all the choices can be made correct by modifying the question. By doing this, four times as much will be learned. For example, the entire thrust of the sample question concerning hypothyroidism could be altered by changing the first few words to read:

"Hyperthyroidism recently discovered in . . ."
"Hypothyroidism prenatally occurring in . . ."
"Hypothyroidism resulting from . . ."

This question can be used to learn and understand thyroid problems in general, not only to memorize the answer to the question.

In the practice exams that follow, every effort has been made to simulate the types of questions and the degree of question difficulty in the USMLE Step 1. While taking these exams, the student should attempt to create the testing conditions that might be experienced during actual testing situations. Approximately 1 minute should be allowed for each question, and the entire test should be finished before it is scored.

Summary

Ideally, examinations are designed to determine how much information students have learned and how that information is used in the successful completion of the examination. Students will be successful if these suggestions are followed:

- Develop a positive attitude and maintain that attitude.
- Be realistic in determining the amount of material you attempt to master and in the score you hope to attain.
- Read the directions for each type of question and the questions themselves closely and follow the directions carefully.
- Bring the paper-and-pencil differential diagnosis approach to each question in the examination.
- Guess intelligently and consistently when guessing strategies must be used.
- Use the test as an opportunity to display your knowledge and as a tool for developing prescriptions for further study and learning.

The USMLE is not easy. It may be almost impossible for those who have unrealistic expectations or for those who allow misinformation concerning the exam to produce anxiety out of proportion to the task at hand. It is manageable if it is approached with a positive attitude and with consistent use of all the information that has been learned.

Michael J. O'Donnell

Test I

QUESTIONS

DIRECTIONS: Each of the numbered items or incomplete statements in this section is followed by answers or by completions of the statement. Select the ONE lettered answer or completion that is BEST in each case.

Questions 1–5

The schematic drawing of a cholinergic synapse in the figure below should be used to answer the following questions.

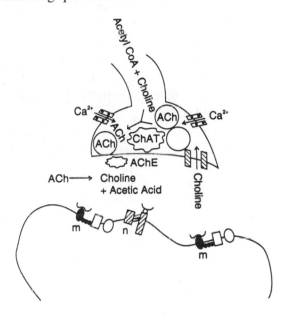

1. All of the following statements about neurons are correct EXCEPT

(A) presynaptic neurons usually do not have receptors for the neurotransmitter that they release

(B) neurons that release acetylcholine (ACh) are found in both the parasympathetic and the sympathetic branches of the autonomic nervous system

(C) cholinergic neurons in the basal nucleus of Meynert selectively degenerate in the brains of patients with confirmed Alzheimer's dementia

(D) the toxin produced by the bacterium *Clostridium tetanae* blocks inhibitory signals to cholinergic motor neurons in the anterior horn

(E) Neurons releasing ACh make connections with cell types other than neurons, including cells found in glands, muscles, and blood vessels

2. All of the following statements about the proteins labeled *m* (i.e., muscarinic) and *n* (i.e., nicotinic) in the diagram are true EXCEPT

(A) muscarinic receptors have been found to carry signals via closely associated G proteins

(B) nicotinic receptors activate the inositol triphosphate (IP_3) pathway leading to the release of stored calcium (Ca^{2+})

(C) drugs that act at muscarinic sites are important in blocking the undesirable side effect of salivation during the administration of inhaled anesthetics

(D) drugs that act at nicotinic sites are important for temporarily paralyzing patients before tracheal intubation

(E) both receptor types bind the endogenous ligand ACh with high affinity

3. With respect to the postsynaptic neuron in the preceding diagram, which one of the following statements best describes signal transduction following the binding of ACh to the postsynaptic membrane?

(A) Nicotinic-type receptor activation leads to rapid influx of potassium (K^+), which causes hyperpolarization and decreased excitability in the postsynaptic neuron

(B) Muscarinic-type receptor activation may be inhibitory or excitatory, because the muscarinic receptors are a class of ligand-gated ion channels that allow the entry of chloride ions (Cl^-) and Ca^{2+}

(C) Muscarine, a mushroom toxin, binds to muscarinic-type receptors, blocking the parasympathetic effects of ACh; the clinical picture includes bradycardia, salivation, flushing of the skin, and bronchoconstriction

(D) Nicotinic-type receptor activation may lead to the influx of Ca^{2+} in the postsynaptic neurons, if the depolarization is great enough to open voltage-gated calcium channels

(E) Muscarinic-type receptor activation does not change the cell's level of excitability because muscarinic receptors are not ligand-gated ion channels and, therefore, cannot affect the neuron's resting potential

4. Which of the following statements about ACh release and deactivation is true?

(A) ACh release is blocked by the toxin associated with *Clostridium tetanae*

(B) Uptake of ACh into the presynaptic receptor is the most important mechanism in terminating the ACh signal

(C) Acetylcholinesterase (AChE) inhibitors, such as pyridostigmine, are not effective in the treatment of myasthenia gravis, because patients with myasthenia have no cholinergic nerve terminals to release ACh

(D) The influx of Ca^{2+} into the depolarized axon terminal is a prerequisite for the release of stored ACh

(E) Inhibitors of the enzyme monoamine oxidase (MAO) are important in the treatment of depression because they inhibit the breakdown of ACh into its constituents, acetic acid and choline

5. All of the following statements about the protein choline acetyltransferase (ChAT) in the preceding diagram are true EXCEPT

(A) ChAT is an enzyme that is synthesized on ribosomes located in the nerve terminal of the presynaptic neuron

(B) ChAT synthesizes ACh from the substrates acetyl coenzyme A (acetyl CoA) and choline

(C) ChAT exists in nerve terminals of both the central and peripheral nervous systems

(D) ChAT is responsible for synthesizing the neurotransmitter ACh before vesicular storage

(E) ChAT levels are decreased in the cerebral cortices of Alzheimer's patients whose brains have been analyzed postmortem

Questions 6–8

A 45-year-old business executive with advanced cirrhosis of the liver and a history of alcohol abuse claims that he does not have a problem with drinking and can quit anytime he wants to.

6. The primary defense mechanism that he is using is

(A) projection

(B) denial

(C) counterphobic behavior

(D) reaction formation

(E) isolation of affect

7. At other times he says that he drinks only because of the constant nagging of his wife. This defense mechanism is best identified as

(A) rationalization

(B) repression

(C) sublimation

(D) reaction formation

(E) isolation of affect

8. Eventually this patient quits drinking but continues to have the symptoms of advanced cirrhosis of the liver. Despite the obvious discomfort caused by his illness, he tells everyone how happy he is to have cirrhosis because it has led to the cessation of his drinking. The defense mechanism he is using is best identified as

(A) projection

(B) denial

(C) counterphobic behavior

(D) reaction formation

(E) isolation of affect

Questions 9–12

A 19-year-old woman presents to the emergency room during her eighth month of pregnancy because of unusual swelling in her hands and face. She denies a history of renal or cardiac disease and states that this is her first pregnancy. She has had no prenatal care and no ultrasonic evaluation of her pregnancy. Her blood pressure is 147/92.

9. Which of the following steps should be taken immediately to diagnose or rule out the most likely possibility?

(A) Human chorionic gonadotropin (hCG) level should be measured because the patient has probably experienced a spontaneous abortion

(B) A urinary dipstick may reveal proteinuria; preeclampsia is a likely possibility and is diagnosed by hypertension and proteinuria in the third trimester

(C) A urinalysis toxicology screen should be performed to confirm a suspicion of benzodiazepine abuse

(D) Rhesus factor (Rh) testing of both the mother and fetus is crucial because pathologic edema is one of the earliest signs of hemolytic disease in the fetus, with the immunologic reaction often causing sympathomimetic effects in the mother

(E) Blood pressure should be monitored because some women experience facial edema as the first sign of pregnancy-related congestive heart failure

10. All of the following statements accurately describe the physiologic regulation of blood pressure EXCEPT

(A) atrial natriuretic factor (ANF) is produced by the right atrium in response to atrial distention, which leads to a subsequent increase in urine production because ANF is a potent diuretic

(B) Angiotensin II is a potent vasoconstrictor

(C) Aldosterone opposes the action of renin by increasing the reabsorption of potassium ions in the kidney

(D) Vasopressin is a potent stimulator of water reabsorption in the medullary collecting duct

(E) Sympathetic nervous system (SNS) activity results in coronary vasodilation but renal and splanchnic vasoconstriction.

11. Which of the following statements correctly pairs an antihypertensive medication with its mechanism of action?

(A) Labetalol (Lopressor) acts at β_1-receptors in the heart to increase stroke volume

(B) Captopril (Capoten) acts in the lung to antagonize the angiotensin-converting enzyme, leaving angiotensin I in its less active state

(C) α-Methyldopa (Aldomet) acts principally in the arterioles, causing vasodilation by blocking peripheral α-adrenergic receptors

(D) Diltiazem (Cardizem) blocks voltage-sensitive calcium channels in the peripheral arterioles, leading to increased peripheral resistance

(E) Thiazide diuretics act in the kidneys by blocking the transport of sodium in the ascending loop of Henle, which leads to an increase in the amount of water reabsorption in the distal tubule and results in diuresis

12. Based on the findings presented previously, which of the following complications would be most likely?

(A) Acute onset of anemia in the mother as a result of Rh incompatibility; the resultant poor tissue oxygenation could lead to multiple organ failure syndrome (MOFS)

(B) Polyuria and hyponatremia caused by mechanisms that attempt to compensate rapidly for the increased peripheral resistance

(C) Severe bleeding and possible shock as a result of spontaneous abortion

(D) Myocardial ischemia and perhaps infarction as a result of the compromised cardiac output in this patient with probable congestive heart failure

(E) Oliguria and seizures indicating a decline in the patient's status from preeclampsia to eclampsia

13. A correct description of the individual curves depicted in the log–dose response relationship below includes which of the following?

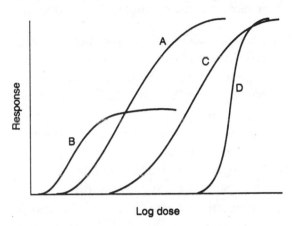

(A) curves A and D: a full agonist (drug A) and a partial agonist (drug D)

(B) curves B and C: an agonist in the absence of a noncompetitive inhibitor (curve B) and in the presence of one (curve C)

(C) curves A, C, and D: three agonists with similar efficacy but different potency

(D) curves A and C: an agonist in the absence of a competitive inhibitor (curve C) and in the presence of one (curve A)

(E) curves A and C: drug A is less potent than drug C

14. The most common type of Ehlers-Danlos syndrome (i.e., type IV) is inherited in an autosomal recessive fashion. Which one of the following extracellular matrix molecules is affected?

(A) Laminin, which is the most abundant glycoprotein in all basement membranes

(B) Type II collagen, which is an important component of cartilage and the vitreous humor

(C) Types I and III collagen, which together have wide distributions in the skin, blood vessels, tendons, and bone

(D) Proteoglycans, which regulate connective tissue structure and permeability

(E) Fibronectin, which is an essential macromolecule secreted by endothelial cells and fibroblasts

15. A 34-year-old woman presented with pelvic pain, and ultrasound revealed a cystic ovarian mass. The multiloculated cyst pictured here was removed. The tumor can best be described as

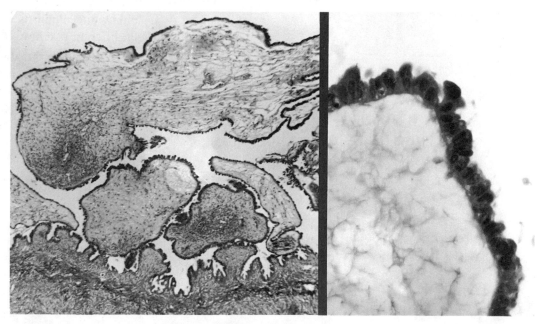

(A) being associated with elevated production of the beta subunit of human chorionic gonadotropin (hCG)

(B) a germ cell tumor requiring interventional chemotherapy

(C) being rare outside of the elderly female population

(D) being an indolent low-grade neoplasm

16. Which of the following pathophysiologic changes may be most useful in documenting, within less than 6 hours, that a patient had a myocardial infarction?

(A) Inverted or biphasic T wave on an electrocardiogram
(B) Elevated serum levels of creatine kinase
(C) Elevated serum levels of myocardial lactate dehydrogenase
(D) Maximal indices of coagulative necrosis
(E) Peak tissue infiltration of neutrophils

17. The incubation period for hepatitis A is

(A) less than 15 days
(B) 15–40 days
(C) 40–60 days
(D) 60–160 days
(E) more than 160 days

18. A healthy person is flying in an airplane that has been pressurized to 10,000 feet (523 mm Hg). Which of the following statements concerning the effects of this barometric pressure is true? It

(A) will not affect alveolar Po_2 because inspired oxygen remains at 0.21
(B) will be associated with significant desaturation of arterial hemoglobin
(C) will shift the subject's oxyhemoglobin dissociation curve to the left
(D) will decrease the vapor pressure of water in the airways
(E) will cause a modest reduction in arterial Po_2

Questions 19–22

A 27-year-old white woman presents with a maculopapular rash confined to her face, most severely on her cheeks. She first noticed the rash about 1 month ago, at which time she also noticed a decline in her energy. She decided to come to the hospital because her chest hurts; the pain is worse when she leans forward from a sitting position. The physician considers a diagnosis of systemic lupus erythematosus (SLE).

19. Which one of the following statements concerning the cause and pathogenesis of SLE is correct?

(A) Evidence from twin and family studies suggests that there is probably not a significant hereditary component to the disease
(B) Sex hormones play little or no role in the occurrence or manifestations of SLE
(C) Antinuclear antibodies are a hallmark of the disease; a variety of different antigens (including histone antigens, double-stranded DNA antigens, and nucleolar antigens) are targeted by antibodies in SLE patients
(D) Immune dysregulation is a problem with self antigens; there is, as yet, no substantial evidence for global immune hyperactivity
(E) Recent evidence suggests that an influenza-like viral infection may precede the symptoms of SLE in as many as half of the patients newly affected by the disease

20. Which one of the following drugs is known to be associated with a drug-induced, lupus-like syndrome?

(A) Piperacillin
(B) Pentamidine
(C) Bleomycin
(D) Lovastatin
(E) Procainamide

21. All of the following clinical features are characteristic of patients with SLE EXCEPT

(A) Proteinuria
(B) Serositis
(C) Photosensitivity
(D) Neurologic disorder
(E) Colonic ulcers

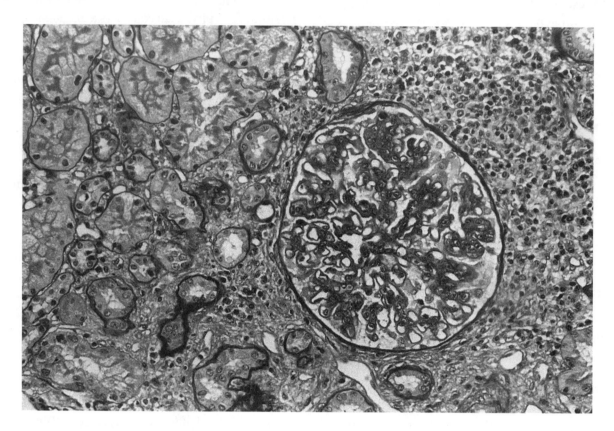

22. The photomicrograph above shows a portion of a renal cortex biopsy from an SLE patient. Which of the following classifications best fits the pathology seen in this biopsy?

(A) Proliferative glomerulonephritis
(B) Membranous glomerulonephritis
(C) Tubular necrosis
(D) Periarterial fibrosis
(E) Interstitial nephritis

Questions 23–25

A 50-year-old man with a history of hemochromatosis presents to the emergency room coughing up bright red blood. He had his most recent phlebotomy yesterday. His blood pressure is 110/85, his pulse 115; his face is flushed, and he is diaphoretic. During the physical examination splenomegaly and a venous pattern on his chest and abdomen are noted. He seems somewhat drowsy and confused but has no focal neurologic signs.

23. What is the most likely cause of this patient's bleeding?

(A) Portal hypertension
(B) Hemoglobin deficiency
(C) Eroded gastric ulcer
(D) Bronchogenic carcinoma
(E) Protein C deficiency

24. What is the probable source of this patient's confusion?

(A) Parkinson's disease
(B) Hepatic encephalopathy
(C) Subarachnoid hemorrhage
(D) Vitamin B_{12} deficiency
(E) Shy-Drager syndrome

25. Which of the following statements concerning the etiology and pathology of hemochromatosis is true?

(A) The excess iron accumulates primarily in cells of the mononuclear phagocyte system
(B) The most severe form of the disease is found in patients with thalassemia and sideroblastic anemia
(C) The iron accumulates due to a failure of renal excretion
(D) Approximately two thirds of patients with hemochromatosis share a common human leukocyte antigen
(E) The organ damage resulting from hemochromatosis is characteristically confined to the liver

26. Which one of the following factors differentiates viruses from *Chlamydia*?

(A) Obligate intracellular parasitism
(B) The need for arthropod vectors
(C) Dependency on the host cell for energy
(D) The presence of a single type of nucleic acid

27. The probability of hepatitis B [$P(D+)$] in a certain patient population is known to be .20 (conversely, $P(D-) = .80$). In a study of a new diagnostic test for hepatitis B, the probability of a positive test result among patients known to have hepatitis, $P(T+|D+)$, is shown to be .90, whereas the probability that a healthy patient will have a negative result, $P(T-|D-)$, is shown to be .95. What is the probability that a new patient with a negative test result is truly healthy?

(A) .95

(B) $\dfrac{(.95)(.80)}{(.95)(.80) + (.10)(.20)}$

(C) $\dfrac{(.90)(.20)}{(.90)(.20) + (.05)(.80)}$

(D) $\dfrac{(.95)(.80)}{(.95)(.80) + (.90)(.20)}$

(E) None of the above

Questions 28–31

The following data were obtained from an arterial blood sample drawn from a hospitalized patient:

$$pH = 7.55$$
$$P_{CO_2} = 25 \text{ mm Hg}$$
$$[HCO_3{}^-] = 22.5 \text{ mEq/L}$$

Recall that $CO_2 = 0.03 \times P_{CO_2}$ (in mmol/L).

28. This patient's arterial blood findings are consistent with a diagnosis of

(A) metabolic alkalosis
(B) respiratory alkalosis
(C) metabolic acidosis
(D) respiratory acidosis

29. These findings indicate that the ratio of [$HCO_3{}^-$] to dissolved CO_2 is

(A) 5:1
(B) 10:1
(C) 20:1
(D) 30:1

30. The data indicate that the CO_2 content is approximately

(A) 22 mmol/L
(B) 23 mmol/L
(C) 24 mmol/L
(D) 25 mmol/L
(E) 26 mmol/L

31. The major compensatory response for this patient's acid–base disorder is

(A) hyperventilation
(B) hypoventilation
(C) increased renal $HCO_3{}^-$ excretion
(D) increased H^+ excretion

Questions 32–36

A 75-year-old woman is admitted to the hospital after suffering a cerebrovascular accident. Her computed tomography (CT) scan shows a focal nonhemorrhagic infarction in the right hemisphere. During the physical examination, no muscular weakness is noted; however, the patient is not responding to any visual, auditory, or tactile stimuli on the left side of her body. The woman also has a deficit involving only the inferior portion of her left visual field in both eyes.

32. Which lobe of the brain has been principally affected by this stroke?

(A) Parietal
(B) Frontal
(C) Occipital
(D) Temporal

33. Which of the sites in the picture below best describes the location of the woman's optic tract lesion?

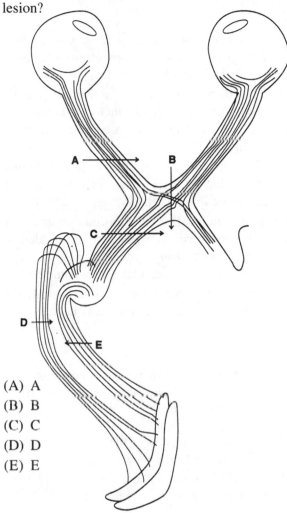

(A) A
(B) B
(C) C
(D) D
(E) E

34. Angiography later showed complete occlusion in a small branch of the middle cerebral artery with no other significant findings. Which one of the following diagnoses best explains the cause of the woman's cerebrovascular accident?

(A) Berry aneurysm
(B) Deep venous thrombosis
(C) Atrial fibrillation with mural thrombus
(D) Congestive heart failure
(E) Arteriovenous malformation

35. All of the following statements concerning the mechanism of clot formation are correct EXCEPT

(A) activation of thrombin by factor V is the final common pathway in converting soluble fibrinogen to insoluble fibrin

(B) the extrinsic pathway is activated by a lipoprotein called tissue factor, whereas the intrinsic pathway is activated by contact with foreign surfaces

(C) thrombin and several other cascade proteins are serine proteases that activate the next molecule in the pathway

(D) antithrombin III is an important regulator of the clotting cascade and acts by covalently cross-linking fibrin monomers into large meshworks in which platelets become lodged

(E) vitamin K is involved in the liver's synthesis of the factors that are calcium chelators

36. Which of the following statements correctly pairs a commonly used anticoagulant with its mechanism of action?

(A) Heparin acts to cleave the covalent linkage between fibrin monomers

(B) Tissue plasminogen activator acts by irreversibly inhibiting thrombin

(C) Dicumarol (warfarin) is a natural product which competitively inhibits the vitamin K–dependent γ-carboxylation of several cascade proteins

(D) Aspirin irreversibly binds fibrinogen, which decreases the pool of available fibrin monomers that can participate in clot formation

(E) Streptokinase is a bacterial product that causes platelet lysis, therefore inhibiting platelet aggregation

Questions 37–38

Five percent of individuals comprising a particular population are known to carry a recessive gene for poliodystrophy, an inherited disorder characterized by the onset of recurrent seizures and dementia in early childhood. A 32-year-old woman who had a brother with this disorder seeks genetic counseling. The patient's husband, an only child, does not know if his family has a history of the disorder.

37. What is the probability that the patient is a carrier of poliodystrophy?

(A) 1/20
(B) 1/10
(C) 3/8
(D) 2/3
(E) 3/4

38. What is the probability that both the patient and her husband are carriers?

(A) 1/30
(B) 1/20
(C) 3/8
(D) 2/3
(E) 3/4

Questions 39–42

A 68-year-old woman who is a volunteer at a church-sponsored kindergarten suddenly develops a fever of 38.2°C and a severe headache one evening. The following morning she also experiences a stiff neck and uncharacteristic drowsiness. At the emergency room, her temperature is 38.8°C, and there are pain and resistance on flexion of her neck. The patient is noted to be mentally competent although lethargic. A cerebrospinal fluid (CSF) sample is obtained by lumbar puncture.

39. On the basis of the history and physical examination of this patient, what is the most probable diagnosis?

(A) Viral meningitis
(B) Fungal meningitis
(C) Bacterial meningitis
(D) Viral encephalitis
(E) Brain abscess

40. On the basis of the patient's age, the probable etiologic agent is

(A) *Staphylococcus aureus*
(B) *Haemophilus influenzae*
(C) *Actinomyces israelii*
(D) *Neisseria meningitidis*
(E) *Streptococcus pneumoniae*

41. Opening pressure on lumbar puncture was slightly elevated, and the diagnosis was acute bacterial meningitis based upon the finding of gram-positive cocci in pairs in the CSF. The cell count was elevated. The prominent cell type most likely was

(A) mononuclear cells
(B) neutrophils
(C) lymphocytes
(D) red cells
(E) segmented neutrophils

42. Protein and glucose concentrations in the CSF probably were

(A) both elevated
(B) elevated and low, respectively
(C) low and elevated, respectively
(D) both low
(E) unaffected

Questions 43–44

The figure below depicts log concentration–time curves for three drugs (X, Y, and Z) after identical amounts of each drug were administered as a bolus at time zero.

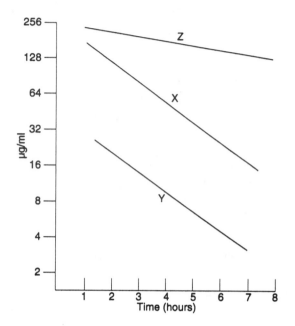

43. Which of the following statements regarding these drugs is correct?

(A) Volume of distribution (V_d) of X = Z < Y
(B) Half-time of elimination ($t_{1/2}$) of X = Y > Z
(C) Clearance of X (CL_X) = CL_Y
(D) CL_Z > CL_X
(E) Elimination rate constant (k) of X < (k) of Y

44. If drugs X, Y, and Z were independently infused in equal amounts at a constant rate, then based on the data from the figure above, which of the following statements is most accurate?

(A) At steady state, [X] > [Z]
(B) At steady state, [X] = [Y]
(C) Z would require more time to reach a steady state than either X or Y
(D) X would reach a steady state faster than Y

45. Which one of the following statements concerning infectious hepatitis is correct?

(A) Hepatitis C infection requires hepatitis B infection
(B) Diagnosis with hepatitis B carries a grave prognosis: Many people die from fulminant hepatitis, and nearly 25% of infected patients progress to hepatocellular carcinoma
(C) Hepatitis B surface antigen (HBsAg) indicates active hepatitis infection
(D) The carrier state is common in patients infected with hepatitis A
(E) Hepatitis A infection accounts for approximately 25% of all hepatitis cases in the United States

46. Of the following cell types, which would contain many mitochondria in the apical portion of the cell?

(A) Smooth muscle cells
(B) Proximal convoluted tubule cells
(C) Steroid-secreting cells
(D) Liver parenchymal cells
(E) Skeletal muscle cells

47. A 29-year-old man whose father died of Huntington's chorea when he was an infant is obsessively worried about developing the disease, symptoms of which appear in one's 30s or 40s. Although he knows little about the genetic disorder, he is aware that there is a 50% likelihood that he has the dominant Huntington's gene. One day, he impulsively rushes to a testing center and demands to initiate presymptomatic testing, making no attempt to hide his intention to commit suicide if he receives positive results. It would be ethically defensible for the testing center staff to

(A) refuse to initiate testing

(B) educate him about the disease and initiate testing

(C) initiate counseling to alleviate his anxieties, educate him about the disease, and defer testing until he is more stable

(D) test him and report negative results regardless of the actual results

(E) test him for other diseases

48. Which one of the following conditions is a characteristic of cirrhosis of the liver?

(A) Degeneration of the cerebral cortex

(B) Ascites

(C) Pulmonary edema

(D) Hemolytic anemia

(E) Gastric ulcer

49. In the general format of the Henderson-Hasselbalch equation:

$$\log\left(\frac{[\text{protonated form}]}{[\text{unprotonated form}]}\right) + pK'_a = pH$$

Phenobarbital is a weak acid. In an emergency situation, a useful maneuver to hasten its elimination in an intoxicated person might be

(A) inhalation of CO_2

(B) infusion of $NaHCO_3$

(C) infusion of NH_4Cl

(D) induction of P_{450} enzymes with a separate barbiturate

(E) infusion of dextrose

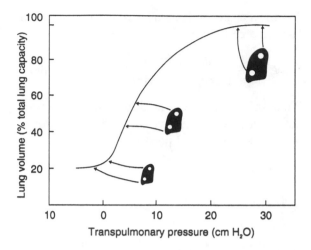

50. Which one of the following statements accurately describes pressure–volume relationships, as shown in the above figure, in the lungs of a healthy individual?

(A) At lung volumes close to functional residual capacity (FRC), alveoli at the base of the lung are smaller than alveoli at the top

(B) At lung volumes close to vital capacity (VC), alveoli at the top of the lung are smaller than alveoli at the base

(C) Alveoli in the base of the lung begin filling first during inspiration from residual volume

(D) Alveoli in the apex receive greater ventilation during inspiration from volumes near FRC

(E) Alveoli in the base of the lung close at volumes near VC

51. Which of the following statements most accurately describes specific features of neuromuscular transmission?

(A) Each muscle fiber contains multiple axon terminals

(B) The end-plate is highly enriched in electrically excitable gates

(C) Enzymatic degradation of the transmitter can terminate transmission

(D) Acetylcholine (ACh) causes chloride channels to open as a result of membrane depolarization

52. Which one of the following statements concerning expiration is correct?

(A) At lung volumes close to vital capacity (VC), expiratory air flow is independent of expiratory effort

(B) At lung volumes close to VC, airway resistance is at its peak

(C) At lung volumes close to VC, expiratory air flow increases with increasing pleural pressures

(D) At 50% of VC, increased expiratory effort results in decreased airway resistance

(E) At lung volumes close to residual volume, the elastic recoil of the chest wall is directed inward

53. A man acquires a "cold sore" from his girlfriend through ordinary kissing. Assuming that this man will exhibit recurrent infections, which nerve axon might this disease traverse during reinfection?

(A) Cranial nerve (CN) VII (upper and lower buccal branches)

(B) CN V and the marginal mandibular branch of CN VII

(C) CN V_2 and CN V_3

(D) CN V_1 only

54. Which one of the following statements about the hormonal regulation of pregnancy is correct?

(A) Human chorionic gonadotropin (hCG) is secreted by the placenta and can first be detected 4 weeks after conception

(B) hCG stimulates the corpus luteum to secrete high levels of estrogen and progesterone

(C) The β subunits of luteinizing hormone (LH), follicle stimulating hormone (FSH), and hCG are identical to one another whereas the α subunits are responsible for their different receptor affinities

(D) Maternal serum hCG levels continue to increase throughout pregnancy

(E) hCG stimulates the pituitary to maintain high LH and FSH levels to keep the corpus luteum functional

55. The process of DNA replication can be best described by which of the following statements? DNA replication

(A) initiates at random sites on the chromosome

(B) of the *Escherichia coli* chromosome begins at multiple origins

(C) is unidirectional for all DNAs

(D) is not dependent on the synthesis of RNA primers

(E) occurs during the S phase of the cell cycle

56. In the figure below, volume–pressure curves from three subjects of the same age, sex, and body size are shown. If subject B is normal, which one of the following statements is most accurate?

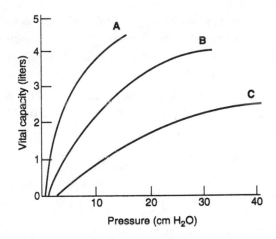

(A) Subject A has a stiff lung (fibrosis)

(B) Subject A has a flabby lung (emphysema)

(C) Subject A has a higher elastic recoil pressure than the other subjects

(D) Subject C is likely to have a higher functional residual capacity

(E) Subject C has the lowest elastic recoil pressure of the three

57. A 20-year-old man has a penile lesion that is crateriform, moist, and indurated. The patient revealed that this lesion has been present for about 20 days and is not painful. Which one of the following groups of tests is most appropriate?

(A) Gram stain, Venereal Disease Research Laboratory (VDRL) test, and culture of the lesion for *Treponema pallidum*

(B) Gram stain and culture of the lesion for *T. pallidum*

(C) VDRL and dark-field examination

(D) Fluorescent treponemal antibody absorption (FTA-ABS) test

58. Which one of the following techniques would be the best way to study a new kind of growth factor that induces proliferation of certain cell types?

(A) Measure uptake of radiolabeled methionine into cells after addition of the growth factor

(B) Measure uptake of radiolabeled thymidine into cells after addition of the growth factor

(C) Measure uptake of radiolabeled uracil into cells after addition of the growth factor

(D) Trypan blue exclusion

Questions 59–60

A 70-year-old woman is brought to the emergency room by her daughter, who noticed that her mother is not as energetic as she previously was. In the emergency room, the patient relates a history of increasing fatigability and shortness of breath over the past several months. On examination, the patient has elevated neck veins, rales in the back, and a third heart sound (S_3 gallop rhythm). Chest x-ray reveals an enlarged cardiac silhouette and increased vascular markings. The patient has a heart rate of 90 and a blood pressure of 150/100.

59. Based on the above history and physical examination, the patient is most likely to have

(A) atrial fibrillation

(B) ventricular paroxysmal tachycardia

(C) congestive heart failure

(D) adult respiratory distress syndrome

(E) rebound hypertensive crisis

60. A hypothetical series of pressure–volume loops of the left ventricle of a control subject and the patient before and after digitalis is shown below. Based on these data, which one of the following groupings is correct?

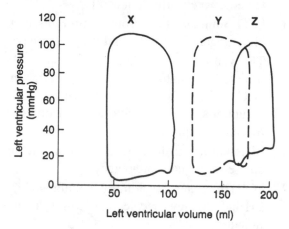

(A) X: control; Y: before digitalis; Z: after digitalis

(B) X: control; Z: before digitalis; Y: after digitalis

(C) Z: control; X: before digitalis; Y: after digitalis

(D) Z: control; Y: before digitalis; X: after digitalis

61. Which of the following areas of the central nervous system (CNS) contains structures that are considered to be phylogenically the oldest parts of the brain?

(A) Frontal lobe

(B) Limbic system

(C) Cerebellum

(D) Visual cortex

62. RNA processing can be best described by which of the following statements? It

(A) occurs in the cytoplasm
(B) results in the addition of nucleotides to the primary transcript of ribosomal RNA (rRNA)
(C) results in the formation of new covalent bonds between RNA and DNA
(D) includes the addition of a tail of polyadenylic acid at the 5' end
(E) includes the methylation of nucleotides in RNA

Questions 63–64

A 10-year-old girl is seen by her pediatrician for flu-like symptoms that were followed (weeks later) by a peculiar expanding skin rash (erythema chronicum migrans) and monarthritis arthritis (months later). Clinical laboratory findings include a positive titer against *Borrelia burgdorferi*.

63. A likely diagnosis for this child includes which one of the following diseases?

(A) Leptospirosis
(B) Lyme disease
(C) Rocky Mountain spotted fever
(D) Relapsing fever
(E) Yaws

64. Assuming a spirochete is the causative agent in this child's syndrome, appropriate pharmacotherapy may include which one of the following drugs?

(A) Rifampin
(B) Penicillin
(C) Chloroquine
(D) Pentamidine
(E) Praziquantel

65. The following sequence is a part of a globular protein. Which of the following statements best describes this peptide?

Ser-Val-Asp-Asp-Val-Phe-Ser-Glu-Val-Cys-His-Met-Arg

(A) At pH 7.4, the peptide has a net negative charge
(B) It has only one sulfur-containing amino acid
(C) The hydrophobic amino acid content exceeds the hydrophilic content
(D) Treatment with chymotrypsin would generate four smaller fragments
(E) Only three of the side chains are capable of forming hydrogen bonds

66. A rational approach for the treatment of ventricular tachycardia associated with myocardial ischemia in a hospitalized patient includes

(A) digitalis
(B) diltiazem
(C) lidocaine
(D) propranolol
(E) verapamil

67. What color would this tumor of the kidney (pictured) be?

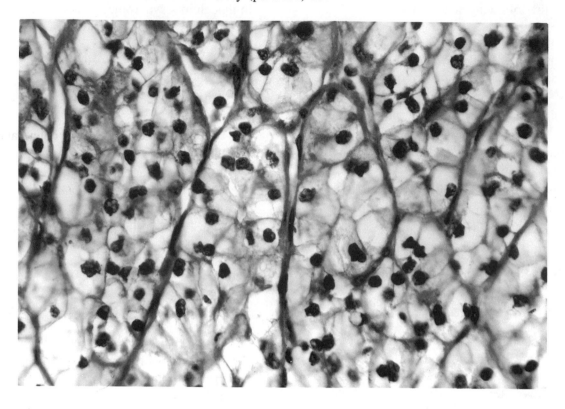

(A) Gray

(B) Translucent, with a pink hue

(C) White

(D) Yellow

68. If an individual has a genetic defect in the enzyme that produces N-acetylglutamate, the most likely clinical finding would be hyperammonemia with

(A) elevated levels of argininosuccinate (the condensation product of citrulline and aspartate)

(B) no detectable citrulline

(C) elevated levels of arginine

(D) elevated levels of urea

(E) no detectable ornithine

69. Which one of the following clinical procedures best demonstrates damage to the cerebellum?

(A) Testing for voluntary weakness by having the patient grasp the examiner's fingers and squeeze as hard as possible

(B) Tapping the patellar tendon and observing the reflex response

(C) Having the patient flex the neck, touching the chin to the sternum, to determine if this action elicits pain

(D) Passively moving the patient's limbs to elicit an increased resistance to motion

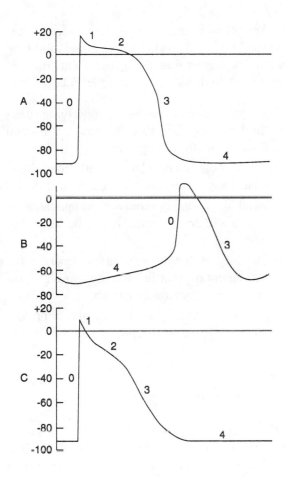

Questions 70–74

Refer to the above traces of action potentials from cardiac cells to answer the following questions.

70. All of the following statements concerning the action potentials illustrated are correct EXCEPT

(A) *trace A* represents the action potential from a myocardial cell in the left ventricle
(B) *trace B* represents the action potential from a cell in the sinoatrial (SA) node
(C) *trace C* represents the action potential from a cell in the atrioventricular (AV) node
(D) in *trace A*, contraction of the cells in the left ventricle correlates with *phase 2*
(E) in *trace A*, the cell is refractory to further stimulation during a portion of *phase 3*

71. Which one of the following statements concerning ionic currents in myocardial cells is correct?

(A) In *phase 0* of the SA node potential, slow, inwardly directed sodium and calcium currents predominate
(B) During *phase 0* in *trace A*, the cell is rapidly depolarized by the influx of potassium
(C) During *phase 3* in *trace B*, the cell is gradually repolarized by an increase in the sodium current
(D) During *phase 3* in *trace A*, calcium-activated sodium currents are important in repolarization
(E) The ionic currents in *phase 3* of the SA node's action potential are the basis for SA node automaticity

72. Which one of the following statements concerning the physiologic regulation of heart rate is correct?

(A) Vagus nerve stimulation causes mild transient depolarization in cells of the SA node
(B) Vagus nerve stimulation increases the slope of *phase 0* depolarization in *trace B*
(C) Vagus nerve stimulation increases the slope of *phase 4* in *trace B*
(D) Stimulation of the sympathetic input to the heart increases the slope of *phase 0* in *trace A*
(E) Stimulation of the sympathetic input to the heart causes an increase in the length of the action potential shown in *trace B*

73. Which one of the following statements correctly pairs a cardiac medication with its direct chronotropic effect and its mechanism of action?

(A) Diltiazem increases heart rate by increasing the slope of *phase 0* in *trace A*
(B) Atropine increases heart rate by increasing the slope of *phase 4* in *trace B*
(C) Nifedipine increases heart rate by increasing the rate of impulse conduction through the AV node
(D) Propranolol decreases the heart rate by decreasing the slope of *phase 3* in *trace A*
(E) Digitalis decreases the heart rate by increasing the slope of *phase 4* in *trace B*

74. Arrhythmias are an important source of cardiac morbidity and mortality. All of the following statements concerning the genesis and maintenance of arrhythmias are correct EXCEPT

(A) arrhythmias can involve an underlying structural abnormality that impairs the normal flow of electrical impulses
(B) bradycardias caused by AV node conduction disturbances can result from digitalis toxicity
(C) atrial fibrillation is a frequent complication of both acute and chronic rheumatic heart disease
(D) Re-entry is the term used to describe the movement of a cardiac impulse through a region that it previously excited
(E) Re-entry usually does not involve a premature beat from an ectopic focus

Questions 75–79

A 42-year-old white woman comes to the emergency room with acute onset of severe abdominal pain following a routine dinner. During a physical examination, the physician notes that she is mildly obese, and her abdominal pain is confined principally to the right upper quadrant. The physician suspects that she may have gallstones.

75. Which of the following symptoms is most specific for cholelithiasis?

(A) Excessive flatulence following a meal
(B) Hemoccult-positive stool
(C) Severe right upper quadrant pain that comes in waves over a period of hours
(D) Rigid abdominal wall with diffuse rebound tenderness
(E) Epigastric pain and nausea following a meal

76. The patient has a fever of 39.4°C and an elevated serum white cell count (12,400/mm³). All of the following organisms are likely pathogens in acute cholecystitis EXCEPT

(A) group D streptococci (enterococci)
(B) *Escherichia coli*
(C) *Klebsiella* species
(D) *Neisseria* species
(E) *Clostridium* species

77. Which of the following statements best characterizes the prevalence of asymptomatic gallstones in western countries?

(A) The prevalence of gallstones in men over 40 years is greater than 60%
(B) The prevalence of gallstones in men over 40 years is between 20% and 60%
(C) The prevalence of gallstones in men over 40 years is less than 3%
(D) The prevalence of gallstones in women over 40 years is greater than 60%
(E) The prevalence of gallstones in women over 40 years is between 20% and 60%

78. All of the following are known predisposing factors for cholesterol and mixed stone formation EXCEPT

(A) diabetes mellitus
(B) alcoholic cirrhosis
(C) obesity
(D) ileal resection
(E) oral contraceptives

79. All of the following statements correctly characterize important contributors to the pathogenesis of cholelithiasis EXCEPT

(A) decreased hydroxymethylglutaryl coenzyme A (HMG CoA) reductase activity and increased secretion of bile acids can markedly increase the stone-forming potential of bile
(B) gallbladder hypomotility leads to the accumulation of biliary sludge, an important precursor to stone formation
(C) Excess unconjugated bilirubin associated with chronic hemolysis leads to the formation of pigmented stones
(D) Chronic infection of the biliary tree leads to pigment stone formation
(E) Decreased lecithin or bile acid synthesis results in a decreased capacity for solubilizing biliary cholesterol

Questions 80–84

A 32-year-old white woman visits her physician because of agitation, weight loss, and the inability to sleep. When questioned further, she reveals an increased appetite and an increased frequency of bowel movements. Previously, she had regular menstrual periods, but now they are less frequent and irregular. During the physical examination, the physician notes that her skin is warm and moist and that she has a fine tremor of the fingers, hyperreflexia, and lid lag. The woman has moderately severe exophthalmos, and her upward gaze seems weak and uncoordinated.

80. Which one of the following disease processes is most likely manifesting itself?

(A) A thyroid adenoma that is secreting thyroxine
(B) Inappropriate hypothalamic secretion of thyrotropin-releasing hormone (TRH)
(C) Graves' disease
(D) Hashimoto's disease
(E) Sick euthyroid syndrome

81. Which other finding would most likely be expected on further physical examination?

(A) Sparse, dry hair that easily falls out
(B) Pericardial effusion
(C) Jaundice
(D) Dermopathy over the dorsum of the leg
(E) Diffuse hyperpigmentation of the skin

82. All of the following laboratory test results are consistent with the clinical picture EXCEPT

(A) Decreased triiodothyronine resin uptake (T_3RU)
(B) Decreased serum thyroid-stimulating hormone (TSH) response to a TRH challenge
(C) Decreased serum TSH concentration
(D) Increased serum thyroxine (T_4) concentration
(E) Positive test for circulating antibodies against the TSH receptor

83. A thyroid radioactive iodine uptake scintiscan is performed and reveals uniform uptake across the gland. Which of the following conditions best describes the histopathology of this woman's thyroid gland?

(A) Multinodular goiter
(B) Multiple adenomas
(C) Single carcinoma
(D) Lymphocytic infiltration (especially plasma cells) with atrophic follicles
(E) Diffuse hyperplasia and hypertrophy

84. All of the following statements correctly pair a useful medication with its mechanism of action EXCEPT

(A) propylthiouracil blocks the coupling reaction in T_4 synthesis
(B) methimazole reduces peripheral conversion of T_4 to T_3
(C) radioactive iodine destroys follicular cells in the thyroid
(D) propranolol blocks the sympathetic components of thyrotoxicosis
(E) prednisone may relieve the mechanical exophthalmos and ophthalmoplegia by reducing inflammation

Questions 85–89

A 64-year-old black man with a 40-year history of smoking 1.5 packs of cigarettes per day visits his physician's office complaining of an unproductive cough of 6 months' duration. When questioned further, the patient discloses hoarseness and generalized muscle weakness. Previously active sexually, he says that he has "lost interest" lately. During a physical examination, the physician notes muscle wasting, an unusual pattern of weight gain in the face and back, and abdominal stria. His serum glucose is 180 mg/dl.

85. Which single set of laboratory tests is best suited to establish a tentative diagnosis?

(A) Serum thyroxine, triiodothyronine resin uptake, and cervical ultrasound
(B) Urinary glucocorticoids, abdominal computed tomography (CT), and chest x-ray
(C) Dexamethasone suppression test and chest x-ray
(D) In-patient hospitalization with water restriction, CT of the head, and chest x-ray
(E) Glucose tolerance, urinary ketones, abdominal ultrasound, and chest x-ray

86. The test results return positive, confirming the suspicion of an endocrine abnormality secondary to a bronchogenic carcinoma. Which of the following hormone or hormone-like substances is the tumor most likely secreting?

(A) Parathyroid or parathyroid-like hormone
(B) Thyroxine
(C) Corticosteroids
(D) Adrenocorticotropic hormone (ACTH) or ACTH-like hormone
(E) Insulin or insulin-like hormone

87. Additional radiology studies to confirm the source of the endocrine abnormalities are desired. Based on the short history presented, which of the following features is most likely expected?

(A) Bilateral hypertrophy of the adrenal gland
(B) Focal enlargement in the thyroid gland
(C) Hypertrophy of a subset of cells in the pituitary gland
(D) Carcinoid tumor
(E) Hypertrophy of a subset of cells in the pancreas

88. Each of the following pieces of evidence relates cigarette smoking to bronchogenic carcinomas EXCEPT

(A) heavy smokers (more than 1 pack/day) have a 20-fold greater lifetime risk of developing bronchogenic cancer
(B) cessation of cigarette smoking for 10 years reduces cancer risk to that of nonsmokers
(C) the bronchial epithelium in more than 10% of cigarette smokers shows atypical or hyperplastic changes on autopsy
(D) tumor-initiating substances (e.g., polycyclic aromatic hydrocarbons), which have caused cancer in mice, are found in cigarette smoke
(E) Lung cancer runs in families in which cigarette smoking is common

89. Each of the following is a potential paraneoplastic syndrome associated with bronchogenic tumors EXCEPT

(A) syndrome of inappropriate antidiuretic hormone (ADH)
(B) hyperaldosteronism
(C) hypercalcemia of malignancy
(D) dermatomyositis
(E) hypertrophic osteoarthropathy

DIRECTIONS: Each of the numbered items or incomplete statements in this section is negatively phrased, as indicated by a capitalized word such as NOT, LEAST, or EXCEPT. Select the ONE lettered answer or completion that is BEST in each case.

90. Of the following types of proteins, all exhibit a protein structure common for physiologic receptors or components of cellular signal transduction systems EXCEPT

(A) ion channels
(B) protein kinases
(C) guanylate cyclases
(D) guanosine triphosphate (GTP)–binding proteins (G proteins)
(E) metallothioneins

91. All of the following statements describe the genetic code EXCEPT

(A) it is nearly identical for all organisms
(B) it is composed of nucleotides containing three nucleotide code letters
(C) it represents all of the nucleotide sequence information within a transcription unit
(D) it contains transcription start and stop sequences
(E) it contains more than one codon for each amino acid

92. All of the following statements about γ-aminobutyric acid (GABA) are true EXCEPT

(A) its receptor is coupled to a benzodiazepine receptor
(B) it is a widely distributed inhibitory neurotransmitter
(C) its activity is increased in hepatic encephalopathy
(D) its activity is increased with antispasticity drugs
(E) its activity is decreased with antiseizure drugs

93. Biologic theory is supported by all of the following EXCEPT

(A) the effects of certain medications on the symptoms of schizophrenia
(B) enlargement of ventricular size in significant numbers of patients with schizophrenia
(C) a strong family history in many cases of manic-depressive disorder
(D) the effect of stimulant medication on the symptoms of ADHD in children
(E) monozygotic twins discordant for schizophrenia

94. All of the following nephritides are associated with hypocomplementemia EXCEPT

(A) immunoglobulin A (IgA) nephropathy
(B) mesangioproliferative glomerulonephropathy
(C) serum sickness
(D) systemic lupus erythematosus (SLE)
(E) vasculitis

95. All of the following statements describing cell–extracellular matrix interactions are correct EXCEPT

(A) integrins are soluble nuclear proteins that directly alter gene transcription
(B) type IV collagen, which is found in basement membranes, stimulates endothelial cells to organize into tubelike structures
(C) fibronectin fragments play a pivotal role in wound healing by promoting migration of endothelial cells and fibroblasts to the damaged area
(D) laminin is a potent stimulus for inducing the replication of endothelial cells
(E) receptor glycoproteins on the surface of platelets are crucial to platelet aggregation at sites of exposed subendothelium

96. All of the following human leukocyte antigen (HLA) associations are matched correctly EXCEPT

(A) rheumatoid arthritis—HLA-DR4
(B) primary Sjögren's syndrome—HLA-DR3
(C) postgonococcal arthritis—HLA-B27
(D) 21-hydroxylase deficiency—HLA-DR4
(E) chronic active hepatitis—HLA-DR3

97. All of the following statements concerning action potentials recorded simultaneously from slow and fast myocardial fibers (illustrated below) are correct EXCEPT

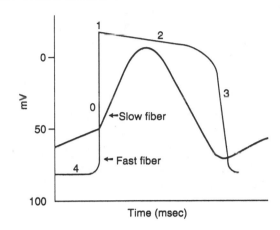

(A) the slow fiber was likely to be present in sinoatrial or atrioventricular nodes
(B) the fast fiber is typical of either atrial or ventricular myocardial cells
(C) in the fast fiber, *phase 0* is caused by opening of Na^+ channels
(D) in the fast fiber, *phase 2* coincides with an increase in conductance to Ca^{2+}
(E) application of acetylcholine (ACh) increases the slope of *phase 4* of the slow fiber

Questions 98–99

A 50-year-old woman complains of increasing fatigue over the past 2 weeks. She has a history of ovarian carcinoma and has received treatment with several courses of cyclophosphamide during the past 3 years; her last course of treatment was given 1 month previously. Physical examination shows slight hepatic enlargement. One examiner thinks the patient has some excess abdominal fluid. Laboratory examination reveals a white blood count of 2000 cells/μl, with 10% polymorphonuclear leukocytes and 90% lymphocytes. The hemoglobin concentration is 9 g/dl, and the platelet count is 50,000/μl.

98. The differential diagnosis of the cause of this patient's pancytopenia includes all of the following EXCEPT

(A) chronic lymphocytic leukemia
(B) acute myelogenous leukemia
(C) recurrent ovarian carcinoma
(D) cyclophosphamide toxicity
(E) aplastic anemia

99. Further evaluation of this patient requires all of the following studies EXCEPT

(A) radiographic studies of the abdomen
(B) cytologic examination of ascites
(C) bone marrow aspiration and biopsy
(D) immunoglobulin gene rearrangement studies
(E) liver function studies

100. Chronic type B (antral) gastritis is characterized by all of the following features EXCEPT

(A) glandular atrophy with the presence of very few short, cystically dilated glands
(B) circulating antibodies to parietal cells and intrinsic factor
(C) excess acid secretion with low intragastric pH and, frequently, duodenal ulcers
(D) low serum gastrin levels
(E) flattened or absent rugal folds

101. Asthma is characterized by an increased responsiveness of the trachea and bronchi to various stimuli and is manifested by widespread narrowing of the airway. Results of pulmonary function tests during an acute asthma attack will demonstrate all of the following EXCEPT

(A) decreased forced expiratory volume in 1 second (FEV_1)
(B) increased forced vital capacity (FVC)
(C) decreased FEV_1/FVC
(D) normal or increased total lung capacity (TLC)

102. All of the following statements about the influence of cardiovascular disease on sexuality are true EXCEPT

(A) some patients have impaired sexual functioning following a myocardial infarction
(B) myocardial infarctions that occur during intercourse are often associated with unusual and stressful circumstances
(C) the most common reason for decreased frequency of intercourse after a myocardial infarction is anginal pain associated with intercourse
(D) there is a higher incidence of return to normal sexual activity by patients who receive exercise training and education than by those who arc not involved in such programs
(E) the spouse of a patient who has had a myocardial infarction needs to be involved in educational programs because his or her fears can interfere with resumption of sexual activity

103. All of the following thalamic nuclei are connected with the basal ganglia EXCEPT

(A) ventrolateral
(B) medial central
(C) pulvinar
(D) ventroanterior

104. All of the following statements concerning hormonal control of the menstrual cycle are true EXCEPT

(A) estradiol causes a proliferation and thickening in the endometrial lining
(B) progesterone induces differentiation of the endometrial lining into a secretory phase
(C) luteinizing hormone (LH) stimulates thecal cells to produce androgens that are aromatized to estrogen by the granulosa cells
(D) the LH surge immediately precedes endometrial shedding and menses
(E) follicle-stimulating hormone (FSH) couples with increasing estrogen levels to induce the synthesis of LH receptors on the granulosa cells

105. A 62-year-old man experiences crushing substernal chest pain. After 4 days of circulatory support in the intensive care unit, he dies. Histologic study of his heart would show all of the following findings EXCEPT

(A) coagulative necrosis
(B) liquefactive necrosis
(C) hypereosinophilic wavy fibers
(D) neutrophilic infiltrate

106. All of the following elements of the adult brain develop from the telencephalon EXCEPT the

(A) corpus striatum
(B) internal capsule
(C) occipital lobe
(D) hippocampus
(E) thalamus

107. Each statement below concerning the contraction of myofibrils in skeletal muscle is true EXCEPT

(A) the size of the A band decreases
(B) the size of the H band decreases
(C) the size of the I band decreases
(D) thin filaments penetrate the A band
(E) Z disks are drawn closer to the A band

108. Each of the following statements concerning intercostal nerves is true EXCEPT

(A) they are the anterior rami of the 12 thoracic spinal nerves
(B) they are connected to the sympathetic trunk by rami communicans
(C) the first intercostal nerve is joined to the brachial plexus
(D) they supply the anterior abdominal muscles
(E) they supply the parietal pleura

109. All of the following statements concerning mammalian chromosomes are true EXCEPT

(A) DNase I can be used to treat chromosomes to determine inactive regions of DNA
(B) approximately 7% of the sequences contained in the eukaryotic genome are ever copied into RNA
(C) heterochromatin is a term used for inactive DNA, and euchromatin is a term used for those regions of DNA that are transcriptionally active
(D) in higher eukaryotic genomes, cytosine is methylated at cytosine–guanine (CG) islands in inactive segments of DNA

110. Psychoanalysis as a form of psychotherapy includes all of the following concepts EXCEPT

(A) free association
(B) resistance
(C) countertransference
(D) interpretation
(E) meditation

111. Serious complications in a patient who has just suffered an acute myocardial infarction include all of the following EXCEPT

(A) cardiac tamponade
(B) peripheral embolism
(C) mitral valve incompetence
(D) aortic aneurysm
(E) rupture of the ventricular septum

112. Which of the following steps is NOT important in the normal synthesis of collagen?

(A) Incorporation of glycine residues into the growing polypeptide
(B) Hydroxylation of proline residues, which adds stability to the mature fiber's triple helix motif
(C) Cleavage of the globular terminal ends of soluble procollagen to make insoluble tropocollagen
(D) Secretion of the cleaved tropocollagen into the extracellular space
(E) Covalent cross-linkage of lysine residues in the nascent collagen fiber, which adds stability to both the intramolecular and intermolecular structures

113. A man is brought to the emergency room after being beaten with a baseball bat. He received one blow to the head that did not fracture the skull. At which of the following locations would a blow cause the LEAST amount of damage to the brain, assuming that all blows were delivered with equal force?

(A) The side of the head
(B) The front of the head
(C) The back of the head
(D) A glancing blow to the back of the head

DIRECTIONS: Each set of matching questions in this section consists of a list of four to twenty-six lettered options (some of which may be in figures) followed by several numbered items. For each numbered item, select the ONE lettered option that is most closely associated with it. To avoid spending too much time on matching sets with large numbers of options, it is generally advisable to begin each set by reading the list of options. Then, for each item in the set, try to generate the correct answer and locate it in the option list, rather than evaluating each option individually. Each lettered option may be selected once, more than once, or not at all.

Questions 114–118

Match each of the following cardiovascular events with its correct place in the cardiac cycle.

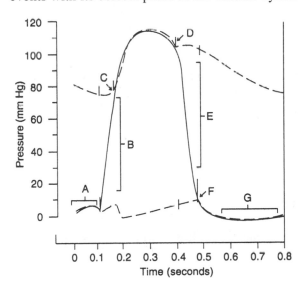

114. Aortic valve opens

115. Left ventricle is filling

116. Isovolumic contraction of the left ventricle

117. Atrial systole

118. Aortic valve closes here, S2 is produced

Questions 119–123

For each case history described below, select the appropriate diagnosis.

(A) Narcissistic personality disorder
(B) Phencyclidine (PCP) ingestion
(C) Schizophrenia
(D) Borderline personality disorder
(E) Bipolar illness

119. Over the past year, Andrew, age 17, has retreated more and more often to his room. He has few friends and never calls anyone. His school performance has deteriorated during this time. His mother finds pieces of paper in his trashcan with unintelligible poems written on them.

120. Margot is brought to the hospital by her husband after she has run through the family bank account by making lengthy long-distance telephone calls and by purchasing expensive jewelry and clothing.

121. George is indignant when his graduate school thesis committee refuses to approve his project. "They're just jealous of me because they know I'll be the most brilliant anthropologist in history," he remarks. This is the attitude he has had all of his life.

122. Sharon's life has always been chaotic. She has a history of fighting and breaking up with her friends. On occasion, she has attempted suicide in an effort to get her boyfriend to reconsider a relationship with her. Last year she contracted gonorrhea and delayed getting medical help.

123. Jean and her friend are discussing a party that they attended several nights before. Jean's friend tells her that she behaved in a bizarre and even threatening manner at the party, in a way that was totally uncharacteristic. Jean is in the habit of smoking marijuana, but she remembers nothing of the party after smoking one joint.

Questions 124–127

Match each biostatistical concept with the definition that best describes it.

(A) Incidence
(B) Prevalence
(C) Specificity
(D) Sensitivity
(E) Validity/accuracy
(F) Reliability/precision

124. Ability of a test to correctly identify a true positive in a patient with a disease

125. Ability of a test to consistently reproduce measurements of the same entity

126. Number of cases of the disease at any moment in time (per 100,000 population)

127. Ability of a test to correctly produce a negative result in a patient without disease

Questions 128–131

Match each of the following descriptions with the appropriate segment or segments of the small intestine.

(A) Jejunum
(B) Ileum
(C) Both
(D) Neither

128. Contains well-developed plicae circulares

129. Contains many arterial arcades

130. May contain Meckel's diverticulum

131. Has appendices epiploicae on its external surface

Questions 132–136

For each statement below, select the tissue culture type most likely to demonstrate the property described.

(A) Organ cultures
(B) Primary cell cultures
(C) Continuous cell lines
(D) Cell strains
(E) None of the above

132. These frequently contain multiple cell types but form monolayers that continue to divide in culture for a few generations

133. These can be subcultured approximately 30 to 50 times before dying out or undergoing spontaneous transformation

134. These will not grow as monolayer cultures but maintain virus sensitivity

135. These maintain some forms of differentiated tissue markers but propagate indefinitely

136. These maintain a very high degree of differentiated cell markers

Questions 137–144

Match each of the following historical, physical, or laboratory findings with the appropriate form of arthritis.

(A) Septic arthritis
(B) Osteoarthritis (degenerative joint disease)
(C) Rheumatoid arthritis
(D) Lyme disease
(E) Systemic sclerosis
(F) Reiter's syndrome
(G) Gout

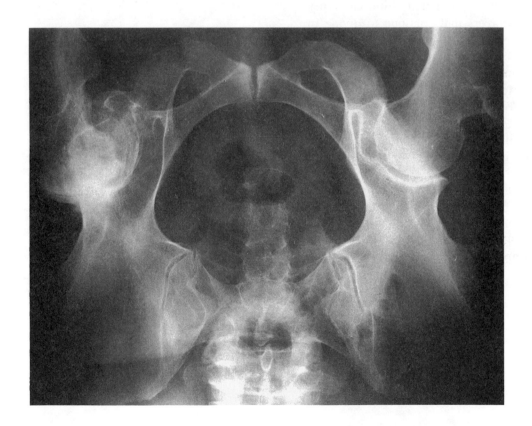

137. The above roentgenogram and the following computed tomography scan of a femoral joint taken from a 40-year-old mail carrier

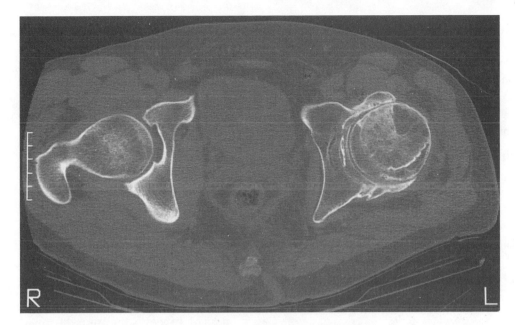

138. The synovial biopsy of the wrist showed invasive pannus tissue eroding the cartilage

139. This condition is associated with human leukocyte antigen B27 (HLA-B27)

140. Obesity predisposes a person to this disease; occurrences are often preceded by gluttonous alcohol consumption and heavy eating

141. Cloudy synovial fluid with a leukocyte count of 110,000/mm^3 (95% polymorphonuclears) was drained from the hip of an elderly woman who experienced acute warmth and tenderness in the joint

142. Cloudy, hypercellular synovial fluid shows negatively birefringent crystals

143. Arthritic symptoms in the knee following an episode of *Chlamydia trachomatis* urethritis

144. Polyarthritis in a 9-year-old girl following a maculopapular erythematous rash

Questions 145–148

Match each visual defect described below with the condition that causes it.

(A) Cataracts
(B) Astigmatism
(C) Presbyopia
(D) Myopia
(E) Hyperopia

145. A progressive decrease in the power of accommodation

146. A progressive loss of lens transparency

147. Focusing point of light rays is in front of the retina

148. Focusing point of light rays is behind the retina

Questions 149–153

Match each characteristic listed below with the most appropriate type of capillary.

(A) Continuous
(B) Fenestrated
(C) Discontinuous
(D) Lymphatic

149. Abundant in skeletal muscle

150. Predominant in areas producing blood filtrates such as urine

151. Line bone marrow sinusoids

152. Present in the choroid plexus

153. Form the blood–brain barrier

Questions 154–157

Match the following patient presentations with the most likely clinical diagnosis.

(A) Cerebrovascular accident in the motor cortex
(B) Guillain-Barré syndrome
(C) Amyotrophic lateral sclerosis (ALS; Lou Gehrig disease)
(D) Neurosyphilis
(E) Duchenne muscular dystrophy
(F) Friedreich's ataxia
(G) Myasthenia gravis

154. A 39-year-old white man presents to his physician because of progressive muscle weakness of 1 week's duration. His medical history is unremarkable, although he reports having had an influenza-like episode approximately 2 weeks ago. He has been sexually active since age 16. During the physical examination, the physician notes a marked decrease in reflexes and a loss of light touch and vibration sensation in the distal extremities.

155. A 6-year-old black boy is brought to the physician's office by his mother. His mother is concerned that he can no longer keep up with his friends, and she notes that he is using his hands to pull himself up from the floor. Medical history reveals that an uncle on her side of the family died in his late teens. During the physical examination, the physician notes that the boy's calf muscles appear enlarged and that his heel tendon is unusually taut. His muscle strength is extremely impaired.

156. A 55-year-old man with no previous medical problems visits a physician because his arms have become progressively weaker over the past 2 months. He is divorced and has been sexually active with more than one partner. The weakness and fatigue began first in one arm and developed later in the other. During the physical examination, the physician notes hyperreflexia, as well as generalized muscle weakness, in all four extremities. The man has no sensory dysfunction, and his gait is normal, considering his weakness.

157. A 34-year-old woman presents with muscular weakness of 3 months' duration and says that she "tires easily" when she's trying to work. After she rests for a while, some of her strength returns. She reports having some trouble with her vision, particularly diplopia; her speech appears to be dysarthric. During the physical examination, the physician notes bilateral facial weakness and a somewhat asymmetric distribution of proximal limb weakness. The woman's tendon reflexes are normal.

Questions 158–161

A drug experiment was conducted, and the figures below show the results, which have been plotted in two different ways. Match each number in the figures with the most appropriate term.

(A) Maximal effect
(B) K_D
(C) $-1/K_D$
(D) 1/Maximal effect
(E) None of the above

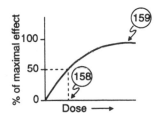 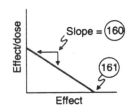

Questions 162–167

For each of the descriptions listed below, select the most appropriate term.

(A) Gene mapping
(B) Linkage
(C) Linkage disequilibrium
(D) Genetic polymorphism
(E) Synteny

162. Usually identified by a lod score of $+3$ or greater at a recombination distance of less than 50%

163. Restriction fragment length polymorphisms (RFLPs) are a commonly used example

164. Can be performed by somatic cell genetic and cytogenetic methods

165. The occurrence of two or more alleles at a locus in frequencies greater than can be maintained by mutation

166. The tendency in a population for specific alleles at two loci to occur together more often than is expected by chance

167. The occurrence of two loci on the same chromosome regardless of how far apart they may be

Questions 168–170

Match each of the following developmental milestone(s) with the appropriate age range in a child who is progressing normally.

(A) 3–12 months
(B) 1–3 years
(C) 4–5 years
(D) 6–9 years

168. Can use two- and three-word phrases

169. Reaches for objects not in the immediate range of grasp

170. Can group objects on the basis of common features; understands that mass or volume is conserved, despite a change in shape or form (i.e., fixed volume of water is the same regardless of whether it is in a tall or short glass)

Questions 171–175

Match each of the following stages of mitosis with the appropriate term.

(A) Anaphase
(B) Early prophase
(C) Late prophase
(D) Telophase
(E) Metaphase

171. Dissolution of the nuclear envelope

172. Separation of the centromeres

173. First appearance of chromosomes

174. Alignment of chromosomes in the equatorial plane

175. Occurrence of cytokinesis

Questions 176–180

Match each of the following clinical presentations with the appropriate spinographic tracing of forced expiration.

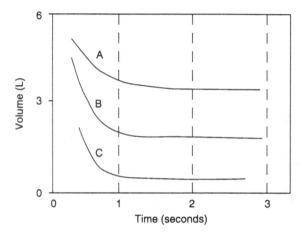

176. A 65-year-old man who has smoked two packs of cigarettes per day for 50 years comes to the office short of breath. His breath sounds are decreased bilaterally.

177. A 58-year-old man presents with a cough that has persisted for 3 months. A chest x-ray shows irregular opacities in the lower and middle lung fields. The man believes he was exposed to asbestos for approximately 5 years when he was in his early forties.

178. A 9-year-old girl with a history of asthma presents to the emergency room with an acute exacerbation, after her albuterol inhaler ran out the day before.

179. A healthy, 30-year-old woman visits the office for a life insurance physical. She has never smoked, and her breath sounds are normal

180. A 30-year-old man has been hospitalized for Guillain-Barré syndrome and is now short of breath.

Questions 181–183

For each cell characteristic or function described below, select the cell with which it is most closely associated.

(A) T cell
(B) B cell
(C) Macrophage
(D) Natural killer (NK) cell
(E) Eosinophil
(F) Basophil
(G) Neutrophil
(H) Mast cell

181. Functions as helper in antibody response

182. Functions as suppressor cell

183. Phagocytizes and processes antigen in the immune response

Questions 184–186

Match each of the following descriptions of developmental theory with the correct researcher.

(A) Piaget
(B) Freud
(C) Maslow
(D) Kohlberg
(E) Erikson

184. Psychosexual development proceeds with different parts of the body serving as the focus of sexual gratification during different stages

185. Development of the ego takes place within a social context across the entire life cycle; each stage is characterized by a struggle that must be resolved before progressing to the next stage

186. Childhood thinking processes develop in stages, with most children passing through each stage in a sequential fashion; reasoning power in each stage is qualitatively different from the previous stage because new skills have been acquired

Questions 187–189

An acutely ill 3-year-old boy is brought to the emergency room. His breathing is extremely labored, and he is producing rust-colored sputum. A Gram stain of the sputum reveals numerous gram-positive cocci in random clusters. A diagnosis of staphylococcal pneumonia is made, and the child is hospitalized and placed on an intravenous methicillin. The mother reports that the child has experienced several such episodes previously that were successfully controlled with antibiotics. Further discussion of the child's medical history reveals that he had experienced a normal recovery from measles approximately 6 months earlier.

187. The most probable diagnosis, based on this history, is

(A) DiGeorge's syndrome
(B) Nezelof's syndrome
(C) Wiskott-Aldrich syndrome
(D) selective immunoglobulin deficiency

Leukocyte function studies are performed and indicate that phagocytosis, intracellular killing, and chemotactic responses are all within normal limits.

188. These features rule out defects in nonspecific resistance, a characteristic of all of the following disorders EXCEPT

(A) chronic granulomatous disease (CGD)
(B) lazy leukocyte syndrome
(C) Job's syndrome
(D) dysgammaglobulinemia

An immunoglobulin profile is ordered. The child has no detectable IgA or IgM in his serum. A small amount of IgG (30 mg/dl) is detected when the assay is repeated with low-level radial immunodiffusion plates.

189. Based on this information, the most probable diagnosis is

(A) selective immunoglobulin deficiency
(B) common variable hypogammaglobulinemia
(C) Wiskott-Aldrich syndrome
(D) Bruton's hypogammaglobulinemia
(E) transient hypogammaglobulinemia of infancy

Questions 190–194

Match the pulse and pressure readings listed below with the most likely diagnosis.

(A) Normal
(B) Isolated systolic hypertension
(C) Autonomic neuropathy (e.g., diabetic neuropathy)
(D) Hypovolemia (dehydration)
(E) Hypertension

	Age	Sex	Pulse, supine	Blood pressure, supine	Pulse, sitting	Blood pressure, sitting
190.	74	F	60	140/80	65	128/85
191.	59	M	62	140/80	85	135/75
192.	68	M	72	138/76	74	124/63
193.	81	F	88	154/86	92	150/88
194.	63	M	64	145/92	66	147/94

Questions 195–200

Match each of the following clinical or historical descriptions with the cellular or biochemical defect underlying the disease.

(A) Defective chloride ion channel regulation throughout the body

(B) Defective sodium channels in excitable tissues

(C) Defective androgen receptors in target tissues

(D) Defective 21-hydroxylase activity in steroid producing tissues

(E) Defective 17-β-hydroxysteroid dehydrogenase activity in steroid producing tissues

(F) Defective hydroxylation of proline residues in collagen

(G) Defective lysyl oxidase activity in fibroblasts

(H) Defective phenylalanine hydroxylase activity in the liver

(I) Defective cystathionine β-synthase activity in the liver

(J) Defective porphobilinogen deaminase activity in the liver

195. An 18-year-old man with moderately severe, diffuse abdominal pain has dark red urine and an increased heart rate. He is nauseated and says that he has been vomiting severely over the last several hours. Deep tendon reflexes are diminished, and he has a generalized muscular weakness. He admits to using barbiturates last night at a party, but says it was his first time.

196. A 2-month-old male infant in the neonatal intensive care unit with microcephaly and severe growth retardation has met few of the developmental milestones for his age. His mother vaguely remembers that she had dietary restrictions as a child.

197. A 3-week-old 46;X,X infant has moderate signs of virilization at birth including clitoral hypertrophy and partial fusion of the labioscrotal folds. Radiographic evaluation indicates normal internal female anatomy. She has been admitted to the neonatal intensive care unit for anorexia, vomiting, and hypotension.

198. A 7-year-old white girl is hospitalized with chronic pulmonary infections and malabsorption. Her development has been retarded secondary to her medical problems, which existed from birth.

199. The sternum of an 8-month-old female infant is sunken inward, and she has not stopped crying since her arrival in the emergency room 2 hours ago. Large ecchymoses are evident all over her body, but a careful examination reveals no signs of abuse. The mother, who is unemployed, and the infant live by themselves.

200. An 18-year-old woman with primary amenorrhea has normal breast development, and her body habitus is clearly female. Pubic hair is scanty but present, and she has no facial hair. Her clitoris and external genitalia are normal. A karyotype reveals that chromosomally she is 46;X,Y.

ANSWER KEY

1-A	29-D	57-C	85-C	113-A
2-B	30-B	58-B	86-D	114-C
3-D	31-C	59-C	87-A	115-G
4-D	32-A	60-B	88-E	116-B
5-A	33-E	61-B	89-B	117-A
6-B	34-C	62-E	90-E	118-D
7-A	35-D	63-B	91-C	119-C
8-D	36-C	64-B	92-E	120-E
9-B	37-D	65-A	93-E	121-A
10-C	38-A	66-C	94-A	122-D
11-B	39-C	67-D	95-A	123-B
12-E	40-E	68-B	96-D	124-D
13-C	41-B	69-B	97-E	125-F
14-C	42-B	70-C	98-A	126-B
15-D	43-A	71-A	99-D	127-C
16-A	44-C	72-D	100-B	128-A
17-B	45-C	73-B	101-B	129-B
18-E	46-B	74-E	102-C	130-B
19-C	47-C	75-C	103-C	131-D
20-E	48-B	76-D	104-D	132-B
21-E	49-B	77-E	105-B	133-D
22-A	50-A	78-B	106-E	134-A
23-A	51-C	79-A	107-A	135-C
24-B	52-C	80-C	108-A	136-A
25-D	53-C	81-D	109-A	137-B
26-D	54-B	82-A	110-E	138-C
27-B	55-E	83-E	111-D	139-F
28-B	56-B	84-B	112-D	140-G

141-A	153-A	165-D	177-C	189-D
142-G	154-B	166-C	178-A	190-A
143-F	155-E	167-E	179-B	191-D
144-D	156-C	168-B	180-C	192-C
145-C	157-G	169-A	181-A	193-B
146-A	158-B	170-D	182-A	194-E
147-D	159-E	171-C	183-C	195-J
148-E	160-A	172-A	184-B	196-H
149-A	161-C	173-B	185-E	197-D
150-B	162-B	174-E	186-A	198-A
151-C	163-D	175-D	187-D	199-F
152-B	164-A	176-A	188-D	200-C

ANSWERS AND EXPLANATIONS

1–5. The answers are: 1-A, 2-B, 3-D, 4-D, 5-A. *(Synaptic pharmacology)*

Acetylcholine (ACh) is among the first of the neurotransmitters to have its synthesis, localization, signal transduction, and pharmacology described. Presynaptic neurons frequently have receptors for the transmitter that they release, and these autoreceptors are often important for regulating the subsequent amount of transmitter release. Cholinergic neurons are found in the cerebral cortex and the anterior horn of the spinal cord. All preganglionic neurons in the autonomic nervous system release ACh, and postganglionic neurons of the parasympathetic branch are also cholinergic. A small subset of postganglionic neurons in the cholinergic sympathetic branch release ACh onto eccrine sweat glands and blood vessels. Alzheimer's dementia is correctly characterized by a relatively focal loss of cholinergic neurons in the basal nucleus of Meynert. Tetanus toxin is rapidly transported in a retrograde fashion from peripheral nerve terminals to the anterior horn cell bodies where it is released; inhibitory interneurons take up the toxin in the spinal cord, and the tetanus protein blocks the inhibitory transmission of these neurons.

Release of inositol triphosphate and diacylglycerol is not a direct result of nicotinic receptor activation. Nicotinic receptors are found in the cerebral cortex and in the neuromuscular junction as well as postsynaptically in the autonomic ganglia. They are complex proteins with an ACh-binding site coupled to a cation-permeable channel. When activated, the receptors conduct sodium and potassium ions. Drugs like succinylcholine produce paralysis during intubation by blocking the nicotinic receptors at neuromuscular junctions. Muscarinic receptors are universally coupled to either excitatory or inhibitory G proteins. They are important in mediating the effects of parasympathetic activation; thus, their blockade with drugs such as atropine results in decreased salivation (as well as other effects). Both receptor types are activated endogenously by ACh.

Nicotinic receptor activation during physiologic conditions principally causes sodium (not potassium) influx, with a resultant depolarization and increase in excitability. Sufficient depolarization leads to the activation of voltage-sensitive calcium channels and an influx of calcium. Muscarinic activation can be inhibitory or excitatory; however, this is not dependent on its function as an ion channel (because these receptors are not ion channels). G proteins can be excitatory or inhibitory, and muscarinic receptors can be coupled to either type of G protein. The particular G protein that is activated determines the effect of muscarinic activation. Different G proteins lead to depolarization or hyperpolarization, and, thus, muscarinic activity can and does change the neuron's resting potential. Muscarinic receptors were initially identified by the muscarine toxin; however, they activate (not inhibit) the receptor and, thus, mimic ACh. The symptoms described (i.e., bradycardia, salivation, flushing of the skin, bronchoconstriction) are the symptoms of mushroom poisoning (parasympathetic activation). The toxin activates the receptors for a longer period because it is not as easily degraded as ACh.

The influx of calcium is a prerequisite for the release of any neurotransmitter from any axonic terminal. ACh release is blocked by the toxin from *Clostridium botulinum*. Whereas high-affinity uptake of choline is important for the synthesis of new ACh, termination of the cholinergic transmission is mainly the function of fast-acting acetylcholinesterase (AChE). Cholinesterase inhibition is an important therapy in patients with myasthenia gravis. Myasthenic patients have an autoimmune disorder directed against their nicotinic receptors, not their nerve terminals. Inhibitors of monoamine oxidase (MAO) are important therapeutics for depression because of their effects on the dopaminergic and adrenergic systems.

All proteins—and, therefore, most enzymes, including ChAT—are synthesized in cell bodies (not axons) of neurons, because ribosomes are confined to the neuronal soma. In the cholinergic neuron, choline acetyltransferase (ChAT) creates a covalent link between choline and acetyl coenzyme A (acetyl CoA) before transport of newly synthesized ACh into storage vesicles. ChAT must be present in all cholinergic nerve terminals. Cholinergic nerve terminals are widely distributed throughout the nervous system in all animals. As mentioned previously, cholinergic neurons selectively degenerate in patients with Alzheimer's dementia, and a subsequent decrease in the ChAT levels of these patients is easily detected.

6–8. The answers are: 6-B, 7-A, 8-D. *(Defense mechanisms)*

Denial, a primitive or infantile defense (i.e., at the lower level of adaptive functioning), has been defined as the disavowing and rejecting of any aspects of internal or external reality, which, if acknowledged, would cause anxiety. The patient is denying his drinking problem despite the associated physical illness. He is thus avoiding the external reality of the cause of his illness. The other defense mechanisms mentioned may play some part in his coping with his alcoholism, but none is the primary mechanism used by this alcoholic patient.

In this instance, the business executive acknowledges his drinking but disavows his own responsibility and justifies his behavior by attributing it to his wife's nagging. The other defense mechanisms, which fall at the middle to the higher levels of adaptive behavior, do not apply in this situation.

It is expected that the patient would feel sad, frightened, angry, or guilty about having developed cirrhosis from his excessive alcohol consumption. To avoid these uncomfortable feelings, he is using the mechanism of reaction formation to push them out of awareness. If the patient were to describe his self-caused serious illness in unemotional terms and claim he felt no anger, sadness, or unhappiness, he would be using the defense of isolation of affect.

9–12. The answers are: 9-B, 10-C, 11-B, 12-E. *(Pregnancy and hypertension)*

Hypertension in pregnancy is a serious but not uncommon complication. The high-output cardiac status of a pregnant woman is principally a result of the decreased peripheral resistance afforded by the addition of the placenta to the maternal circulation. Thus, by the third trimester some women actually show decreased blood pressure. The historical factors of greatest importance in this case include the woman's relatively young age, her first pregnancy, and the fetal age (third trimester). All of these factors characterize a woman with pre-eclampsia, a disorder of unknown etiology that is diagnosed by proteinuria and hypertension. The physical finding of pathologic edema in the face and hands is common but not diagnostic. Spontaneous abortion in the third trimester might result in substantial bleeding, and passage of the fetus would almost certainly be noted by the mother. Benzodiazepine abuse in this young mother would certainly be of concern but would probably not lead to the physical findings described (especially not hypertension in a woman without renal disease). Hemolytic disease of the newborn is a complication of Rhesus factor (Rh) incompatibility in the second and subsequent pregnancies, when there is Rh incompatibility in a previous pregnancy. An Rh-negative mother is "inoculated" with the incompatible Rh antigen during delivery of her Rh-positive child, and later the mother mounts an anamnestic response against other Rh-positive pregnancies. Congestive heart failure is not likely in this young woman who has no history of cardiac or renal disease. In any case, congestive heart failure usually produces dependent edema of the lower extremities.

The role of atrial natriuretic factor (ANF) in physiologic maintenance of blood pressure has not been ascertained, but it is a potent diuretic (as its name indicates). The role of angiotensin II is complicated but includes peripheral vasoconstriction and the enhancement of vasopressin [i.e., antidiuretic hormone (ADH)] release by the hypothalamus and aldosterone secretion by the adrenal cortex. The activity of vasopressin in the medullary collecting duct is critical, as can be seen in patients with both inappropriate as well as insufficient ADH production [i.e., syndrome of inappropriate ADH (SIADH) and pituitary stalk section, respectively]. Vasopressin increases water permeability of the tubules so that the large osmotic gradient can facilitate water reabsorption. Sympathetic nervous system (SNS) activity (e.g., release of norepinephrine and epinephrine) causes vasoconstriction in most arteriole beds, but vasodilation in the coronary circulation. This is mainly because of the increased number of β-adrenergic receptors on coronary vessels. Aldosterone increases tubular reabsorption of sodium (not potassium) ions in the distal tubule at the expense of potassium and hydrogen ions. Spironolactone, an important aldosterone antagonist, is known as a potassium-sparing diuretic principally because of its inhibition of aldosterone-mediated losses in potassium. Renin increases aldosterone production, and its actions augment the effects of aldosterone.

Labetalol acts principally by blocking β_1-receptors, therefore decreasing cardiac contractility as well as conduction velocity through the A node. Labetalol is both a negative inotrope and chronotrope, and it is best used in hypertensive patients who also have ischemic heart disease. Methyldopa acts (after being converted to methylnorepinephrine) by stimulating α_2-adrenergic autoreceptors in the brainstem (i.e., central effect), causing a diminished sympathetic outflow from the central nervous system (CNS). Diltiazem and other calcium channel blockers (e.g., verapamil, nifedipine) act principally by decreasing smooth muscle tension and, thus, lowering arteriolar resistance. Thiazide diuretics act in the distal tubule to decrease sodium reabsorption by reducing sodium–chloride cotransport. This results in increased urine volume because more sodium is delivered to later segments of the tube that cannot adequately compensate. Renin cleaves angiotensinogen to angiotensin I; captopril competitively inhibits the angiotensin-converting enzyme, which is found in the lung. The enzyme normally converts angiotensin I to the more active angiotensin II.

The best answer is the decline from preeclampsia to eclampsia. Clinical criteria for eclampsia include seizure activity, which can lead to coma; oliguria often precedes this decline. As described earlier, the mother is not the target of antibodies in hemolytic disease of the newborn (or fetus). The rapidly occurring compensations for hypertension involve the SNS; polyuria and hyponatremia, both of which are kidney mechanisms, do not occur rapidly. In any case, the close regulation of both plasma volume and plasma sodium would not be compromised to regulate this degree of blood pressure elevation. As stated earlier, cardiac output is actually increased in most pregnant women because of the decreased peripheral resistance afforded by the placenta; neither congestive heart failure nor myocardial ischemia are likely in this woman. Bleeding and shock can accompany spontaneous abortion; however, the woman in this case did not present with these clinical signs.

13. The answer is C. *(Log–dose response relationships)*
Curves A, C, and D all reach approximately the same maximal response and, thus, are similar in efficacy. However, curve A is more potent than C, which, in turn, is more potent than D. Potency is based on the relative positions of the curves along the X axis. A competitive inhibitor would shift the curve to the right. For instance, curves A and C might be responses to an agonist in the absence (curve A) and presence (curve C) of a competitive inhibitor. Noncompetitive inhibitors decrease the efficacy (like a partial agonist might do). Thus, curves A and B might be the response to an agent in the absence (curve A) and the presence (curve B) of a noncompetitive inhibitor.

14. The answer is C. *(Ehlers-Danlos syndrome)*
Ehlers-Danlos syndrome represents a spectrum of disordered collagen biosynthesis. The clinical features of Ehlers-Danlos syndrome depend on the exact underlying abnormality but can include hyperextensible skin, hypermobile joints, large vessel fragility, and vulnerability to retinal detachment. The defect in type VI Ehlers-Danlos syndrome involves the collagens that predominate in the skin, bone, tendons, and vessels (i.e., types I and III). The syndrome results from decreased lysyl hydroxylase activity. Since hydroxylysine residues are critical to proper crosslinking, the structural stability of collagen in patients with Ehlers-Danlos syndrome is compromised. There are no common Ehlers-Danlos syndromes that principally involve the cartilage and vitreous humor, which are structures that contain type II collagen. The characteristics describing laminin, proteoglycans, and fibronectin are all correct; however, none of these macromolecules are implicated in any of the Ehlers-Danlos syndromes.

15. The answer is D. *(Serous intermediate ovarian tumor)*
The papillary tumor pictured is a serous intermediate (borderline) tumor of the ovary, which is commonly seen in young women. The tumor behaves in an indolent fashion, with repeated recurrences but rare metastases outside of the abdominal cavity, resulting in a high incidence of intestinal obstruction and long survival. The tumor is characterized by edematous papillae lined by stratified cuboidal to columnar cells, which have atypical cytology. Unlike serous adenocarcinomas, serous intermediate tumors do not invade ovarian stroma.

16. The answer is A. *(Myocardial infarction)*
Immediately after a person suffers a myocardial infarction, changes are often evident on an electrocardiogram. Alterations in electrical events in the ventricles, including prolonged depolarization, are common and are manifested by abnormalities in the T wave. Although changes in circulating enzyme levels are helpful for diagnostic and prognostic purposes, they usually occur 6 hours or more after the attack and are more helpful 24 to 72 hours after the myocardial infarction.

17. The answer is B. *(Hepatitis A)*
Hepatitis A has a short incubation period of between 15 and 40 days. The infection is transmitted by the fecal–oral route and takes hold very quickly. The virus replicates in the gastrointestinal tract and is shed in the feces during both the incubation and acute phases of the disease.

18. The answer is E. *(Gas exchange and partial pressure of oxygen)*
The change in cabin air pressure will cause a modest reduction in arterial Po_2. The partial pressure of a gas is proportional to the fractional concentration of the gas and total gas pressure. Predictably, Po_2 would decrease from the normal range of 97 to 100 mm Hg to approximately 67 mm Hg following decreases in alveolar Po_2. This decrease is partially due to water vapor pressure, which remains constant at 47 mm Hg, and Pco_2, which may decrease slightly due to stimulation from ventilation. This modest decline in Po_2 would not be associated with a decrease in oxygen saturation of arterial hemoglobin. A compensatory response would shift the oxyhemoglobin dissociation curve to the right because of the production of 2,3-diphosphoglycerate (2,3-DPG); however, this response usually takes more time than the average plane flight.

19–22. The answers are: 19-C, 20-E, 21-E, 22-A. *(Systemic lupus erythematosus)*
Many types of antinuclear antibodies are found in lupus patients, and the presence of antinuclear antibodies is an American Rheumatology Association (ARA) criterion for systemic lupus erythematosus (SLE). Histone antigens, double-stranded DNA antigens, and nucleolar antigens, as well as several others, are targeted in SLE. Interestingly, histones seem to be the primary target in greater than 95% of drug-induced lupus patients. Antinuclear antibodies are also found in other autoimmune connective tissue diseases including polymyositis and systemic sclerosis. Evidence from large family trees and concordance studies among monozygotic twins indicate a strong genetic component in the etiology of SLE, and there is a possible association between SLE and the human leukocyte antigen haplotypes DR2 (HLA-DR2) and DR3 (HLA-DR3). Sex hormones clearly influence the pathophysiology and progression of SLE: Women are nine times more likely to be affected by SLE than are men. Exacerbation of SLE during pregnancy is relatively common, and there is even a link between estrogen metabolism and antibody synthesis. Patients with SLE have global immune hyperactivity that manifests as increased antibody response to both self and foreign antigens. This immune dysregulation can be demonstrated both in vivo and in vitro: B-cell hyperactivity may be fundamental to SLE pathology. Although viruses have long been suspected in the cause of SLE, there is, as yet, no hard evidence linking infectious agents with human SLE.

Drug-induced lupus is caused by a variety of drugs including cardiac medications (e.g., procainamide, labetalol, minoxidil, quinidine, hydralazine), several antiepileptic medications (e.g., carbamazepine, phenytoin, valproic acid), some anti-inflammatory medications (e.g., sulfasalazine, penicillamine), an antimycobacterial agent (i.e., isoniazid), and a hyperthyroidism medication (i.e., propylthiouracil). The clinical picture of drug-induced SLE is characteristically void of the typical renal or central nervous system involvement; it is frequently confined to arthralgias, fever, and serositis. In these patients, a deficiency may exist in the liver's capacity to metabolize drugs requiring N-acetyltransferase. [The "slow acetylator" hypothesis proposes that the nonacetylated metabolites accumulate and couple with haptens to become antigenic.] Most drug-induced SLE patients recover completely following withdrawal of the drug. Bleomycin is associated with pulmonary fibrosis; lovastatin with cataracts, myopathy, and hepatitis; pentamidine with hypoglycemia and acute hypotension; and piperacillin (like all penicillin derivatives) with idiopathic hypersensitivity.

The 11 diagnostic criteria established by the ARA include: antinuclear antibodies, malar (i.e., butterfly) facial rash, serositis (i.e., pleuritis, pericarditis, peritonitis), oral ulcers, photosensitivity, renal disorder (i.e., proteinuria or cellular casts), neuropsychiatric disorder (i.e., seizure or psychosis), hematologic dyscrasia (i.e., anemia with reticulocytosis, leukopenia, thrombocytopenia), LE cell or false-positive Venereal Disease Research Laboratory (VDRL) tests. Any four of these criteria met at any time (serially or simultaneously) constitute adequate evidence for an SLE diagnosis.

Renal failure is a common cause of death in SLE patients, and the extent of renal inflammation frequently determines the intensity of anti-inflammatory therapy. It is rare for a person with confirmed SLE to have a normal renal biopsy if immunofluorescence and electron microscopy are performed. The most benign of lesions is mesangial lupus glomerulonephritis, which is characterized by minor histologic changes and immunoglobulin and complement deposits in the mesangial cells. The photomicrograph demonstrates proliferative glomerulonephritis, which is found in over 80% of renal biopsies taken from SLE patients. The histopathology shows fibrinoid deposits; mesangial and endothelial cell proliferation; and basophilic inflammatory cells in and surrounding the glomerulus. A critical feature is the paucity of patent capillary loops because the loops have been squeezed shut by the hypercellularity. In focal proliferative glomerulonephritis, not all glomeruli are affected, and only portions of each glomerulus show gross histologic changes. Diffuse proliferative glomerulonephritis is a more advanced stage; there is hypercellularity throughout the glomerulus, and most glomeruli are involved. Clinically, patients with proliferative glomerulonephritis have symptoms ranging from a nephrotic syndrome with mild proteinuria to overt nephritis with gross hematuria and a compromise in glomerular filtration rate (GFR). Membranous glomerulonephritis accounts for fewer than 10% of cases. It appears as a distinct thickening of the capillary walls with symptoms of nephrosis resulting. Periarterial fibrosis is a lesion of the spleen which is characteristic of SLE. Tubular necrosis is the lesion most commonly seen following shock-induced hypoperfusion of the kidneys; inflammation and necrosis are confined to the tubules and interstitium and, for the most part, spare the glomeruli. Interstitial nephritis is encountered in a number of different renal disease processes, most notably diabetic nephropathy. As with tubular necrosis, the hypercellularity and inflammatory cells are mainly associated with the area between the glomeruli. In the photomicrograph shown, the interstitium is comparatively normal, and the glomerulus is the obvious target of a tremendous number of inflammatory cells.

23–25. The answers are: 23-A, 24-B, 25-D. *(Hemochromatosis and clinical findings in cirrhosis)*
Identification of hemochromatosis in its early stages facilitates effective treatment of this otherwise relentlessly progressive disease. Although he is being treated, this patient has already progressed to late stages of the disease, and he is now displaying the classic signs of cirrhosis. The bleeding is most likely the result of ruptured esophageal varices. Portal hypertension chronically diverts blood through the esophagus veins, and those vessels dilate to support the increased flow. Portal hypertension causes the development of several collateral circulations; these other vessels offer less resistance to flow, and they enlarge over time to accommodate the increased volume. The rectal and esophageal veins dilate to become varices, which may allow significant blood loss if they tear. The caput medusae vascular pattern over the abdomen represents the enlargement of another collateral circulation. Portal hypertension also causes blood flow to back up in the spleen, which results in splenomegaly. Hemoglobin synthesis is limited by iron availability. A hemochromatosis patient has excess iron and will probably not be hemoglobin deficient. Protein C is an anticoagulant whose exact mechanism of action remains unknown. Deficiency of protein C has been demonstrated in some cases of disseminated intravascular coagulation. Although neither eroded gastric ulcer nor bronchogenic carcinoma is excluded by hemochromatosis, hemochromatosis does not predispose to either of those conditions. The patient's bleeding is more likely the result of portal hypertension.

Hepatic encephalopathy is an important complication in cirrhosis of the liver. It causes no irreversible pathology, and clinical symptoms recede as soon as metabolic corrections are made. The clinical findings can range from mild disturbances in consciousness to frank coma. The flapping tremor of asterixis (i.e., rapid extension–flexion movements of the head and arms) is most distinctive. Parkinson's disease is primarily confined to the motor system. Alterations in consciousness are rarely attributable to Parkinson's pathology. Shy-Drager syndrome is a degenerative disease characterized by autonomic neuropathy and Parkinsonian-like motor abnormalities; the man would not be showing signs of sympathetic activation. The neuronal degeneration in vitamin B_{12} deficiency is characterized by demyelination in the spinal cord and leads to peripheral sensorimotor deficits without changes in consciousness. Patients usually characterize subarachnoid hemorrhage as the "worst headache of my life."

Hemochromatosis is an autosomal recessive disorder that is five times more common in men, and it is related to the human leukocyte antigen A3 in 70% of cases. Renal excretion of iron is inherently limited to approximately 1 mg/day. Thus, in developed countries, the regulation of iron homeostasis requires absolute control of absorption. Unfortunately, the normal mechanisms of regulation are not well understood. The iron buildup seen as a physiologic response to anemia is almost entirely confined to phagocytic cells of the reticuloendothelial system. Yet, in hemochromatosis patients, parenchymal cells of the liver, pancreas, and heart accumulate large amounts of iron, whereas phagocytes remain normal. Thus, although there is clearly a regulatory problem at the absorptive stage, the reticuloendothelial system is also functioning improperly. Patients with various erythropoietic difficulties, and a resultant physiologically normal iron accumulation, almost never experience the extensive pathology seen in patients with primary hemochromatosis. Involvement of the pancreas commonly leads to diabetes mellitus, and skin pigmentation is a routine finding.

26. The answer is D. *(Structure of viruses)*
Viruses have either RNA or DNA, not both. Bacteria in the genus *Chlamydia* contain both types of nucleic acid. Both *Chlamydia* and viruses are obligate intracellular parasites, which depend on the host cell for energy. Because some viruses require arthropod vectors, but other viruses (and *Chlamydia*) do not need arthropod vectors, this is not a dependable differentiating characteristic.

27. The answer is B. *(Probability of hepatitis B)*
Given that $P(D+) = .20$, $P(D-) = .80$, $P(T+|D+) = .90$, and $P(T-|D-) = .95$, the probability that a patient with a negative test result does not have hepatitis B, $P(D-|T-)$, is

$$P(D-|T-) = \frac{P(T-|D-)P(D-)}{P(T-|D-)P(D-) + P(T-|D+)\,P(D+)}$$

$$= \frac{(.95)(.80)}{(.95)(.80) + (1 - .90)(.20)}$$

28–31. The answers are: 28-B, 29-D, 30-B, 31-C. *(Acid–base physiology)*
The blood findings indicate that this patient has a respiratory alkalosis, an acid–base disturbance characterized by increased arterial pH (or decreased $[H^+]$), decreased $Paco_2$ (hypocapnia), and decreased plasma $[HCO_3^-]$. It should be noted that both $[H^+]$ and $[HCO_3^-]$ are decreased in this patient, which is consistent with the axiom that $[H^+]$ and $[HCO_3^-]$ change in the same direction in respiratory acid–base imbalances. The decline in $[HCO_3^-]$ indicates that renal compensation has begun.

In alkalotic states, the $[HCO_3^-]/S \times Pco_2$ ratio exceeds the normal 20:1, because of either an increase in $[HCO_3^-]$ (metabolic alkalosis) or a decrease in Pco_2 (respiratory alkalosis). S is a solubility constant. The normal ratio of 20:1 is derived as

$$\frac{[HCO_3^-]}{S \times Pco_2} = \frac{24 \text{ mmol/L}}{0.03 \times 40 \text{ mm Hg}} = \frac{24 \text{ mmol/L}}{1.2 \text{ mmol/L}} = \frac{20}{1}$$

In this alkalotic patient, the $[HCO_3^-]/S \times P_{CO_2}$ ratio is 30:1. This ratio can be determined by substituting the patient's blood data into the preceding equation, as

$$\frac{[HCO_3^-]}{S \times P_{CO_2}} = \frac{22.5 \text{ mmol/L}}{0.03 \times 25 \text{ mm Hg}} = \frac{22.5 \text{ mmol/L}}{0.75 \text{ mmol/L}} = \frac{30}{1}$$

The total CO_2 content for this patient is approximately 23 mmol/L. Total CO_2 equals the sum of all forms of CO_2 in the blood (i.e., HCO_3^-, H_2CO_3, dissolved CO_2, and CO_2 bound to proteins). Dissolved CO_2 content ($[CO_2]$) is calculated as

$$\begin{aligned} [CO_2] &= 0.03 \times P_{CO_2} \\ &= 0.03 \times 40 \text{ mm Hg} \\ &= 1.2 \text{ mmol/L} \end{aligned}$$

Because $[H_2CO_3]$ is negligible, the total CO_2 content normally exceeds the $[HCO_3^-]$ by 1.2 mmol/L and, therefore, equals 25.2 mmol/L when normal plasma $[HCO_3^-]$ and P_{CO_2} values exist, as

$$\begin{aligned} \text{total } CO_2 \text{ content} &= [HCO_3^-] + (S \times P_{CO_2}) \\ &= 24 \text{ mmol/L} + 1.2 \text{ mmol/L} \\ &= 25.2 \text{ mmol/L} \end{aligned}$$

Total CO_2 content is decreased in respiratory alkalosis. From this patient's blood data, the CO_2 content is calculated as

$$\begin{aligned} \text{total } CO_2 \text{ content} &= [HCO_3^-] + (S \times P_{CO_2}) \\ &= 22.5 \text{ mmol/L} + 0.75 \text{ mmol/L} \\ &= 23.25 \text{ mmol/L} \end{aligned}$$

Respiratory alkalosis decreases the renal reabsorption of HCO_3^-, causing a transient HCO_3^- diuresis and a decline in net acid secretion. Because the major change in respiratory alkalosis is a decrease in Pa_{CO_2}, the compensation will be in the alternate variable (kidney) and in the same direction as the primary event. Thus, there is a decline in plasma $[HCO_3^-]$, which is indicative of a partial renal response (i.e., increased HCO_3^- excretion).

32–36. The answers are: 32-A, 33-E, 34-C, 35-D, 36-C. *(Stroke, neuroanatomy of vision, anticoagulation)*
The absence of motor defects rules out much of the frontal lobe, and the presence of partial visual field defects (as well as the striking cognitive disturbance) indicates temporal or parietal lesions. The patient is displaying signs of lateral neglect syndrome, in which lesions to the nondominant parietal lobe cause severe disturbances in a person's ability to respond to any stimuli contralaterally. Thus, sensory stimuli administered to the left side are attributed to the homologous region on the right side of the body; persons or objects in the left visual field are ignored. However, there is clearly no primary sensory loss—the deficit is purely perceptual (i.e., secondary and tertiary processing are dysfunctional). The visual deficit described is commonly referred to as "pie-on-the-floor" because the two homologous lower quadrants are lost. This pattern of visual loss coupled with the features of lateral neglect strongly suggest a parietal lesion, because half of the optic radiations from the thalamus proceed upward through the parietal lobe before reaching the calcarine cortex.

The correct localization of optic tract lesions can be instrumental in isolating tumors, infarctions, and other sources of neurologic disorders. Lesions of the optic nerve (A) result in unilateral blindness and are generally not difficult to identify. Severance of the chiasm at B results in the unique finding of bitemporal hemianopsia. There is complete loss of the nasal visual fields because the temporal retinal fibers cross over to the other hemisphere at this point. Section of the fibers at *C* results in a unilateral visual loss of the contralateral visual field (again, retinal arcas always "look at" the contralateral field). The fibers at *D* and *E* are the optic radiations that relay information from the thalamus to the calcarine cortex. Cutting the fibers at *D* causes a "pie-in-the-sky" lesion opposite to the one described because the two homologous upper quadrants are lost. Information from the lower half of the retinal ganglion cells projects through the temporal lobe—the lower retina "looks at" the upper visual field. The correct lesion interrupts the parietal optic radiation, which conducts information from the superior retinal ganglia and causes pie-on-the-floor deficits. Thus, the characteristic visual deficit coupled with the lateral neglect syndrome give adequate reason to suspect a parietal lobe lesion.

Perhaps the most important reason for identifying the cause of a cerebrovascular accident (CVA) is to prevent the next one from happening. Berry aneurysms in the circle of Willis cause a different set of symptoms (most commonly, subarachnoid hemorrhage and what patients describe as "the worst headache of my life"). Berry aneurysms would have been detected by angiography. In some cases, deep venous thrombosis might indicate a coagulopathy, which could also cause local thrombosis in the cortex. However, in this 75-year-old woman, it is more likely that deep venous thrombosis is the result of decreased physical activity. Thrombi breaking off of a deep venous thrombosis would most directly give rise to a pulmonary (not cerebral) embolus and infarction. Congestive heart failure can cause low-flow ischemia and infarction, especially in patients with severe atherosclerotic disease. However, low-flow ischemia generally targets the areas of the brain that are most susceptible to hypoxia—the large pyramidal cells of the motor cortex (i.e., Betz cells) and the large hippocampal neurons. This woman has neither focal motor deficits nor memory dysfunction. Arteriovenous malformations would have been found on routine angiography, and they usually cause frank hemorrhage or hemorrhagic infarction, which were not seen on a computed tomography (CT) scan. Atrial fibrillation with mural thrombosis is the likely cause of this woman's thromboembolic event. Thrombi breaking off of a large clot in the left atrium have easy and direct access to the vessels of the cerebral cortex. Areas without collateral circulation are quickly infarcted after embolic occlusion of the small vessel serving that region of tissue. Multi-infarct dementia is often related to a large clot in the left atrium, the common carotid, or one of the major branches of the carotids. The clot serves as a ready source of tiny emboli, which continually break off and cause focal lesions in the tissue served by the small vessel that they occlude. The region of tissue is often small enough that the deficit is not immediately noted; instead, a large number of individual deficits produce substantial functional loss over time. This woman needs to be evaluated as a candidate for anticoagulant and antiarrhythmic therapy.

The liver synthesizes most of the substances in the clotting cascade as zymogen (inactive) proteins, which are either cofactors or enzymes. Many of the enzymes are members of a class known as serine proteases, because a serine residue forms the active site and cleaves the ester or amide linkage on the substrate. Tissue factor, which is derived from endothelial cells, is released after tissue damage to activate the extrinsic pathway. High molecular weight kininogen, prekallikrein, and Hageman factor interact to activate the intrinsic cascade. The final common pathway is activation of the serine protease thrombin by factor V; thrombin cleaves platelet-bound fibrinogen to create the fibrin monomer. Vitamin K is essential in the liver synthesis of γ-carboxyglutamate. The large negative charge afforded by the extra carboxylic acid is critical in the calcium-binding properties of several clotting factors. Antithrombin III is an important regulatory protein, but, as its name implies, it antagonizes the clotting cascade by irreversibly binding to activated thrombin. Antithrombin III is similar to the protein α_1-antitrypsin, which inhibits elastase in the lung.

Heparin, a large, negatively charged polysaccharide, acts by increasing the speed of binding of antithrombin III to thrombin (i.e., increasing the effectiveness of antithrombin III). Because it directly affects the clotting cascade, heparin's onset of action is relatively acute. Tissue plasminogen activator and urokinase both cleave plasminogen to plasmin, the active form. Plasmin cleaves the cross-linked fibrin clot in the connector rod regions, converting the clot into a multitude of fibrin monomers. Thus, tissue plasminogen activator and urokinase act in an extremely direct fashion to dissolve established clots (which may be growing); therefore, they are the mainstay in the treatment of acute myocardial infarction. Aspirin irreversibly inhibits cyclooxygenase in all the cells of the body. For platelets, this irreversible enzyme inhibition means irreversible platelet inhibition since platelets have no protein synthesis machinery. Because platelet activation depends on enzymatic release of arachidonic acid metabolites, such as thromboxane, inhibition of the enzyme permanently inactivates the platelet. Streptokinase acts by aiding the enzymatic cleavage of inactive plasminogen to active plasmin. Its action is similar to urokinase and tissue plasminogen activator; however, it is much less specific, markedly antigenic, and no longer the drug of choice. Dicumarol (warfarin) competitively inhibits vitamin K from binding to the liver enzymes that are responsible for carboxylation. Vitamin K antagonists like dicumarol have a slow onset of action, are easily overcome by vitamin K injections, and are important therapeutics in patients with a need for chronic anticoagulation.

37–38. The answers are: 37-D, 38-A. *(Biostatistical analysis of genetic disorders)*
The patient had a brother with poliodystrophy; therefore, the patient's mother and father must be carriers of the disorder. The patient herself may be heterozygous or homozygous for the dominant allele of the poliodystrophy gene. The probability that a child born to two known carriers will be healthy is 3/4; the probability that such a child is also a carrier is 1/2. Thus,

$$P(\text{patient carrier}|\text{patient healthy}) = \frac{P(\text{patient carrier and patient healthy})}{P(\text{patient healthy})}$$
$$= (1/2) \div (3/4)$$
$$= 2/3$$

In the absence of information on his family history of poliodystrophy, the probability that the patient's husband is a carrier is assumed to equal that of the general population (i.e., 1/20). The probability that both the patient and her husband are carriers is, therefore,

$$P(\text{patient carrier and husband carrier}) = P(\text{patient carrier}) \, P(\text{husband carrier})$$
$$= (2/3) \, (1/20)$$
$$= 1/30$$

39–42. The answers are: 39-C, 40-E, 41-B, 42-B. *(Bacterial meningitis)*
The findings of fever, headache, nuchal rigidity, and lethargy with an acute onset and the lack of dramatic neurologic manifestations suggest acute bacterial meningitis. Viral meningitis causes much of the same symptomatology, but the onset typically is more insidious and the patient usually is less acutely ill. Patients with viral encephalitis display the same general symptomatology as those with viral meningitis, but encephalitis is differentiated by dramatic neurologic manifestations and a much poorer prognosis. Fungal meningitis is more chronic and frequently is seen with other systemic signs of mycotic disease. Brain abscess usually is seen with other foci of infection, and the patient typically has deficits that reflect the location of the lesion.

Streptococcus pneumoniae is the most common cause of bacterial meningitis among the elderly. *Haemophilus influenzae* type b is the most common cause of bacterial meningitis overall. Its incidence is highest in children 6 to 12 months old and decreases with age; the incidence of meningitis caused by *H. influenzae* is low in adults. Meningococcal meningitis occurs primarily among young adults, and *Neisseria meningitidis* serogroups A, B, C, and Y cause most cases. *Staphylococcus aureus* occasionally causes meningitis but is a common cause of brain abscess. *Actinomyces israelii* is a rare cause of meningitis associated with trauma to the jaw and gingiva or gastrointestinal tract.

The cell count in the cerebrospinal fluid (CSF) is elevated during acute bacterial meningitis to 1,000–10,000 cells/mm^3; neutrophils are the predominant cell type. Normal cell counts are 0–5 cells/mm^3 CSF. Mononuclear cells are predominant in the CSF late in viral meningitis and in patients with late manifestations of neuro-syphilis; lymphocytes are prominent in early manifestations of neurosyphilis. A few erythrocytes may contaminate the CSF during the lumbar puncture; many erythrocytes can indicate brain hemorrhage. Segmented neutrophils are predominant in the CSF during viral meningitis, but the count rarely exceeds 1,000 cells/mm³.

CSF chemistry is an important tool in determining the general diagnosis of meningitis. During bacterial meningitis, CSF protein characteristically is increased in relation to the cell count; glucose levels are low with a concentration of approximately 40% of simultaneous serum glucose levels. Elevated protein and a very low glucose level usually are found in fungal meningitis. In viral meningitis, protein levels are moderately elevated and glucose concentrations are normal or slightly decreased.

43–44. The answers are: 43-A, 44-C. *(Pharmacokinetics)*
The volume of distribution (V_d) is the ratio of the amount injected to the extrapolated concentration (C_0) at time zero. Because equal amounts of X, Y, and Z were injected, V_d is inversely related to C_0. Therefore, X and Z have an identical V_d, and $V_d Y > V_d X$ or $V_d Z$. Clearance is proportional to the ratio of V_d to half-time ($t_{1/2}$). Because $V_d Y > V_d X$, clearance of Y > clearance of X. Because $t_{1/2}Z > t_{1/2}X$ (which is identical to $t_{1/2}Y$), clearance of Z < clearance of X.

The time to reach steady state is purely a function of $t_{1/2}$. Because $t_{1/2} Z > t_{1/2} X$ or $t_{1/2} Y$, it will take Z longer to reach a steady state than either X or Y. However, X and Y will reach a steady state at precisely the same time. The steady-state concentration (C_{SS}) is a function of the ratio of infused rate to clearance. The infused rates are constant; therefore, C_{SS} is inversely related to clearance. Because clearance of Y > clearance of X or clearance of Z, steady-state concentrations will be [Z] > [X] > [Y].

45. The answer is C. *(Infectious hepatitis)*
Hepatitis B surface antigen (HBsAg) is the earliest serologic marker of the hepatitis B virus (HBV) infection. It indicates active infection (acute or chronic) and usually appears before the onset of symptoms. By the end of 6 months, HBsAg has declined to undetectable levels in most patients. Hepatitis C (HCV; also called non-A, non-B, or transfusion-associated hepatitis) progresses to chronic hepatitis in as many as 60% of infected individuals; as many as 2%–3% of the general population may be HCV carriers. Hepatitis D infection requires coexisting hepatitis B infection because it needs the HBV encapsulation (i.e., surface antigen). Hepatitis B causes subclinical disease in two thirds of infected individuals; fulminant hepatitis occurs in fewer than 1% of affected individuals, and progression to hepatocellular carcinoma occurs in fewer than 5%. Hepatitis A is not common in the United States but is very common in developing countries because it is spread by the fecal–oral route. The carrier state does not exist for hepatitis A infections.

46. The answer is B. *(Mitochondrial intracellular localization)*
Mitochondria typically exist in cell areas that use substantial amounts of adenosine triphosphate (ATP). They are abundant in the apices of ciliated cells because the beating action of cilia consumes ATP. They also exist in apices of cells that have a microvillous brush border such as the cells lining the proximal thick segment of the kidneys, because solute transport and pinocytosis of proteins in the glomerular filtrate consume energy and, therefore, require ATP. Mitochondria are distributed evenly throughout the cytoplasm of smooth muscle cells, steroid-secreting cells, skeletal muscle cells, and liver parenchymal cells rather than existing in apical concentrations.

47. The answer is C. *(Huntington's chorea; medical ethics)*
The man's highly emotional state indicates that he might not be competent. Providing counseling and educating him about his options make a reasoned decision possible. Until he appears competent, his demand for testing is overridden by the physician's duty to prevent a suicide (beneficence). Lying to him about test results would disrespect his autonomy, as would refusing to test him without attempting to facilitate a state of mind in which he could make a reasoned decision. Testing for other diseases would be irrelevant as well as impractical.

48. The answer is B. *(Cirrhosis of the liver)*
Cirrhosis of the liver is an important contributor to morbidity and mortality in the United States. Ascites, the collection of excess fluid in the peritoneal cavity, is caused by portal hypertension, and, for obscure reasons, renal retention of sodium and water. Other important features of cirrhosis include pathologic development of collateral circulations, leading to esophageal varices, hemorrhoids, and caput medusae; decreased estrogen metabolism with concomitant gonadal atrophy, gynecomastia, and amenorrhea; splenomegaly (congestion of the spleen occurs secondary to portal hypertension); impaired liver synthesis of albumin and clotting factors; and hepatic encephalopathy. Gastric ulcers are common in alcoholics, but this is related to the alcohol, not the cirrhosis. Dependent edema can be related to insufficient albumin and general sodium retention in cirrhosis, but pulmonary edema is not characteristic. The mental status changes often seen in cirrhosis are the result of hepatic encephalopathy, which is an important complication in a patient with cirrhosis. The encephalopathy is completely reversible following metabolic correction, and, even when fulminant, the pathologic changes are negligible. There are no signs of chronic or acute degeneration of the cerebral cortex. Hemolytic anemia is also not commonly associated with cirrhosis. The jaundice seen in cirrhosis patients is not due to hemolysis but rather to ineffective bilirubin excretion.

49. The answer is B. *(pH partitioning)*
A weak base such as phenobarbital tends to be in its ionized form at a higher pH. Therefore, alkalinizing the urine with $NaHCO_3$ has the desired effect of hastening renal elimination. In addition, urine flow increases in an alkaline situation, further increasing the amount of phenobarbital that is eliminated. Alkalinization of plasma also tends to move un-ionized phenobarbital out of the central nervous system (CNS) and into the plasma by creating a transient gradient in which movement can occur. Phenobarbital and other barbiturates tend to induce P_{450} enzymes, which should aid the elimination of these drugs. However, the induction of P_{450} enzymes is somewhat slower than desired in an emergency situation.

50. The answer is A. *(Pulmonary mechanics)*
Pleural pressure is not equally distributed from the base to the apex. For a variety of reasons, the pleural pressure is more negative at the apex and, therefore, the transpulmonary pressure (i.e., alveolar–pleural pressure) is greater at the apex. The pressure–volume relationship shown is dependent on the lung's elastic properties, which are constant from base to apex. If it is correctly interpreted, the graph answers the question. The alveoli at different places in the lungs experience different pressures and thus have different volumes. At lung volumes close to functional residual capacity (FRC), which is the resting lung volume, the pressure–volume relationship is steep. Thus, the alveoli at the base, which have slightly smaller pressures, have much smaller volumes. At volumes close to VC, the transluminal pressure has reached the flat portion of the curve, so that the small pressure differences from base to apex no longer matter; alveoli are uniformly inflated. The transluminal pressure is actually negative (therefore closing the alveoli) at the base when the lungs are near residual volume. Not until the lungs have begun filling elsewhere do these alveoli open up again. Alveoli in the apex are more full at FRC than are alveoli at the base; therefore, they receive less ventilation than the alveoli at the base. In other words, alveoli that are already full do not have much room for more ventilation.

51. The answer is C. *(Neuromuscular transmission)*
Motoneurons innervate many skeletal muscle fibers. In large muscles, thousands of fibers may be innervated by one neuron. However, each fiber receives only one axon terminal. Depolarization of the nerve terminal releases acetylcholine (ACh) into the synaptic cleft, where it binds directly to Na^+ channels, causing an end-plate potential. The end-plate itself is not electrically excitable, but passive spreading of end-plate potential to a nearby membrane leads to propagation of the action potential and contraction of all muscle fibers innervated by the motoneuron. When ACh is the neurotransmitter, termination of transmission is accomplished by hydrolysis via acetylcholinesterase.

52. The answer is C. *(Pulmonary mechanics)*
According to the equal pressure point theory, expiratory effort increases flow until airways are actually closed off by the pressure of the effort. Inspiratory efforts that lead to vital capacity inflate the lungs to a large end-inspiratory pressure. Therefore, there is sufficient positive alveolar pressure to maintain patency through all airways, even with a large expiratory effort. Thus, from vital capacity, increased expiratory efforts (i.e., increased positive pleural pressures) are rewarded with increased flow. However, at 50% of VC, increased expiratory efforts only increase the resistance of the airways because the pleural pressure exceeds the alveolar pressure and closes the airways. Because airway resistance decreases with increasing size of the airway, resistance is lowest at vital capacity, where the airways are at their largest calibre. At residual volume, the elastic properties of the chest wall are directed outward. (Try holding your lungs at residual volume for a moment to see how much elastic recoil exists.)

53. The answer is C. *(Herpes simplex virus infection of the nervous system)*
"Cold sores" are caused by the herpes simplex virus (HSV), which usually infects the lips, philtrum, and the areas around the nares of affected individuals. After the primary infection, HSV establishes a latent state in the ganglia of cranial nerve (CN) V where the second (CN V_2) and third (CN V_3) branches of this nerve innervate the areas described above. CN VII is not infected by this virus.

54. The answer is B. *(Hormonal regulation of pregnancy)*
Human chorionic gonadotropin (hCG) can be detected within 10 days of conception, providing a rapid and specific test for pregnancy. Human chorionic somatomammotropin (hCS) directs maternal metabolism to maintain a continuous nutrient flow to the fetus and is first detected 4 weeks after conception. Luteinizing hormone (LH), follicle-stimulating hormone (FSH), and hCG [as well as thyroid-stimulating hormone (TSH)] share α subunits; their β subunits have approximately 70% homology. The first function of hCG is to maintain the corpus luteum steroid production. Without hCG, the corpus luteum dies from lack of LH, and menses begin. After the first 8–12 weeks of gestation, placental production of steroids is sufficient, and the corpus luteum is no longer needed. The hCG level declines somewhat to a plateau, where it remains for the remainder of pregnancy. The hCG actually suppresses pituitary LH secretion, which is already low by the time of conception (i.e., 1–3 days after ovulation).

55. The answer is E. *(DNA replication)*
DNA replication begins at specific sites. In *Escherichia coli*, DNA replication starts at a unique origin and proceeds sequentially in opposite directions. Because of the size of the eukaryotic genome, multiple replication origins are important for timely DNA replication. DNA polymerase cannot start chains de novo; all known DNA polymerases add mononucleotides to the 3' hydroxyl end of an RNA primer, or, as in the case of adenovirus replication, DNA synthesis begins from a serine residue on a protein primer. DNA replication occurs during the S phase of the cell cycle.

56. The answer is B. *(Pulmonary mechanics)*
Compliance is defined as a change in volume over change in pressure. The steeper the curves of the static volume–pressure relationships shown in the figure, the more compliant the lungs. A compliant, or flabby, lung is typical of emphysema, in which recoil pressures are lower at any given lung volume and the functional residual capacity tends to be higher. In contrast, a fibrotic, stiff lung (subject C) has decreased compliance and increased elastic recoil and tends to have a lower functional residual capacity. This increased elastic recoil pulls the chest wall in until the outward recoil of the chest wall equals (but is opposite) the inward recoil of the lung, therefore lowering functional residual capacity.

57. The answer is C. *(Diagnosis of syphilis)*
A Venereal Disease Research Laboratory (VDRL) test and dark-field examination would be the most appropriate combination of tests for determining the cause of the penile lesion. A painless penile lesion that

is crateriform, moist, and indurated is suggestive of primary syphilis. The organism responsible, *Treponema pallidum,* cannot be cultured or detected by Gram stain. It can, however, be visualized by dark-field observation of scrapings from the lesion. Some, but not all, patients with primary syphilis have serologic evidence of infection, readily detected by the VDRL test. The fluorescent treponemal antibody absorption (FTA-ABS) test is only used to confirm diagnosis and is not appropriate here.

58. The answer is B. *(Radiolabeled nucleic acid uptake)*
One of the best methods for measuring cellular proliferation is measuring the uptake of radiolabeled nucleic acid. Dividing cells require nucleotides for DNA synthesis, and the uptake of labeled thymidine and its incorporation in DNA are excellent indicators of cell proliferation. Uracil, which is only used in RNA synthesis, except for some reconstituted through a salvage pathway, would not be indicative of cell division, only of messenger RNA (mRNA) synthesis. Likewise, uptake and incorporation of radiolabeled methionine would involve protein synthesis, not cell division. Trypan blue exclusion is used for quantitating viability and would not be useful in this experiment.

59–60. The answers are: 59-C, 60-B. *(Cardiac mechanics and congestive heart failure)*
The major signs of congestive heart failure are fatigue and dyspnea. Vascular congestion confirmed by physical examination (i.e., neck veins, rales) and third heart sounds due to abnormally high diastolic flow to a normal ventricle or normal flow into a dilated ventricle are also consistent with congestive heart failure. The enlarged cardiac silhouette with pulmonary vascular markings is strongly suggestive of left-sided heart failure. Neither the heart rate nor blood pressure is elevated significantly enough to consider this a malignant arrhythmia or emergency hypertensive crisis.

In the control subject (X), end-diastolic pressure is low, and ejection is well-maintained during systole. In the failing heart, end-diastolic pressure and volume are greatly elevated, and ejection is poorly maintained (stroke volume is reduced). Digitalis (Y) exerts a positive inotropic effect by inhibiting Na^+-K^+ ATPase and indirectly elevating intracellular Ca^+. The effect is to decrease diastolic pressures and volumes and increase stroke volume.

61. The answer is B. *(Neuroanatomy)*
The limbic system is concerned with unconscious biologic drives and emotions and, therefore, is considered the most primitive part of the brain. It contains the limbic lobe, hippocampus, anterior thalamic nucleus, hypothalamus, and the amygdala.

62. The answer is E. *(RNA structure and function)*
In eukaryotes, messenger RNA (mRNA) is formed in the nucleus and must be exported into the cytosol for translation. The initial product of transcription includes all of the introns and flanking regions, which must be removed by splicing before correct translation can occur. The splicing reaction involves hydrolysis of phosphodiester bonds and formation of new phosphodiester bonds within the mRNA molecule. Other processing reactions include additions at both the 5' and 3' ends. A guanosine triphosphate (GTP) molecule is added in reverse orientation to form a cap at the 5' end, and the cap is further modified by the addition of methyl groups. A polyadenylate tail is added at the 3' end.

63–64. The answers are: 63-B, 64-B. *(Lyme disease)*
Lyme disease is a recently described tick-borne disease in which the infectious agent is a spirochete, *Borrelia burgdorferi.* Erythema chronicum migrans and positive antibody to the spirochete are presumed to be diagnostic for this condition, which may be manifested by flu-like symptoms that may ultimately progress towards arthritic, cardiac, and central nervous system (CNS) symptoms. The causative spirochete is sensitive to several antibiotics, including penicillin, tetracycline, and erythromycin.

65. The answer is A. *(Structure and function of amino acids in proteins)*
The physical and chemical properties of the peptide reflect the properties of the constituent amino acids. At pH 7.4, the positive and negative charges of the α-aminó and α-carboxyl terminal groups cancel one another. The side chains of the two aspartate and one glutamate residues are negatively charged; the side chain of arginine is positively charged. Cysteine and methionine both contain sulfur atoms. Any of the amino acids that contain a hydrogen atom attached to a sulfur, nitrogen, or oxygen atom, or containing an atom with an unshared pair of electrons, could form hydrogen bonds. The amino acids valine, phenylalanine, methionine, and cysteine contribute hydrophobic character to the peptide. The specificity of chymotrypsin is for peptide bonds in which the carboxyl group is donated by an aromatic amino acid.

66. The answer is C. *(Pharmacologic treatment of arrhythmias)*
Lidocaine is often the drug of choice for the treatment of ventricular arrhythmia. It suppresses Na^+ currents in the infarct area that have abnormal resting membrane potentials and elevated K^+ levels. If lidocaine fails, the most frequently chosen agent is another Na^+-channel blocker, procainamide. The Ca^{2+}-channel blockers (diltiazem, verapamil) and β-blockers (propranolol) have a greater effect on supraventricular disturbances in which slow Ca^{2+} channels are involved more significantly than Na^+ channels.

67. The answer is D. *(Renal cell carcinoma)*
The renal mass pictured is classic clear cell carcinoma of the kidney. The cells have round to oval nuclei and inconspicuous nucleoli. The cytoplasm is abundant; it is clear because of the large amounts of glycogen and lipid within these cells (the glycogen accounts for the yellow color). Renal cell carcinomas may be hemorrhagic, and they tend to invade the renal veins and inferior vena cava, from which they may metastasize to the bones and lungs.

68. The answer is B. *(Urea cycle)*
Urea is the principal compound by which ammonia is excreted from the body. The nitrogens in urea come from ammonia and aspartate. Ammonia reacts with carbon dioxide and adenosine triphosphate (ATP) to form carbamoyl phosphate in a reaction catalyzed by carbamoyl phosphate synthetase (ammonia). This enzyme requires N-acetylglutamate as a positive allosteric effector. Without this reaction, urea would not be formed, and ammonia levels would be high. The next step in the urea cycle is the reaction of carbamoyl phosphate with ornithine to form citrulline. In the absence of carbamoyl phosphate, ornithine levels are high, citrulline is undetectable, and neither argininosuccinate nor arginine is formed.

69. The answer is B. *(Neurologic assessment)*
Cerebellar disease manifests as dystonia to palpation but does not alter grip strength. Pain elicited by touching the chin to the chest is known as Brudzinski's sign and usually indicates inflammation of the meninges. Cerebellar disease is indicated by decreased resistance of the limbs to passive movement. Deep tendon reflexes continue for longer than usual; in the patellar tendon this is known as the ''pendular knee jerk'' due to the motion of the limb when the reflex is elicited. Patients with cerebellar disease also show voluntary ataxia, dysdiadochokinesia, nystagmus, and dysarthria of the larynx. Cerebellar lesions usually affect the ipsilateral body.

70–74. The answers are: 70-C, 71-A, 72-D, 73-B, 74-E. *(Electrical activity of the heart)*
The traces shown in *A, B,* and *C* are of cells from the left ventricle, sinoatrial (SA) node, and left atrium, respectively. The refractory period, during which the cell cannot fire another action potential, occurs during the first one half to two thirds of *phase 3* in each of the traces. Contraction of the left ventricle occurs during the calcium plateau (*phase 2*) of myocytes in the left ventricle.

  Phase 0 of cells in the ventricles and atria is marked by the opening of voltage-gated, tetrodotoxin-sensitive sodium channels. These ''fast'' sodium channels are responsible for the rapid upstroke of action potentials in the contractile cells; however, these channels do not seem to play a role in the action potentials of cells in the SA or atrioventricular (AV) nodes. The fast sodium channels inactivate almost as rapidly as they activate, so that the increase in sodium conductance, which leads to depolarization, is soon terminated. No sodium currents are activated until the next action potential. The resting potential of contractile myocytes is maintained by a large potassium conductance. An increase in the potassium conductance does not result in rapid depolarization but rather mild hyperpolarization caused by a small potassium efflux. However, during the action potential, repolarization (*phase 3* of both traces *A* and *B*) is characterized by an increase in the potassium conductance, leading to an outward potassium current (efflux). Because the cell is depolarized at this time, the increase in potassium current quickly moves the cell toward the resting potential. Calcium-activated potassium currents seem to be particularly important in the ventricular repolarization (*phase 3*); these currents may be the site at which the calcium increases result in an increased heart rate (staircase effect). SA node automaticity (the unique pacemaker potential) occurs in *phase 4* (slow depolarization).

The physiologically important sites of heart rate regulation are the SA node and the AV node. Whereas the SA node plays the critical role as pacemaker, the conduction velocity through the AV node determines the rate at which SA node impulses hit their target in the left ventricle. Vagus (parasympathetic) stimulation of the intact heart results in long-lasting decrease in the slope of the pacemaker potential (*phase 4*); transient, mild hyperpolarization of the SA nodal cell; decrease in the slope of the SA node upstroke (*phase 0*); and a decrease in the conduction velocity through the AV node. Sympathetic stimulation from the cells in the stellate ganglion results in lasting increase in the slope of *phase 4;* increase in the upstroke velocity (*phase 0*); and an increase in the AV node conduction speed. Sympathetic stimulation also has a significant role in regulating ventricular cells (a greater role than the parasympathetic system); a protein known as phospholamban is activated by β-adrenergic receptors in the cardiac myocytes. Once activated, this protein produces a variety of effects that collectively supercharge ventricular cells. *Phase 0* upstroke velocity increases, the plateau is reached more quickly, and the speed of repolarization increases; all of these actions prepare the myocyte to efficiently handle an increased heart rate.

Each of the cardiac medications listed has a number of effects, but this discussion serves only to highlight the drug's direct effect on heart rate. Diltiazem and nifedipine are different classes of L-type, voltage-gated calcium channel blockers; the net effect of both drugs is to reduce conduction velocity through the AV node and decrease heart rate. There are no clinically useful drugs whose isolated effect is to increase *phase 0* upstroke velocity. Atropine is a muscarinic antagonist; most of the actions of vagally released acetylcholine are mediated in cardiac cells through muscarinic receptors. Thus, atropine blocks parasympathetic tone in the heart and results in faster SA node impulses and faster AV node conduction. Propranolol is the prototype β-adrenergic receptor blocker; it is not particularly specific for either β_1 or β_2. Most of the sympathetically mediated effects described above can be ascribed to the β_1 receptor. Thus, propranolol blocks the "supercharging" of ventricular cells; it also blocks the sympathetic tone on the heart. It is true that propranolol's direct effect, then, is to decrease heart rate. However, this effect is primarily achieved through the SA and AV nodes as well as the effects on *phase 0* and *phase 2* in ventricular cells. In addition, the reduction in cardiac output caused by the powerful β blockade generally results in reflex tachycardia. Finally, the effects of digitalis (a prototype cardiac glycoside) on the heart are quite complicated, but its principal effect on heart rate is achieved at the AV node. In any case, increasing the slope of *phase 4* (pacemaker potential) in the SA node increases the heart rate.

Structural abnormalities, whether congenital or acquired through inflammation and ischemia, are common sources of conduction problems. Ultimately, the structural defect may give rise to ectopic beats or to unidirectional block, either of which may contribute to arrhythmia. As alluded to above, the principal chronotropic actions of digitalis are effected at the AV node. Digitalis toxicity gives characteristic electrocardiogram abnormalities accompanied by bradycardia. Inflammation in the endocardium is frequently responsible for the atrial fibrillation seen in patients with acute and chronic rheumatic fever. In patients with chronic rheumatism, serious structural problems can cause an atrial fibrillation that is refractory to therapy.

Re-entry almost always involves ectopic beats. Additionally, a condition of unidirectional block is generally required. Finally, the effective refractory period of the re-entered region must be shorter than the travel time through the re-entry loop.

75–79. The answers are: 75-C, 76-D, 77-E, 78-B, 79-A. *(Cholecystitis and cholelithiasis)*

Fat, forty, and female are the features of a patient with a classic case of symptomatic gallstone disease. The pain is correctly described as biliary colic; that is, severe pain lasting for up to 20 minutes and then subsiding, only to return several more times in the hours following. Such a characterization is highly specific to cholelithiasis. Nausea and vomiting frequently accompany biliary colic, and mild elevation of serum bilirubin occurs in 25% of these patients. However, none of these are specific signs for biliary calculi. Ultrasonic radiography is diagnostic in more than 90% of cases and, if available, it is the evaluation of choice. Abdominal rigidity and rebound tenderness are the signs of "acute abdomen," a surgical emergency that is frequently the result of visceral perforation. Hemoccult positive stool is a nonspecific indicator of a more emergent problem that requires additional workup. Excessive postprandial flatulence needs to be evaluated with other more specific signs of abdominal disease. Steatorrhea and lactose intolerance are two fairly common conditions associated with a tremendous amount of abdominal gas.

The fever and elevated white blood cell count are explained by an acute infection in the patient's gallbladder. Enterococci, *Escherichia coli, Klebsiella,* and *Clostridium* are commonly occurring enteric pathogens. *Neisseria* species are not commonly found in the gut, but rather cause urinary tract infections and meningitis.

In autopsies performed in the United States, more than 20% of women and 8% of men over the age of 40 are found to have had asymptomatic gallstones. There has been substantial debate over the appropriate management of asymptomatic gallstones found incidentally when imaging the abdomen for other problems. Currently, surgical intervention is not indicated for asymptomatic disease.

Cholesterol and mixed stones account for more than 80% of biliary calculi, with the remaining 20% being pigment stones. The risk factors for the more common cholesterol stones fall into two groups: factors that increase cholesterol output and factors that decrease bile salt secretion. Clofibrate therapy, obesity, pregnancy, and diabetes mellitus all tend to increase cholesterol output. Oral contraceptive use and ileal disease or resection result in fewer bile salt secretions (the ileum is the principal site of bile salt recycling, which is a major source of secreted bile salts). Alcoholic cirrhosis and chronic hemolysis are examples of disease processes that result in elevations of unconjugated serum bilirubin. Insoluble bilirubin can be converted to calcium bilirubinate, which is the major component of pigment stones.

Cholesterol stones are formed when an imbalance between bile acid secretion and cholesterol output occurs. Increases in cholesterol output or decreases in the cholesterol-solubilizing bile acids result in an increased likelihood of stone formation. HMG CoA reductase performs the rate-limiting step in cholesterol synthesis and, therefore, it is the target of a family of cholesterol-reducing drugs (e.g., lovastatin). Hence, decreases in the activity of HMG CoA coupled with increased bile acid secretion markedly decrease the stone-forming potential. Gallbladder hypomotility associated with severe trauma, total parenteral nutrition, and oral contraceptives is an important factor in the genesis of bile calculi. Infection of the biliary tree with certain pathogens can result in cleavage of the conjugation moieties, turning soluble, conjugated bilirubin into insoluble, unconjugated forms.

80–84. The answers are: 80-C, 81-D, 82-A, 83-E, 84-B. *(Graves' disease and hyperthyroidism)*

Severe illness or physical trauma can cause changes in thyroid hormone regulation that are referred to as sick euthyroid syndrome (SES). Euthyroid indicates that the patient has sufficient but not excess thyroid hormone function. Clinically, the patient appears normal; however, the different thyroid laboratory tests return values that indicate hypo- or hyperthyroidism, depending on the variant of SES. Hashimoto's thyroiditis is characterized in the chronic phase by thyroid insufficiency. Symptoms common in hypothyroidism include lethargy, constipation, cold intolerance, menorrhagia, and weight gain. Dry skin and patchy hair loss emerge as the disease progresses. Graves' disease, thyroid adenomas, and the extremely rare overproduction of thyrotropin-releasing hormone (TRH) by the hypothalamus all result in the hyperthyroid symptoms described. However, the ocular pathology described (i.e., exophthalmos, extraocular ophthalmoplegia) is characteristic of the autoimmune disorder known as Graves' disease. The inflammatory reaction against the muscles and connective tissue in the orbit causes edema, muscular weakness, and fibrosis leading to the symptoms described.

The complete triad of Graves' disease also includes pretibial myxedema, an inflammatory thickening of the dermis most often found over the dorsum of the legs and feet. The skin is raised and thickened; it may be itchy and often has a peau d'orange appearance. Pericardial effusion and patchy loss of hair are both consistent with hypothyroidism. Diffuse hyperpigmentation is often found with adrenal insufficiency (e.g., Addison's disease) or pituitary adrenocorticotropic hormone (ACTH)-producing adenomas. Jaundice is not a finding commonly related to Graves' disease.

The TRH challenge is particularly useful in demonstrating thyrotoxicosis. The pituitary thyroid-stimulating hormone (TSH) response to TRH is significantly blunted by high serum T_3 levels. Serum TSH is a less useful indicator but should be low or undetectable in this woman. Thyrotoxicosis coupled with the ocular signs described gives strong evidence for Graves' disease, in which autoantibodies against the TSH receptor provide unregulated stimulation of the thyroid gland. The triiodothyronine resin uptake (T_3RU) test is useful in describing the relation between total and free T_3. In this in vitro test, excess radiolabeled T_3 is introduced into the patient's serum, and a particulate resin is used to collect any unbound T_3 (labeled or unlabeled). The resin uptake is inversely proportional to the number of available binding sites on the patient's thyroid-binding globulin (TBG). If the patient's own T_3 occupies most of the available sites (as it has in this case), much of the labeled T_3 remains for the resin to "soak up." If, on the other hand, there is an excess of available TBG-binding sites (i.e., in patients with low serum T_3), the labeled T_3 first binds the sites, and less labeled T_3 is left for the resin (decreased T_3 resin uptake).

Multinodular goiter, autonomous adenomas, and single carcinoma all have distinctive scintiscan results that are inconsistent with the description given (i.e., uniform radioiodine uptake). Multinodular goiter and autonomous adenomas show areas of particular brightness or dullness on a scintiscan; the carcinoma is often nonfunctional and dark. Lymphocytic infiltration with atrophic follicles usually shows up on a scintiscan as uniformly dull, but the radiographic description alone does not rule out this condition. However, follicular atrophy is characteristic of Hashimoto's disease (i.e., thyroid insufficiency), not Graves' disease. Lymphocytic infiltration is common to Hashimoto's disease and Graves' disease, although it is much more striking in Hashimoto's disease.

Propylthiouracil (PTU) and methimazole share a common mechanism of action in inhibiting the synthesis of thyroxine, but methimazole is more potent. However, PTU offers the advantage of reducing the peripheral conversion of T_4 to T_3; it is, therefore, equipped to give faster relief from the symptoms of thyrotoxicosis because T_3 has substantially more biologic activity. Radioactive iodine is a useful alternative to surgery in the patient who might have perioperative complications (e.g., the elderly, those with severe thyrotoxicosis). No carcinogenic effects have been documented, but radioactive iodine may be contraindicated in women who want to become pregnant in the future. Because the mechanical components of the ocular pathology in Graves' disease are inflammatory in nature, they are relieved with large doses (120 mg/day) of prednisone. Propranolol provides the fastest symptomatic relief of the nervousness, tachycardia, lid lag, and other sympathetic manifestations.

85–89. The answers are: 85-C, 86-D, 87-A, 88-E, 89-B. *(Paraneoplastic syndromes)*
Paraneoplastic syndromes represent an important source of morbidity in the spectrum of cancer pathophysiology. The varied signs and symptoms that fall into this category cannot be directly related to the physical tumor but are instead a result of the tumor's presence in the body. Although the mechanisms involved are not completely understood, in some cases the tumor produces a substance and, in other cases, the signs and symptoms are probably related to the body's immunologic reaction against the tumor.

This patient presents with the classic symptoms of Cushing's syndrome, which is indicated by an excess of corticosteroids. In this case, the lack of libido is the result of cortisol suppression of the pituitary's secretion of gonadotropin releasing hormone (GnRH). The muscle wasting and abdominal stria are caused by deranged protein metabolism, which results in degradation of the connective tissue. The characteristic patterns of weight gain (e.g., buffalo hump, moon facies) are due to ill-defined effects of excess steroids on lipid metabolism. The signs and symptoms of a paraneoplastic syndrome can often present at the same time as (or earlier than) the symptoms associated with the tumor (e.g., hoarseness, cough). The two sets of signs together are a strong indicator of a bronchogenic tumor.

The best confirming tests are a chest x-ray and dexamethasone suppression test. The suppression test helps to differentiate between endocrine dysregulation and completely autonomous steroid production (i.e., no regulation). Although urinary glucocorticoids can indicate that steroids are being produced in excess, physical examination is needed to confirm a diagnosis. The water restriction is useful for diagnosing syndrome of inappropriate ADH (SIADH), which is characterized by hyponatremia and water retention. The other tests are useful for diagnosing primary thyroid and glucose abnormalities, which are not likely given this clinical scenario.

When Cushing's syndrome coexists with a bronchogenic tumor, it is almost always a result of tumor ACTH production. Tumors almost never produce steroids—the synthesis pathway is too complex for a dysfunctional cell. Autonomous secretion of parathyroid hormone causes a syndrome known as hypercalcemia of malignancy, which is associated with hypercalcemia and lytic lesions of the bone. There is no indication of thyroid dysfunction. Although glucose metabolism is almost certainly altered, the glucose derangement is a result of the excess steroids; insulin alone could not be responsible for the other metabolic abnormalities.

Ectopic, unregulated ACTH production causes bilateral hypertrophy of the adrenal cortices. Focal enlargement in any organ indicates neoplasia. Carcinoid tumors are nonbronchogenic lung tumors that cause a paraneoplastic syndrome associated with serotonin and histamine release. Pituitary hypertrophy is the result of excess hypothalamic secretion of corticotropin-releasing hormone (CRH), and it may indicate the presence of an ACTH adenoma. Such an excess gives rise to Cushing's syndrome, but tumor production of CRH is uncommon.

Lung cancer occurring in families with members who smoke is not definitive epidemiologic evidence for either a genetic or an environmental hypothesis of lung carcinoma. In trying to establish a correlation between a variable (cigarette smoking) and a disease (lung cancer), one needs to look for a confounding relationship (i.e., a positive family history for both).

With the exception of hyperaldosteronism, the other signs and symptoms listed are all common in various bronchogenic carcinomas. Squamous cell carcinomas are most frequently associated with hypercalcemia; small cell carcinomas tend to cause Cushing's syndrome or SIADH. The dermatomyositis is less common and is thought to be related to an immunologic reaction against the tumor. Hypertrophic osteodystrophy with clubbing involves unknown mechanisms but is a common manifestation of lung cancer.

90. The answer is E. *(Protein structure; receptors)*
Known receptors for physiologic growth factors and effectors display a small group of structures that are shared among different proteins and are found on either the external or internal domain of the protein. These structures are recognizable at a primary amino acid sequence level. This allows receptors to be classified into groups that resemble ion channels; groups that resemble kinases, especially tyrosine, serine, and threonine kinases; and cyclases. Several plasma membrane receptors require interactions with guanosine triphosphate (GTP)–binding proteins (G proteins) to function in signal transduction. Metallothioneins are good acceptors for zinc and heavy metal, but have not been reported to be receptors or elements in signal transduction systems.

91. The answer is C. *(Genetic code; nucleotides)*
Three nucleotides are required to specify the insertion of an amino acid into a polypeptide chain. These groups of three nucleotides comprise a codon that is represented in the 5′ to 3′ direction. Because there are four different bases in RNA, the maximum number of codons is sixty-four. Sixty-one of these codons specify the twenty amino acids; some amino acids have more than one. The triplet AUG serves as a start signal, and three triplets that do not code for any amino acid serve as stop signals. The genetic code is virtually universal; all organisms use the same codons to translate their genomes into proteins. A transcription unit can be influenced by promoter and enhancer elements as well as methylation of nucleotides.

92. The answer is E. *(Neurotransmitters; excitatory amino acids)*
Decreased GABA-ergic activity is associated with increased seizure activity, and antiepileptic drugs are GABA-ergic. Baclofen, used for multiple sclerosis, reduces muscle spasms. Benzodiazepines have agonist activity at a macromolecular receptor complex that includes a γ-aminobutyric acid (GABA) receptor, and the activity of this receptor appears to be overactive in hepatic encephalopathy.

93. The answer is E. *(Biologic theory)*
Biologic theory proposes some alteration of brain function as underlying mental disorder. If schizophrenia is considered a genetic disorder, monozygotic twins would be concordant for the disorder.

94. The answer is A. *(Hypocomplementemia-associated renal disease)*
Complement levels are normal in immunoglobulin A (IgA) nephropathy and diffuse proliferative glomerulonephritis (poststreptococcal glomerulonephritis). Nephritides associated with hypocomplementemia include cryoglobulinemia, membranoproliferative glomerulonephropathy, and a variety of visceral infections, including infections of peritoneal and central nervous system (CNS) shunts ("shunt" nephritis).

95. The answer is A. *(Extracellular matrix)*
Cell–cell interactions and cell–matrix interactions are essential for normal development and wound healing. The integrins are part of the supergene family, which also includes leukocyte adhesion molecules and receptors on the platelet membrane surface. These transmembrane glycoproteins have extracellular domains that bind matrix molecules (e.g., fibronectin) and intracellular domains that interact with cytoskeletal elements to activate signals in the cytosol and nucleus. The integrins do stimulate gene transcription indirectly as a result of their mobilization of cytosolic signal-transducing pathways. Platelet aggregation requires a fibrinogen bridge between two transmembrane receptors. Adhesion to the damaged surface requires that a different receptor interacts with von Willebrand factor and the subendothelium. Laminin is thought to be important in the developing nervous system, and several extracellular matrix molecules are crucial to the formation of proper relationships between cells (e.g., endothelial cells making tubes).

96. The answer is D. *(Immunologic disorders)*
The major histocompatibility complex, which is also known as the human leukocyte antigen (HLA) complex, has been associated with a variety of diseases. Probably the best known association is between HLA-B27 and ankylosing spondylitis. All of the HLA associations in the question are matched correctly except for 21-hydroxylase deficiency, which is associated with HLA-BW47, not HLA-DR4.

97. The answer is E. *(Membrane physiology)*
Application of acetylcholine (ACh) or vagal stimulation decreases the slope of phase 4 of a slow fiber (or pacemaker cell) that is likely to be found in the sinoatrial or atrioventricular nodal tissue. This is due to increased permeability to K^+ and causes a decrease in heart rate in situ. Fast fibers like those found in non-nodal atrial or ventricular tissue have a rapid depolarization (phase 0) caused by the opening of fast Na^+ channels, followed by a plateau (phase 2) secondary to the opening of slow Ca^{2+} channels.

98–99. The answers are: 98-A, 99-D. *(Diagnosis and pathology of acute leukemia)*
The presence of pancytopenia is not associated with chronic lymphocytic leukemia. Patients with acute myelogenous leukemia, recurrent ovarian carcinoma, and aplastic anemia can have pancytopenia. Cyclophosphamide, which is used to treat some patients with ovarian carcinoma, does cause bone marrow depression, and recovery can be delayed.

An immunoglobulin gene rearrangement analysis would not be useful for this patient unless she had shown evidence of a lymphoproliferative disorder. Radiographic and cytologic studies could confirm the presence of ascites and possible recurrent ovarian carcinoma. Bone marrow aspiration is essential to establish the diagnosis. With hepatic enlargement, it is necessary to evaluate the patient for evidence of liver damage. Some agents that damage the liver can also damage the bone marrow.

100. The answer is B. *(Characteristics of chronic type B gastritis)*
Chronic type B gastritis is four times more common than type A (fundal) gastritis, the form of chronic gastritis in which there are circulating antibodies to the parietal cells and intrinsic factor. Type B gastritis may result from chronic alcohol or aspirin use, bile reflux, ulcer disease, or postgastrectomy states. Type A is found in elderly individuals and individuals with pernicious anemia. Levels of gastrin tend to be low, and there may be antibodies to gastrin-producing cells in type B gastritis, in contrast to type A gastritis. In type B gastritis, the stomach wall loses its rugal folds and becomes flattened, glazed, and red.

101. The answer is B. *(Asthma; pulmonary mechanics)*
The forced vital capacity (FVC) is unchanged or decreased during an acute asthma attack. An important spirometric manifestation of asthma is a decrease in forced expiratory volume in 1 second (FEV_1) by itself or normalized to FVC. Total lung capacity (TLC) will be normal, or elevated possibly, because of loss of elastic recoil.

102. The answer is C. *(Cardiovascular disease and sexuality)*
The most common reasons for a decreased frequency of sexual intercourse after a myocardial infarction are psychological. Patients who have had a myocardial infarction can have decreased self-esteem and concerns about impotence. The stress associated with an unusual circumstance (e.g., an atypical sexual activity, inebriation, a new sexual partner) is often responsible for myocardial infarction during intercourse. Exercise and educational programs have been effective in helping cardiac patients resume a normal life, but the involvement of the partner in these programs is important.

103. The answer is C. *(Thalamic connections)*
The pulvinar nucleus receives input from the superior colliculus and pretectal areas and projects to visual cortex areas 18 and 19. It does not connect with the basal ganglia.

104. The answer is D. *(Endocrinology of menstruation)*
A detailed understanding of the hormonal control of menstruation is especially important to evaluate vaginal bleeding and the choice of oral contraceptives. The surge of luteinizing hormone (LH) immediately precedes ovulation; LH, estradiol, and progesterone levels are all declining at the beginning of menses, whereas follicle-stimulating hormone (FSH) is rising to recruit the follicle for the subsequent cycle. Early in the cycle, FSH renders cells sensitive to LH, which later causes ovulation. The follicles that were not sufficiently sensitive to FSH to mature do not develop sensitivity to LH for ovulation.

105. The answer is B. *(Histology of liquefactive necrosis)*
Coagulative necrosis follows hypoxic death in most body tissues except those of the central nervous system (CNS). For example, the necrotic process that ensues following a myocardial infarction is coagulative

necrosis, due to occlusion of the coronary vessels. Liquefactive necrosis occurs only in the CNS, as a result of vascular occlusion. It is more commonly caused by pyogenic bacterial infection or septic emboli.

106. The answer is E. *(Telencephalon)*
Elements that develop from the telencephalon, which includes the internal capsule and the area lateral to it, include the forebrain; parietal, temporal, and occipital lobes; the hippocampus; and the corpus striatum. The thalamus is considered part of the diencephalon.

107. The answer is A. *(Skeletal muscle contraction)*
The length of the A band remains constant during the contraction of myofibrils in skeletal muscle. The sarcomere of the myofibril is composed of thick and thin filaments. According to the sliding filament hypothesis, thick and thin filaments slide past one another during contraction, increasing the amount of overlap between them; they do not change length. The H band contains only thick filaments; the A band contains thin and thick filaments. The I band contains only thin filaments, which are anchored in the middle of the I band by components of the Z disk. During contraction, thin filaments slide into the A band, reducing the size of both the H band and I band and drawing the Z disks closer to the A band.

108. The answer is A. *(Intercostal nerves)*
Intercostal nerves are the anterior rami of the first 11 thoracic spinal nerves; the twelfth thoracic nerve gives rise to the subcostal nerve.

109. The answer is A. *(Transcriptional activation of chromosomes)*
Mammalian DNA utilizes only about 7% of the genome to transcribe RNA. Inactive DNA is referred to as heterochromatin, and it is tightly wound in an organized fashion in conjunction with nucleosomes. Inactive DNA is also methylated at cytosine–guanine (CG) islands, but the exact relation between inactivation and methylation is not clear. Active segments of DNA are referred to as euchromatin. Euchromatin is not wound as tightly and is less protein bound than heterochromatin. Because it is less organized, euchromatin also happens to be more sensitive to enzymatic digestion by DNase I, which can be used to determine active regions of DNA.

110. The answer is E. *(Psychoanalysis)*
Free association is the major method of communication in psychoanalysis. Interpretation is a method of intervention, and resistance and countertransference are processes that develop during the treatment. Meditation is not involved in the psychoanalytic process.

111. The answer is D. *(Acute myocardial infarction)*
Aortic aneurysm is usually related to peripheral atherosclerotic disease; therefore, it is related to coronary atherosclerotic disease. Cystic medial necrosis can cause a dissecting form of aortic damage without much aortic dilation. Syphilis can cause aneurysmal dilation, especially in the ascending aorta. However, there is no common relationship between acute myocardial infarction and any of these aortic diseases. Cardiac tamponade, mitral valve incompetence, and rupture of the ventricular septum represent serious complications following damage to the myocardial wall or the papillary muscles. Peripheral embolism can occur as a result of mural thrombosis after infarctions involving the cardiac endothelium. Not mentioned are cardiac arrhythmias, which account for 75% of complications in acute myocardial infarction.

112. The answer is D. *(Collagen formation)*
Collagen, which is widely distributed in all animals, is important because it has been studied extensively as a model of the relationship between protein structure and function. Glycine is critical to collagen's structure because of glycine's small size: The triple helix motif could not contain a large side chain on the inside, so the

Gly-X-Y repeat puts a small glycine in the center of each turn. The degree of hydroxylation on proline residues is directly correlated with the thermodynamic stability of the collagen fiber. Because the strength of the triple helix is largely dependent on hydrogen bonding and other weak cooperative interactions, it is important to have a large number of these weak interactions to achieve high overall stability. Cleavage of the globular ends is important in making the insoluble tropocollagen molecule. However, this step must occur after secretion. Otherwise, secretion of the insoluble molecule would be much more difficult. Thus, it is the uncleaved procollagen molecule that is secreted. Cross-linkage of lysyl and hydroxylysyl residues occurs both within and between the collagen monomers. As discussed previously, ineffective cross-linkage can lead to disease.

113. The answer is A. *(Cranial injury)*
The amount of injury to the brain is proportional to the amount of distance the brain moves within the skull before being forcibly halted by fixed structures within the skull. Blows to the front or back of the head cause more displacement of the brain and, hence, more trauma than blows directed to the side of the head. A blow that glances off the head causes considerable rotation of the brain within the skull and, thus, is potentially more dangerous than blows to the sides, front, or back of the head.

114–118. The answers are: 114-C, 115-G, 116-B, 117-A, 118-D. *(Cardiac cycle)*
The cardiac cycle illustrated shows the simultaneous measurement of three entities. At the *top* is aortic pressure, left ventricular pressure is the *solid bold line,* and left atrial pressure is the *dashed line* at the bottom. At the end of the phase marked *A* (atrial systole), the mitral valve closes, giving rise to the S1 sound. Mitral valve closure marks the beginning of isovolumic left ventricular contraction. When ventricular pressure is equal to aortic pressure, the aortic valve is forced open (*C*), and the rapid ejection phase begins. Ejection then begins to slow and later ends abruptly with aortic valve closure (*D*); the S2 sound is generated at this time. *E* marks the phase of isovolumic relaxation in the left ventricle, until pressure is low enough that the mitral valve opens (*F*). The left ventricle can then begin refilling (*G*).

119–123. The answers are: 119-C, 120-E, 121-A, 122-D, 123-B. *(Personality disorders)*
Andrew's deterioration in performance, his social withdrawal, and his apparent difficulties in cognition have lasted longer than 6 months. These symptoms, as well as his age, suggest a diagnosis of schizophrenia.

Spending sprees and grandiosity that extend to energetic dysfunctional actions are characteristic of manic episodes. Although acute states such as these can be present in patients with narcissistic personality disorder, they usually are of brief duration.

The type of reaction to major disappointments that is exhibited by George is typical of individuals with narcissistic personality disorders. These individuals are given to a sense of self-importance and entitlement. Fantasies concerning success and infinite capabilities also are characteristic.

"Stable instability" is characteristic of borderline personality disorder. It is evidenced by instability of interpersonal relationships (i.e., difficult relationships punctuated by anger, threats, and even suicidal manipulations). Borderline personality disorder is associated with fluctuating moods and potentially self-damaging acts.

Jean is amnestic regarding her behavior. PCP often is inhaled by smoking marijuana laced with the drug and, therefore, can be taken unknowingly.

124–127. The answers are: 124-D, 125-F, 126-B, 127-C. *(Biostatistics and clinical reasoning)*
Understanding definitions is crucial to reading and critically evaluating the literature. Sensitivity and specificity are terms frequently used to describe clinical tests. A test with high sensitivity finds the abnormality if it is there; however, many tests with a high sensitivity have a low specificity (i.e., they are often positive in the absence of disease). A test with high specificity is very useful as a confirmation (because it is rarely positive in the absence of disease), but it may not be useful as a screening tool (where false positives are usually better than false negatives).

Validity reflects a test's ability to accurately assess a given element. For example, if urine glucose is below normal, a valid test reveals low urinary glucose. Sometimes a test's validity must first be established by active research. This is often true of tests that seek to assess psychiatric disease or cognitive development. Reliability refers to the test's ability to reproduce values that it already measured. A reliable test delivers relatively constant values when measuring the same entity. Again, tests of more nebulous entities must be examined for reliability before their results can be meaningfully interpreted.

Incidence and prevalence are essential concepts for the clinician to understand. Incidence is the number of new cases of a disease diagnosed in a given year (per 100,000 population). Prevalence is the number of diagnosed cases at any given moment in time (per 100,000 population). The prevalence of chronic diseases (e.g., rheumatoid arthritis) is generally higher than the incidence. Similarly, the incidence of diseases that can be rapidly lethal (e.g., disseminated intravascular coagulation) is usually higher than the prevalence.

128–131. The answers are: 128-A, 129-B, 130-B, 131-D. *(Small intestine)*
Differences between segments of the small intestine are subtle; however, several distinguishing features aid identification. The jejunum contains well-developed plicae circulares, tall arteriae rectae, and few arterial arcades. The ileum has rudimentary plicae circulares, short arteriae rectae, and many arterial arcades. Meckel's diverticulum, a remnant of the embryonic vitelline duct, is present in the ileum in approximately 3% of the population. Appendices epiploicae (fat-filled tags) are diagnostic for the large bowel only.

132–136. The answers are: 132-B, 133-D, 134-A, 135-C, 136-A. *(Tissue culture types)*
Because viruses are obligate intracellular parasites, living cells are needed for virus propagation. Animal cells propagated in culture, regardless of their origin, have complex nutritional requirements, many of which are not defined. The need for these trace-level undefined nutrients is met best through the inclusion of serum in the tissue culture medium.

Primary cell cultures are derived directly from tissues. Primary cell lines often contain multiple cell types but are capable of only limited growth in culture (i.e., a few subcultures). Primary and secondary cell cultures are referred to as diploid.

Some secondary cell cultures are capable of surviving many (approximately 30–50) subcultures before a natural aging process ensues, leading to senescence and eventual death of the cell lines. In some cases, the cell strains undergo spontaneous transformation to become continuous cell lines.

Organ culture permits the maintenance of differentiated cells of several types in a single culture and is required for the propagation of some viruses. Although the cells in organ cultures usually do not divide, they may be maintained for long periods of time.

Tumor cells, when established in culture, frequently maintain a few of the differentiated characteristics of the stem cell of the tumor. In addition, tumor cells are transformed and become immortal continuous cell lines.

The most effective way to maintain maximal differentiation of cells is to leave them in their surrounding tissue matrix and culture them in their original organ configuration.

137–144. The answers are: 137-B, 138-C, 139-F, 140-G, 141-A, 142-G, 143-F, 144-D. *(Differential diagnosis of arthritis)*
Osteoarthritis is a degenerative disease that most commonly affects the large weight-bearing joints. Osteoarthritis is related to use; therefore, mail carriers are more susceptible than office administrators. The x-ray shows classic radiographic findings in osteoarthritis including asymmetrical involvement of joints (i.e., only the left), segmental narrowing of the medial and superior joint space, subchondral sclerosis of the bone, and osteophyte formation. The osteophyte formation is striking and can be best seen on the computed tomography scan: The normal femoral head has been completely dislodged from the joint space by the large femoral osteophyte, and the acetabulum is covered with its own distinct osteophyte. This is an advanced case, and these radiographs were taken immediately prior to total joint replacement. Generally speaking, inflammatory changes are not a feature of osteoarthritis.

Rheumatoid arthritis is an autoimmune disease in which cellular inflammation and antibody complex formation destroy normal synovial tissue and articular cartilage. The disease has a propensity towards small joints of the wrists, hands, ankles, and feet. The lymphokines and hydrolytic enzymes found in the synovial fluid of a patient with rheumatoid arthritis combine with activated inflammatory cells to destroy articular cartilage. Chronic rheumatoid arthritis is characterized by the formation of pannus, which is a form of granulation tissue with inflammatory cells, proliferating fibroblasts, and small blood vessels. This destructive tissue ultimately replaces articular cartilage with a fibrous scar, which frequently results in joint ankylosis. Two other histopathologic features of rheumatoid arthritis are large lacunae in the cartilage (the result of invasive pannus) and inflammatory cells in the marrow, which can destroy bone. Rheumatoid arthritis is associated with the DR4 haplotype of the human leukocyte antigen (i.e., HLA-DR4).

Reiter's syndrome is a seronegative arthritis following an episode of infectious urethritis, cervicitis, or dysentery. When initially described, the complete triad also included noninfectious conjunctivitis. The inflammation associated with the ocular and joint symptoms is reactive and probably related to an autoimmune phenomenon triggered by the urethritis. Other documented symptoms include hyperkeratotic lesions of the skin and painless shallow ulcers of the penis, urethral meatus, and mouth. Human leukocyte antigen B27 (HLA-B27) occurs in approximately 80%–90% of all patients with Reiter's syndrome. The knee and ankle joints are commonly involved, and sacroiliitis occurs in about 25% of patients. Most episodes of Reiter's arthritis last less than 6 months and are rarely debilitating.

Gout is a poorly understood disease that results from urate crystal formation in joints (i.e., arthritis), renal tubules (i.e., gouty nephropathy, urate renal calculi), and soft tissues (i.e., tophi). Although hyperuricemia is usually necessary for the manifestations of gout, it is not sufficient; hyperuricemia can exist without the clinical findings of gout. Two common characteristics are described in the questions. The first association pairing gout with diet and alcohol intake is well documented. Obesity and hyperlipidemia are much more common in patients with gout, and excess intake of ethanol during the course of a heavy meal may be adequate to incite a painful attack. The second question describing synovial fluid from the wrist is diagnostic for gout. Being negatively birefringent, urate crystals produce a bright yellow color under polarized light. The cellular infiltrate seems to be a response to the crystals, and leukocyte counts between 2000 and 75,000/mm^3 are routine.

Septic arthritis is most common in elderly people and individuals who are immunocompromised. It is most frequently caused by *Staphylococcus aureus,* although *S. epidermidis* and group A streptococci are also encountered. People with connective tissue diseases and those with chronic arthritis are more inclined to develop coincidental septic arthritis. Disseminated gonococcal infection is the most common bacterial arthritis in urban populations and complicates as many as 0.5% of all gonococcal infections. However, disseminated gonococcal infection is usually distinguished from other forms of septic arthritis because of its route of transmission. In general, infectious arthritis is characterized by the acute onset of a warm, swollen joint, most commonly the knee (involvement of more than one joint is indicative of disseminated gonococcal infection). A synovial leukocyte count greater than 50,000 with 80% (or more) polymorphonuclears is strongly suggestive of septic arthritis. Although other inflammatory arthritides can elevate synovial cell counts to that level, the high percentage of polymorphonuclears is relatively specific to infections. A Gram's stain or culture is necessary for definitive diagnosis. Treatment of infectious arthritis requires immediate and complete drainage of the synovial fluid. Intravenous antibiotics administered without delay can help reduce the potentially irreversible joint damage associated with such a large inflammatory response. Even with prompt therapy, complete functional recovery following *S. aureus* arthritis is less than 60%, and infectious arthritis remains a significant cause of joint deformity.

Lyme disease is an infectious process caused by the tick-borne spirochete *Borrelia burgdorferi*. The first stage of the illness occurs within 1 month of exposure and is characterized by erythema migrans at the site of the tick bite. Flu-like symptoms can accompany the rash, and the rash frequently spreads to other sites. In about 10% of patients, neurologic or cardiac involvement occurs within weeks to months. As many as 67%

of patients develop frank arthritis following the initial rash. Intermittent attacks of arthritis in the large joints, particularly the knee, are typical. Synovial fluid examination reveals an average leukocyte count of 25,000 (predominantly PMNs), which is similar to the chronic inflammatory arthritides. The clinical symptoms of Lyme disease have a slower onset than do the symptoms of acute infectious arthritis. Lyme disease can cause irreversible damage if the disease is not discovered until its later stages (weeks to months after the initial rash). However, most patients respond to oral tetracycline in the early stages, and complete recovery is not uncommon.

Systemic sclerosis is another disorder that has an unknown cause. Convincing evidence has implicated the overproduction of collagen as a factor, but the trigger for this disease continues to elude investigators. Two variants, CREST (i.e., *c*alcinosis cutis, *R*aynaud's phenomenon, *e*sophageal dysfunction, *s*clerodactyly, *t*elangiectasia) syndrome and diffuse cutaneous scleroderma, have been described, and usually Raynaud's phenomena or polyarthritis of the small joints is the presenting complaint. Laboratory and clinical findings are usually much different than those provided in the questions. Synovial fluid often contains less than 10,000 leukocytes/mm^3. In most cases, the radiographic findings show atrophy of disuse and osteopenia. Finally, fibrin deposition and chronic inflammatory cell infiltration are the only significant changes in synovium biopsy. Later, fibrosis of the connective tissue can occur, but rarely does one see the erosion that is characteristic of rheumatoid arthritis in a patient with systemic sclerosis.

145–148. The answers are: 145-C, 146-A, 147-D, 148-E. (*Neurophysiology and visual science*)
Presbyopia (impairment of vision due to old age) is caused by a decrease in the elasticity of the lens. As a result, the eyes are unable to accommodate for near vision. Another condition associated with aging is cataracts, in which the lens becomes progressively less transparent. Myopia is caused by an overall refractive power that is too great for the axial length of the eyeball. It causes distant objects to be focused in front of the retina and can be corrected by a diverging lens. In hyperopia, the overall refractive power is too low for the axial length of the eyeball, therefore the eyes must continuously accommodate to see distant objects clearly.

149–153. The answers are: 149-A, 150-B, 151-C, 152-B, 153-A. (*Types of capillaries*)
Continuous capillaries are present in skeletal muscle, the lungs, and the brain. They form a continuous epithelial barrier that restricts diffusion of materials from the blood into the tissues.

Fenestrated capillaries are present in renal glomeruli. The fenestrations are holes through the walls of capillary endothelial cells.

Discontinuous capillaries are present in the liver, bone marrow, and spleen. Gaps large enough to allow passage of cells exist between the endothelial cells of discontinuous capillaries. In the bone marrow, for example, mature erythrocytes move from the hematopoietic compartment into the blood through intercellular gaps in the discontinuous capillaries.

Cerebrospinal fluid (CSF), a blood filtrate containing some of the proteins found in whole blood, is produced in the choroid plexus. Fenestrated capillaries in the choroid plexus allow a select subset of blood proteins to enter CSF.

Continuous capillaries in the brain form the blood–brain barrier by restricting the flow of some substances in blood into the brain parenchyma.

154–157. The answers are: 154-B, 155-E, 156-C, 157-G. (*Differential diagnosis of neuromuscular disease*)
The differential diagnosis of muscular weakness is an essential skill for both a neurologist and a general practitioner. In ascertaining a diagnosis, it is important to distinguish between purely motor difficulties and sensorimotor difficulties, and to localize the problem (i.e., upper versus lower motor neuron disease, neuromuscular junction, muscular atrophy). Cerebrovascular accidents in the motor cortex almost always give rise to two distinct phases: flaccid paralysis of the affected areas, followed by distinct upper motor neuron

signs (e.g., hyperreflexia, hypertonia, minimal muscular atrophy). Generally, the affected areas are well demarcated and most cerebrovascular accidents do not cause bilateral symptoms. Furthermore, only the 55-year-old man would be in the age range in which cerebrovascular accidents would be high in the differential.

Guillain-Barré syndrome is an autoimmune disorder frequently triggered by a preceding viral infection or surgery. Herpes-type viruses are thought to be involved in an unusually large percentage of cases. The principal feature of the disease is peripheral demyelination, and the clinical presentation is generally gradual at first, leading later to fulminant symptoms that require hospitalization (many patients need ventilatory support). Early clinical findings are related to the demyelination, including hyporeflexia, hypotonic paralysis (especially in the distal extremities), and loss of light touch and vibration sensation. Although the motor symptoms mimic upper motor neuron disease, the findings are actually related to the decreased muscle spindle fiber (i.e., inhibitory) input to the anterior horn cells. Recovery is usually complete within 1 month.

Duchenne muscular dystrophy is a primary myopathy whose clinical course is severe, resulting in death from respiratory failure by the middle to late teens. Age of onset is usually 3 to 7 years. The mother observed all of the common symptoms of Duchenne muscular dystrophy. Earlier difficulties are noticed in children who are more active (e.g., difficulty running, frequent tripping, difficulty climbing). The pseudo-hypertrophy seen principally in the calf is nearly pathognomonic at the age of 6, and biopsy reveals significant fibrosis with almost no normal muscle fibers. Most children are confined to a wheelchair by age 12.

Amyotrophic lateral sclerosis is slightly more common in men than in women and rarely has its onset before age 50. It is a relentlessly degenerating disease that attacks both upper and lower motor neurons. One of the cardinal features of amyotrophic lateral sclerosis, as is seen in this man, is that it occurs in the complete absence of any sensory loss. The cause of this disease is unknown, and there is currently no treatment. The clinical onset includes weakness and fatigue that generally begin in one extremity and progress to include the entire body. Hyperreflexia is usually apparent early and is a sign of upper motor neuron disease. Babinski sign is often present (i.e., upgoing). As the underlying disease progresses, the lower motor neuron degenerates so that areflexia and flaccid paralysis predominate in the later stages. Muscle wasting eventually leads to the amyotrophy that gives the disease its name.

Myasthenia gravis is much more common in women than in men and is an autoimmune disorder with antibodies directed against nicotinic cholinergic receptors of the neuromuscular junction. Treatment is available and somewhat effective, so that early diagnosis of this disease is critical. The features described, particularly weakness that subsides after rest, are cardinal symptoms of the disease. The characteristic distribution of fatigue that affects facial musculature earlier is a hallmark of the myasthenia pathology. Because this is not an upper motor neuron disease, reflexes are maintained. Also, it should be clear that there are no sensory deficits.

Neurosyphilis, or tabes dorsalis, is the tertiary (late) stage of the sexually transmitted syphilis organism. It appears in patients 20 to 30 years following infection and was, at one time, part of every differential diagnosis of muscular weakness. Sensory manifestations are almost universally reported, so that only the 39-year-old man had signs even remotely related to neurosyphilis. Severe gait disturbances (caused by loss of proprioception) and recurrent fleeting pains radiating down the legs are common presentations. Hyporeflexia, impaired light touch and vibration sensation, and bladder disturbance occur in many patients. The Argyll Robertson pupils, which accommodate but do not react to light, are also a frequent sign.

Friedreich's ataxia (i.e., spinocerebellar degeneration) is characterized by degeneration of the spinocerebellar tracts, with accompanying loss of the peripheral neurons that synapsed with the now dead spinocerebellar neurons. In its true form, Friedreich's ataxia is generally inherited as a recessive trait (although it is sometimes dominant), and the clinical picture first appears in the legs. Clumsiness in the hands follows later, and general weakness marks the final stages. Survival beyond early adulthood is rare, and death is frequently the result of an associated cardiomyopathy.

158–161. The answers are: 158-B, 159-E, 160-A, 161-C. *(Quantitative dose–response curves)*
The figure on the *left* represents an ideal concentration–response curve for a drug and shows the typical hyperbolic effect. The concentration that gives the half-maximal effect (K_D) can be estimated from the figure, but the maximal effect cannot easily be determined because of the hyperbolic nature of the data. The figure on the *right* is a mathematical transformation of these data to a linear form that is more useful—a Scatchard plot that allows the maximal effect to be determined from the intercept at the X axis. The concentration of K_D is the reciprocal of the slope.

162–167. The answers are: 162-B, 163-D, 164-A, 165-D, 166-C, 167-E. *(Genetics)*
Lod scores are the usual statistical method of measuring linkage. Loci that are separated by recombination less than 50% of the time are said to be linked. This recombination fraction corresponds to a genetic distance of 50 cM.

Common examples of genetic polymorphisms include restriction fragment length polymorphisms (RFLPs), variable number of tandem repeats (VNTRs), chromosome heteromorphisms, inherited enzyme variants, and antigenic variants of proteins.

Several methods are available for the assignment of genetic loci to specific chromosomes (i.e., for gene mapping). Family studies to demonstrate linkage are widely used, but somatic cell genetic methods are often easier to perform when there is no knowledge of the location of the gene. Cytogenetic methods of gene mapping are particularly useful for regional localization within a chromosome.

Genetic polymorphism is defined as the occurrence of two or more alleles at a locus in a frequency greater than can be maintained by mutation alone. In practice, polymorphism is often said to exist when the most common allele at a locus accounts for less than 99% of all alleles. Many genes exhibit polymorphism of their coding regions, but polymorphic DNA variation in noncoding regions is even more common.

Linkage describes the close physical proximity of two or more loci on a chromosome, but the specific alleles present at each locus are irrelevant to the identification of linkage. If a certain allele at one locus tends to be found more often than expected by chance with a certain allele at another locus linked to the first, linkage disequilibrium is said to be present. Linkage disequilibrium is specific for a given population, and the same alleles may or may not be similarly associated in a different population.

Synteny occurs when two or more loci are on the same chromosome. Syntenic loci may or may not be linked, but linked loci are always syntenic. Syntenic loci may be far enough apart on a chromosome for crossing over to occur between them. By definition, linked loci are so close that recombination usually does not occur between them.

168–170. The answers are: 168-B, 169-A, 170-D. *(Childhood development)*
Effective monitoring of childhood developmental milestones is critical for the early detection and management of developmental delay. A number of helpful charts are available to allow the primary care physician to make an assessment of normal cognitive development. Infants reach for objects outside of their immediate grasp as early as 3 months but should certainly have achieved this task by 8 months. Similarly, some precocious toddlers use intelligible phrases by 2 years of age, but the sole use of single words in a child of 3 years is clearly abnormal. Piaget described the concrete operations phase, during which children learn to categorize and mentally manipulate tangible objects. Before this stage, they are easily fooled by the short glass–tall glass trick. For some children, achievement of this milestone marks their final cognitive development, as some adults never become proficient at abstract thinking.

171–175. The answers are: 171-C, 172-A, 173-B, 174-E, 175-D. *(Cell division)*
The beginning of prophase is marked by the appearance of chromosomes within the nucleus. Throughout prophase, the chromosomes condense further; dissolution of the nuclear envelope marks the end of this phase.

During metaphase, the kinetochore becomes attached to tubulin, the major component of the mitotic spindle. Metaphase is marked by the alignment of chromosomes along the equatorial (metaphase) plane. The next stage of cell division is anaphase, and it is marked by the separation of the centromeres. By the addition of tubulin to the mitotic spindle, the chromosomes are drawn toward opposite poles of the cell. Anaphase ends when the chromosomes are clustered at opposite poles of the cell. During the final stage, telophase, the chromosomes uncoil, the nuclear envelope reforms, and the cell divides. As the cell divides, the cytoplasm also divides by a process known as cytokinesis; these processes continue until two daughter cells are produced. During telophase, cell division is thought to occur by the constriction of a ring of actin filaments.

176–180. The answers are: 176-A, 177-C, 178-A, 179-B, 180-C. *(Pulmonary function tests in disease)*
Forced expiration spirometry provides valuable information for the classification of pulmonary disease. Specific variables assessed include forced vital lung capacity, forced expiratory volume in the first second (FEV_1), forced expiratory volume between 25% and 75% of total lung capacity (FEV_{25-75}; also called maximum midexpiratory flow rate), and residual capacity. The traces shown represent classic spirometric results for people with (*A*) obstructive disease, (*B*) normal function, and (*C*) restrictive disease.

The hallmarks of obstructive disease are increased forced vital capacity, decreased FEV_1 and substantially increased residual volume. The most striking feature is usually the increased residual volume, for which obstructive disease is named. The increase in residual volume is responsible for the characteristic "barrel-chested" appearance of someone with chronic obstructive pulmonary disease. The hallmarks of restrictive disease are reduced forced vital capacity, normal to increased FEV_1, and decreased residual volume.

To correctly answer the question, the classic clinical features of two different manifestations of each broad disease type must be recognized. More than 20% of life-long, heavy smokers progress to emphysema or chronic bronchitis (chronic obstructive pulmonary disease). Decreased breath sounds are a result of the substantial increase in residual volume coupled with a decrease in tidal volume and vital capacity.

A child with an active asthma exacerbation produces a spirometric tracing that also has the features of obstructive disease. Although only directed at the symptoms, the bronchodilation afforded by a β_2-selective adrenergic agonist (e.g., albuterol) results in a more normal spirometric tracing. Effective treatment of the disease process requires the use of inhaled or systemic corticosteroids.

Progressive pulmonary fibrosis can follow chronic exposure to a variety of environmental and industrial hazards, including asbestos. The clinical picture of dyspnea on exertion, unproductive cough, and diffuse radiographic opacities, which are first apparent in the lower lung fields, is characteristic of the interstitial fibrosis process that occurs following chronic exposure to any one of the known irritants.

Although particulars about the spirometric tracing may vary, disorders associated with diaphragmatic weakness produce the picture of restrictive disease. Guillain-Barré, muscular dystrophy, myasthenia gravis, and impingement of the phrenic nerve all can result in diaphragmatic weakness and a spirometric picture of restrictive lung disease in an individual with normal lungs.

181–183. The answers are: 181-A, 182-A, 183-C. *(Cell characteristics and function)*
The T cell—specifically the helper T (Th) cell—can help with the B-cell proliferation and differentiation to an antibody-secreting plasma cell that occurs in the antibody response. If antigen on an accessory cell (e.g., a macrophage) interacts with its homologous receptor on a T-cell surface, this will trigger lymphokine release from the Th cell, as well as proliferation and differentiation of the B cell, if both the cells are identical at the class II major histocompatibility complex (MHC). The Th cells that participate in B-cell maturation also show this MHC restriction.

There are several functional subsets of T cells. Cytotoxic T (Tc) cells cause lysis of antigen-bearing target cells (virally infected cells, tumor cells, transplanted allogeneic cells). Besides being important in B-cell maturation, Th cells also function in Tc-cell development. The suppressor T (Ts) cell has an opposing function: It serves to down-regulate (depress) the immune response. Ts cells suppress directly, or via suppressor factors, the function of other immunologically active cells (e.g., Th cells). Ts cells and Tc cells bear the CD8 membrane antigen but not the CD4; therefore they are $CD8^+$, $CD4^-$, and are easily distinguished from Th cells, which are $CD8^-$, $CD4^+$.

Macrophages and the dendritic cells of the spleen and the Langerhans cells of the skin are responsible for the initial processing of an antigen as it enters the spleen or lymph nodes. The processed antigen is complexed with class II MHC molecules in the cytoplasm and is presented to the lymphocytes on the membrane of the antigen-presenting cell. Peripheral blood neutrophils are phagocytic, as are the macrophages, but do not process antigen effectively.

184–186. The answers are: 184-B, 185-E, 186-A. *(Developmental theories)*
A broad range of thinking has contributed to our understanding of personal, moral, and cognitive development. Freud is best known for his classic description of the "superego" conscience and its battle of the immoral, irreverent, and aggressive "id." The unconscious battle results in the "ego," which is the outward manifestation of both components of our subconscious personality. According to Freud's theory, the development of the ego is a progression through a series of phases, during which different parts of the body serve as the focus of an individual's sexual gratification.

Erikson elaborated on Freud's thinking but maintained a similar structure. He emphasized the development of individuals as being a series of crises within a societal context. For example, an infant interacts with its mother and learns either to trust or distrust the world. In each stage a decision is made (i.e., to trust or to mistrust), and subsequent development is influenced by the outcome of earlier crises.

The French psychologist Piaget studied young children throughout their development. He asked them to explain commonplace events (e.g., what happens to the sun when it sets) and created a series of simple experiments to let them demonstrate their mode of reasoning. What he found was that most children in fact do proceed through a standard set of phases using qualitatively different intellectual tools at each stage.

Maslow was interested in "self-actualization" and motivation. What he described was the classic pyramid of goals for which people universally strive. In general, people cannot have altruistic goals and motives until their more basic needs are met. They do not seek companionship, for example, until they have sufficient food; nor will they look for intellectual stimulation until shelter has been found.

Kohlberg was primarily interested in moral development, and he described a series of stages through which people progress as they shape their behavior. Fear of punishment initially promotes children to obey their parents. Later, behaviors are based on "what others will think." Ultimately, some people achieve a moral character in which the needs of others are considered equal to their own when they make decisions.

187–189. The answers are: 187-D, 188-D, 189-D. *(Bruton's hypogammaglobulinemia)*
Normal recovery from viral diseases suggests an intact thymus-dependent immune system, thus eliminating DiGeorge, Nezelof's, and Wiskott-Aldrich syndromes, all of which feature variable or total deficits in T-cell immunity. Selective immunoglobulin deficiency is a possible diagnosis because of its characteristic of normal T-cell function.

Dysgammaglobulinemia is a selective immunoglobulin deficiency, in which one or more, but not all, immunoglobulins show a decrease in serum levels; nonspecific immunity is normal in this disorder. Normal leukocytic function would not be characteristic of chronic granulomatous disease (CGD) [impaired intracellular killing], Job's syndrome (faulty chemotactic response), or the lazy leukocyte syndrome (defective chemotactic response and abnormal inflammatory response).

The patient has Bruton's hypogammaglobulinemia. The presence of a small amount of IgG is consistent with this diagnosis. Common variable hypogammaglobulinemia resembles Bruton's disease, except that symptoms first appear in patients 20 to 30 years of age. Selective immunoglobulin deficiency is characterized by a decrease in serum levels of one or more immunoglobulin class; in selective IgA deficiency, the most common form, there is little serum IgA but normal or increased levels of IgG and IgM. Wiskott-Aldrich syndrome features low IgM levels, elevated IgA and IgE, but normal IgG levels. Transient hypogamma-globulinemia of infancy is self-correcting by age 30 months, and thus would be an unlikely diagnosis by age 3 years.

190–194. The answers are: 190-A, 191-D, 192-C, 193-B, 194-E. *(Systemic blood pressure)*
Normal blood pressure is 140/90 or less in adults. If only the systolic pressure is elevated, this is called isolated systolic hypertension; if the word "hypertension" is used without further qualification, it is presumed that both the systolic and the diastolic elements are high. The normal response to standing upright is a slight rise in pulse rate, a small drop in systolic pressure, and a small rise in diastolic pressure. With volume depletion, both the systolic and the diastolic pressure often drop more considerably; however, if the host has intact vascular reflexes, the pressures may be maintained, or nearly so, by a marked increase in heart rate. This is the situation depicted in the 59-year-old man, where the pressures are almost steady, but at the cost of a 23-beat rise in heart rate. If the pressures drop and there is no compensatory increase in heart rate, the autonomic response is dysfunctional, as shown in the 68-year-old man.

195–200. The answers are: 195-J, 196-H, 197-D, 198-A, 199-F, 200-C. *(Biochemical basis of disease)*
The diagnosis of acute intermittent porphyria is rarely made before puberty, but the description given is classic. The disease is transmitted in an autosomal dominant fashion, but it has a variable degree of heterozygous expression. Generally, hemoglobin synthesis by the erythrocytes is normal, but the liver's ability to synthesize heme is impaired. Most attacks are brought on by the introduction of a drug that is metabolized through the cytochrome P_{450} oxidase system. Diffuse abdominal pain, dark red urine, increased heart rate, nausea, and vomiting reflect a buildup of γ-aminolevulinic acid and porphobilinogen, which are the precursors of porphyrin synthesis. Because there is not a serum buildup of preformed porphyrin rings, the cutaneous photosensitivity seen in erythrogenic porphyrias does not occur. The abdominal pain and vomiting are thought to be related to an autonomic neuropathy induced by the deranged metabolism. The other neuropathies described are mild in the spectrum; more striking presentations might include paraplegias, delirium, and seizures.

The description of maternal phenylketonuria has become all too common. Women who were diagnosed and treated in childhood may have forgotten their disease because effective control is important only until growth and sexual development are complete. The disease reappears strikingly when they bear children. The extremely high maternal levels of phenylalanine and alternative phenylalanine metabolites diffuse across the placenta to the fetus. Effects on the fetus include retarded myelination, impaired synthesis of catecholamines, and reduced transport of other amino acids (thus reducing their availability for protein synthesis). Mental retardation in these children is almost uniform; congenital heart defects and microcephaly occur in many. Now that treated women are able to live and function as normal adults, it is critical to identify and treat them during pregnancy to prevent this alarming outcome. If a mother is effectively managed with dietary modifications during pregnancy, the fetus is not subjected to the toxic effects of the mother's disease. Generally, the infant is heterozygous for the disorder and will have normal phenylalanine metabolism and normal development after birth.

The 21-hydroxylase deficiency is inherited in an autosomal recessive fashion and is the most common cause of congenital adrenal hyperplasia (CAH). CAH occurs in both males and females with a spectrum of severity that roughly corresponds to the underlying defect in the steroid synthesis pathway. The earlier and more complete the defect, the less able the body is to compensate. In this case, normal female anatomy has developed because of a lack of müllerian inhibiting substance, whose expression is Y-chromosome dependent. However, estrogen-dependent development (e.g., urogenital sinus differentiation) is ambiguous, and in some cases can be strikingly male, resulting in misassignment of sex. As many as two thirds of these children inherit a defect severe enough that the body is unable to compensate despite adrenal hyperplasia. In this subset of children, secretion of cortisol and aldosterone are impaired enough to produce salt-wasting, volume depletion, anorexia, and vomiting within the first few weeks of life. In the remaining cases, the hyperplasia is sufficient to compensate for the synthetic defect, and the adrenal glands produce enough glucocorticoids and mineralocorticoids so that the signs of salt-wasting are not seen. Ambiguous genitalia or virilization is common to both the salt-wasting and the non–salt-wasting cases.

Cystic fibrosis is the most common X-linked disease among white children. The malabsorption is a result of diminished secretion of digestive enzymes by both the exocrine pancreas and the liver. The chronic pulmonary infections (usually *Pseudomonas aeruginosa*) are generally the earliest manifestations and often the cause of death. Dysregulation of chloride channels results in viscous secretions from all exocrine organs, and diagnosis is made following a chloride sweat test. Better antibiotics, supplemental enzyme therapy, and earlier intervention can extend the average lifespan into the third decade, but the diagnosis still carries a grim prognosis.

Vitamin C deficiency (i.e., scurvy) is now a disease largely confined to the urban poor and elderly edentulous persons, both of whom are susceptible to a variety of malnourishment syndromes. The underlying biochemical defect of vitamin C deficiency involves the impairment of the hydroxylation of proline residues; ascorbic acid is required to maintain the enzyme in its reduced (active) form. Capillary fragility, poor wound healing, and abnormal joint and bone development result because the stability of the collagen triple helix is largely dependent on the hydroxyproline content. Bleeding into the periosteum of long bones can cause painful swellings, which are probably the source of the infant's incessant crying. All of the processes are reversible if the hemorrhage and resulting inflammation in the bones do not remain unchecked for long.

The complete testicular feminization syndrome is the third most common cause of primary amenorrhea. Prepubertal inguinal hernia would be the only other reason for otherwise normal phenotypic females to present. The vagina is often short and blind-ending in these women, and all internal genitalia are absent except for normal but undescended testes. Physical growth and bone age are normal, although late epiphyseal closure frequently results in rather tall women. As with all cryptorchidism, the major long-term complication is the development of testicular tumors. The physician can generally elicit a family history of a disorder of sexual development. The defective androgen receptor is a typical member of the steroid hormone receptor super-family with DNA-binding properties; it is encoded on the long arm of the X chromosome. Testosterone levels are high as a result of lack of feedback inhibition on luteinizing hormone (LH), and estradiol levels are intermediate between normal females and normal males. However, because the normal expression of female characteristics is dependent on an estrogen–androgen balance, these androgen-insensitive, genotypic men tend to have a greater degree of feminization than do normal women (who are sensitive to the low levels of testosterone that they have).

Defective sodium channels, which do not inactivate like their normal voltage-gated sodium channel counterparts, are implicated in the pathophysiology of periodic paralysis, a relatively rare disorder of muscle tissue.

Defective 17-β-hydroxysteroid dehydrogenase in the testis results in a lack of virilization in 46; X,Y males (male pseudohermaphroditism), without any symptoms of congenital adrenal hyperplasia. Because this enzyme is only important for the final step in testosterone synthesis, there are no glucocorticoid or miner-alocorticoid deficiencies. The lack of complete male development in male pseudohermaphroditism is different from the seemingly normal female development seen in testicular feminization syndrome.

Defective oxidation of lysyl residues in collagen is the underlying problem in the most common variant (type VI) of Ehlers-Danlos syndrome.

Defective cystathionine β-synthase activity is the most common cause of homocystinuria, a defect in the metabolism of sulfur-containing amino acids (i.e., methionine, cysteine).

Test II

QUESTIONS

DIRECTIONS: Each of the numbered items or incomplete statements in this section is followed by answers or by completions of the statement. Select the ONE lettered answer or completion that is BEST in each case.

1. In patients with Barrett's esophagus, factors responsible for the morphologic changes in the distal portion of the esophagus from normal squamous cell epithelium to columnar epithelium include all of the following EXCEPT

(A) incompetence of the lower esophageal sphincter

(B) the ingrowth of immature pluripotent stem cells

(C) increased exposure to acid and pepsin

(D) the absence of inflammatory processes

(E) increased exposure to bile acids and lyso-lecithin

2. Of the following effects, drug binding to plasma proteins generally

(A) limits glomerular filtration

(B) is highly drug-specific

(C) is an interaction between drug and immuno-globulins

(D) is irreversible

(E) limits renal tubular secretion

Questions 3–5

A 36-year-old woman is brought to the emergency room because a friend found her unresponsive on the floor at home. Her friend relates a recent history of depression. An empty prescription bottle for thirty 100-mg amitriptyline tablets was found nearby. The woman's amitriptyline level is 2300 ng/ml, and her serum ethanol level is 250 mg/100 ml.

3. The physician's first step would be to

(A) prepare involuntary commitment documents

(B) order an immediate electroencephalogram

(C) insert a nasogastric tube

(D) administer physostigmine

(E) place the patient on a respirator

The patient is placed on a cardiac monitor, the results of which are shown below.

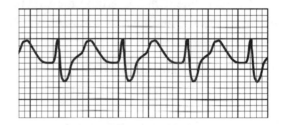

4. This electrocardiogram reveals which of the following patterns?

(A) Widened QRS complexes consistent with quinidine-like effects of tricyclics

(B) Bradycardia consistent with the cholinergic effects of tricyclics

(C) Premature ventricular contractions consistent with the toxic effects of ethanol

(D) S-T segment elevation consistent with the ischemic effects of ethanol

(E) Shortened P-R interval consistent with the toxic effects of tricyclics

5. The patient is now alert, her electrocardiogram is normal, and her total serum amitriptyline level is 128 ng/ml. The physician should next

(A) lecture her about the dangers of toxic doses of tricyclics
(B) elicit information about the suicide attempt
(C) interpret her behavior as an angry reaction
(D) discuss the paternalism of involuntary psychiatric hospitalization

6. The plasma membrane is composed of lipids and proteins with the basic structure of a lipid bilayer. Correct statements regarding the structure and function of the plasma membrane include all of the following EXCEPT

(A) phospholipids are amphipathic
(B) proteins may penetrate either portion of or the entire bilayer
(C) phospholipids promote free diffusion of ions and small water-soluble molecules
(D) proteins are amphipathic
(E) some large proteins are free to diffuse laterally in the plane of the membrane

7. A polymerase chain reaction can increase the sensitivity of certain genetic tests. Necessary components of a polymerase chain reaction include all of the following EXCEPT

(A) the DNA to be amplified is denatured in the presence of an equimolar ratio of primers
(B) a heat-resistant DNA polymerase is used for strand synthesis
(C) multiple heating and cooling cycles are required for amplification of the DNA
(D) the sequence of the segment of DNA to which the primers will bind must be known

8. Of the following statements about messenger RNA (mRNA) transcription, the most accurate is that it

(A) proceeds by synthesis of the RNA in the 3′ to 5′ direction
(B) involves the removal of internal regions of DNA from the genome
(C) only occurs in the cytoplasm of the human cell
(D) may be regulated by hormones
(E) involves the post-transcriptional addition of adenylate nucleotides to the 5′ end of the molecule

9. An individual with a gastric carcinoma is likely to present with any of the following skin lesions EXCEPT

(A) seborrheic keratosis
(B) acanthosis nigricans
(C) erythema nodosum
(D) amyloidosis
(E) Paget's disease

10. Which sequence below is the correct order of epidermal maturation?

(A) Stratum basale, stratum spinosum, stratum lucidum, stratum granulosum, stratum corneum
(B) Stratum basale, stratum spinosum, stratum granulosum, stratum lucidum, stratum corneum
(C) Stratum basale, stratum granulosum, stratum spinosum, stratum lucidum, stratum corneum
(D) Stratum basale, stratum lucidum, stratum spinosum, stratum granulosum, stratum corneum
(E) Stratum basale, stratum lucidum, stratum granulosum, stratum spinosum, stratum corneum

11. A 25-year-old sexually active woman is evaluated for her fourth acute urinary tract infection during the past 12 months. Her infections are characterized by frequency, urgency, dysuria, and *Escherichia coli* bacteriuria. Her recurrent infections are most likely due to

(A) overgrowth of highly resistant *E. coli* in her fecal reservoir

(B) passage of an infected renal calculus

(C) resistance of the bacteria to the drugs selected for treatment

(D) presence of a foreign body within the genitourinary tract

(E) colonization of the vaginal introitus with fecal Enterobacteriaceae

12. A 2-year-old child is hospitalized with splenomegaly, anemia, hypersplenism, hepatomegaly, and progressive nervous system dysfunction. Enzyme studies show an absence of glucocerebrosidase with an accumulation of β-glucosylceramide in macrophages and hepatocytes. The lipid storage disease most likely to be diagnosed in this child is

(A) Niemann-Pick disease

(B) Gaucher's disease, type II

(C) Krabbe's disease

(D) Tay-Sachs disease

Questions 13–15

The micrograph below is of the male reproductive system.

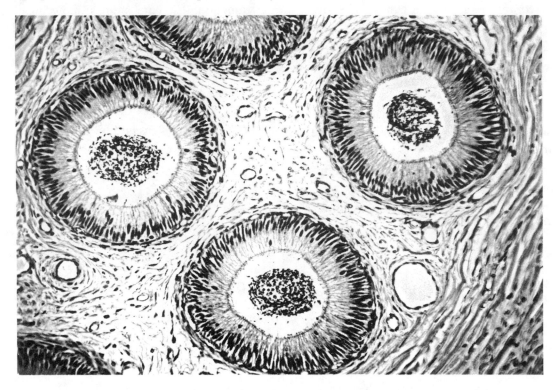

13. Which of the following organs is pictured in the micrograph?

(A) Testis
(B) Epididymis
(C) Vas deferens
(D) Seminal vesicle
(E) Bulbourethral gland

14. The epithelium of the organ pictured in the micrograph can best be described as

(A) simple cuboidal
(B) simple columnar
(C) stratified columnar
(D) pseudostratified columnar with stereocilia
(E) stratified squamous

15. Which adjective below best describes the function of the epithelium in the micrograph?

(A) Gametogenic
(B) Proliferative
(C) Secretory and absorptive
(D) Inactive
(E) Apoptotic

16. What condition is marked by formation of a malignant pustule?

(A) Enteritis necroticans
(B) Lockjaw
(C) Cutaneous anthrax
(D) Pseudomembranous colitis
(E) Woolsorter's disease

17. A 52-year-old man presented with painless swelling of his right testis. An orchiectomy was performed. A sample of the tissue is pictured in the photomicrograph below. The correct diagnosis is

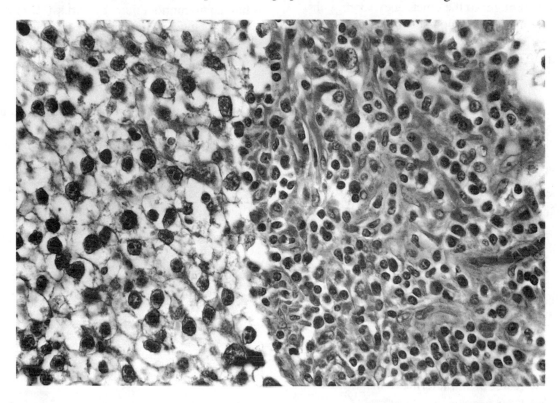

(A) seminoma

(B) mumps orchitis

(C) immature teratoma

(D) choriocarcinoma

18. A patient must be evaluated because of thrombocytopenia. The patient is a 55-year-old, previously well man, who was admitted to the hospital yesterday because of pneumonia. Antibiotic therapy was started; and, although his temperature continues to spike, it is lower than it was on admission. On admission, his hemoglobin was reported to be 13 g/dl, his white blood cell count was 9000/µl, and his platelet count was 70,000/µl. The next laboratory study that should be done is

(A) bone marrow examination

(B) bleeding time

(C) examination of the peripheral smear

(D) platelet aggregation studies

(E) antiplatelet antibody detection tests

Questions 19–21

An infant is brought to the emergency room with severe oral thrush and hypocalcemia. A complete blood count shows a white cell count within normal limits. The mother admits to being an intravenous drug user.

19. What is the most likely diagnosis in this case?

(A) Chronic mucocutaneous candidiasis
(B) Severe combined immunodeficiency disease
(C) DiGeorge syndrome
(D) Chronic granulomatous disease

20. Which of the following statements concerning this child's condition is true?

(A) It is an autosomal recessive disorder
(B) It is an X-linked disorder
(C) It is the result of intrauterine damage
(D) The mode of inheritance is unknown

21. The most appropriate treatment for this patient would be

(A) transplantation of a fetal thymus
(B) infusion with white cells genetically engineered to produce adenosine deaminase
(C) administration of antifungal agents
(D) administration of corticosteroids

22. After osmotic equilibrium, infusion of several liters of a hypertonic saline solution will

(A) decrease intracellular osmolality
(B) not affect intracellular volume
(C) increase extracellular fluid volume
(D) decrease the plasma osmolarity

23. The Food and Drug Administration (FDA) has announced that it will test the vaccines against human immunodeficiency virus (HIV) with the least potential for causing the disease and the best chance of inducing protective immunity. Which of the vaccination reagents listed is most likely to be tested?

(A) An attenuated virus that does not cause disease in monkeys
(B) A recombinant HIV DNA in a vaccinia virus to induce host cells to produce only the HIV p24 protein, and then antibodies to p24 protein
(C) A denatured, purified CD4 (T4) protein to cause the host to mount an immune response to the HIV-infected CD4$^+$ cells
(D) A human monoclonal antibody that reacts with the intact CD4 (T4) receptor

24. All of the following statements concerning immunogenicity are true EXCEPT

(A) compounds with a molecular weight greater than 6000 daltons are generally immunogenic
(B) haptens become immunogenic only when coupled to high molecular weight carriers
(C) a homopolymer of lysine with a molecular weight of 30,000 daltons would not be immunogenic
(D) a polymer of lysine, methionine, and glutamate with a molecular weight of 10,000 daltons would not be immunogenic

25. The most important allosteric activator of glycolysis in the liver is which one of the following compounds?

(A) Fructose 2,6-bisphosphate
(B) Acetyl coenzyme A (acetyl CoA)
(C) Adenosine triphosphate (ATP)
(D) Citrate
(E) Glucose 6-phosphate

26. Ingestion of 150 mEq Na^+/day is usually balanced by excretion of a similar amount in urine. Because the glomerular filtrate normally contains 26,000 mEq Na^+/day, several important Na^+-reabsorbing mechanisms have evolved, including all of the following EXCEPT

(A) active transport of Na^+ from inside proximal epithelial cells to interstitial spaces
(B) passive cotransport of Na^+ with glucose or amino acids in the proximal tubular epithelium
(C) active transport in the thick segment of the loop of Henle
(D) hormone-independent passive reabsorption in the distal tubular epithelium

27. The thyroid tumor pictured here was removed from a 60-year-old woman whose medical history likely includes

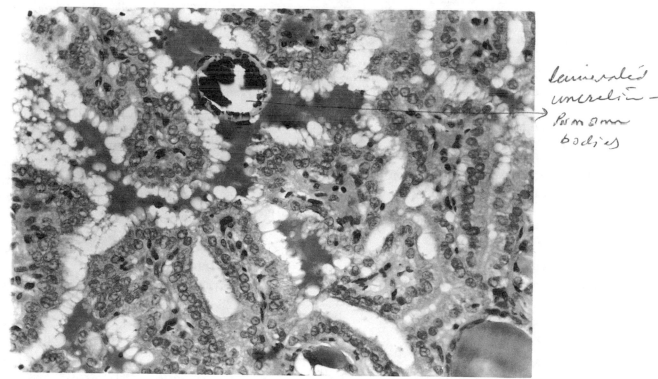

(A) hyperthyroidism
(B) hypothyroidism
(C) irradiation to the head and neck
(D) a pituitary adenoma

28. When comparing pertussis and diphtheria, true statements include which one of the following?

(A) Both pertussis and diphtheria are caused by bacteria that must adhere to respiratory tract cells

(B) Diphtheria symptoms are caused by an exotoxin, but no symptoms of pertussis result from an exotoxin

(C) The bacteria responsible for diphtheria and pertussis both produce endotoxin

(D) Pertussis is caused by an intracellular pathogen, but diphtheria is caused by an extracellular pathogen

(E) The neurologic problems observed with the current DTP (diphtheria-tetanus-pertussis) vaccine are caused by the diphtheria component of this vaccine

Questions 29–31

A 68-year-old widower complains of headaches, forgetfulness, decreased appetite, weight loss, insomnia, constipation, and anhedonia. An electrocardiogram shows first-degree heart block; he also has prostatic hypertrophy.

29. Considering side effect profiles, the best choice of medication would be

(A) imipramine
(B) phenelzine
(C) lithium carbonate
(D) clonazepam
(E) chlorpromazine

The patient's psychiatric symptoms improve with treatment, but his headaches persist. They occur daily and are bifrontotemporal, nonthrobbing, and bring him to tears when the pain is severe, but they do not disrupt his sleep. Physical examination reveals tenderness near the eye ridges.

30. The most appropriate test would be

(A) computed tomography scan of the head
(B) biopsy of the temporal artery
(C) electroencephalogram
(D) examination of the cerebrospinal fluid

31. Medication for migraine headache includes all of the following agents EXCEPT

(A) lithium carbonate
(B) ergotamine
(C) methysergide
(D) amitriptyline
(E) propranolol

32. Which of the following statements concerning the maturation of T cells is true?

(A) It occurs earliest in the thymic medulla
(B) It is independent of thymic epithelial cells
(C) It is independent of antigen
(D) None of the above

33. Each condition below is a diagnostically significant abnormality in Zellweger syndrome EXCEPT

(A) absent or grossly reduced numbers of peroxisomes
(B) catalase in the cytosol of hepatocytes
(C) overproduction of platelet activating factor (PAF)
(D) elevated plasma C26:0/C22:0 ratio
(E) accumulation of phytanic acid in central nervous system (CNS) tissues

34. A 24-year-old man presented to his family practitioner with a purulent penile discharge. Gonorrhea was diagnosed based on the finding of intracellular gram-negative cocci in his discharge. He was given amoxicillin and probenecid. The infection improved, but 1 week later the patient still complained of a persistent urethral discharge and pain on urination. On a visit to a local clinic for sexually transmitted diseases, a diagnosis of postgonococcal urethritis was made. What is the most likely cause of his latest syndrome?

(A) A common side effect of probenecid administered during the initial treatment

(B) A lingering gonococcal infection caused by a penicillin-resistant strain of *Neisseria gonorrhoeae*

(C) An improper therapy regimen, which did not treat a coinciding chlamydial infection

(D) A side effect of the correct therapy regimen, which suppressed the patient's normal flora and allowed the establishment of a secondary infection

35. A 38-year-old man with AIDS develops meningitis. Microscopic examination of his spinal fluid shows yeast cells. India ink staining of these yeasts shows a visible clear halo surrounding each cell. Which one of the following pathogens is responsible for the man's meningitis?

(A) A virus

(B) *Cryptococcus neoformans*

(C) *Haemophilus influenzae*

(D) *Neisseria meningitidis*

(E) *Candida albicans*

36. All of the following properties are shared by acetylsalicylic acid (aspirin) and acetaminophen EXCEPT

(A) inhibits lipoxygenase activity

(B) analgesic activity

(C) antipyretic effects

(D) anti-inflammatory activity

37. Captopril is useful in the treatment of systemic hypertension because it

(A) blocks the effect of angiotensin II at its receptor in the central nervous system (CNS)

(B) directly relaxes vascular smooth muscle

(C) inhibits the movement of extracellular calcium into myocardial cells

(D) decreases the activity of angiotensin-converting enzyme (ACE)

(E) inhibits the production of renin

38. All of the following statements concerning insulin-dependent diabetes mellitus (type I; IDDM) are correct EXCEPT

(A) sulfonylureas may be a useful adjuvant to insulin therapy

(B) use of recombinant "human" insulin has eliminated problems of immunologic toxic effects

(C) insulin levels are routinely monitored

(D) ingestion of carbohydrates may be required to offset undesired hypoglycemia

(E) insulin therapy usually reverses the course of the disease

39. All of the following statements about allosteric enzymes are true EXCEPT

(A) positive cooperativity sensitizes the enzyme to small changes in substrate concentration
(B) they frequently catalyze the slowest step in a metabolic pathway
(C) the allosteric site can be located on a different subunit from the catalytic site
(D) the binding of a ligand to the allosteric site induces a conformational change in the active site
(E) they have substrate saturation curves that frequently show first-order kinetics

40. A patient presents with a torn medial collateral ligament of the left knee. Which of the following signs may be elicited on physical examination?

(A) Posterior displacement of the tibia
(B) Abnormal lateral rotation during extension
(C) Abnormal passive abduction of the extended leg
(D) Inability to lock the knee on full extension

41. The female reproductive viscera are best characterized by which of the following statements?

(A) The mesosalpinx contains the tubal branches of the uterine vessels
(B) The ovarian veins drain directly into the inferior vena cava
(C) Lymph from the cervix drains into the inguinal nodes
(D) Visceral afferent nerves from the body of the uterus course along the pelvic splanchnic nerves

42. The uterine cervical tissue shown in the photomicrograph below shows features of which one of the following infections?

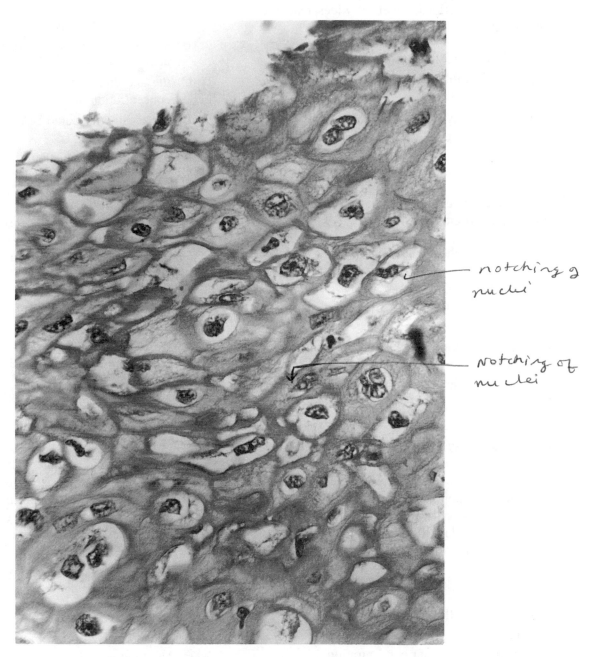

notching of nuclei

notching of nuclei

(A) Papillomavirus
(B) Herpes genitalis
(C) Gonorrheal cervicitis
(D) Carcinoma in situ

43. Tetracycline, a broad-spectrum antibiotic used in treating rickettsial, mycoplasmal, and chlamydial infections, receives widespread use because it

(A) is particularly useful in children
(B) causes minimal gastrointestinal side effects
(C) is bactericidal
(D) is selectively toxic to prokaryotes
(E) inhibits DNA-dependent RNA polymerase

44. Hepatic gluconeogenesis from alanine requires the participation of

(A) glucose 6-phosphatase and pyruvate kinase
(B) phosphofructokinase and pyruvate carboxylase
(C) pyruvate carboxylase and phosphoenolpyruvate carboxykinase
(D) fructose 1,6-diphosphatase and pyruvate kinase
(E) transaminase and phosphofructokinase

Questions 45–47

A resident has been assigned to the operating room for a 2-month rotation. The staff surgeon under whom he will work is a stickler for theory, and on the first day of the new rotation, he asked the resident the following questions.

45. With regard to anesthetics, MAC refers to

(A) maximum allowable concentration
(B) minimum alveolar concentration
(C) maximum alveolar concentration
(D) minimum arterial concentration
(E) maximum arterial concentration

46. If an anesthetic has a high blood:gas partition coefficient, it means that

(A) recovery will likely be prolonged
(B) lean patients should receive a lower dose than heavy patients
(C) the anesthetic should be delivered at a low concentration initially
(D) the anesthetic should be mixed with an inert gas or oxygen
(E) none of the above should occur

47. Nitrous oxide cannot be used alone to produce surgical anesthesia but is often used in conjunction with a more powerful agent, such as halothane, because nitrous oxide is

(A) explosive
(B) slow in onset of action due to a low blood:gas partition coefficient
(C) not very potent (i.e., has relatively low lipid solubility)
(D) rapidly metabolized

48. A 52-year-old middle school teacher has chronic peptic ulcer disease that has been treated for several years with ranitidine (Zantac) and metoclopramide (Reglan). On examination, the physician notes that the patient has involuntary, irregular chewing movements and repetitive tongue protrusion. The most likely cause of these movements is

(A) dystonic reaction
(B) Wilson's disease
(C) Huntington's disease
(D) cerebellar degeneration
(E) tardive dyskinesia

Questions 49–54

A mildly obese 20-year-old man presents to the emergency room at 5:00 A.M. He had ingested several six-packs of beer the evening before and had awakened at home with a sharp pain in his wrist at the radial–carpal articulation. The wrist is swollen and tender. The patient is slightly disoriented and ataxic but does not remember falling. X-rays of the wrist are negative. A slight fever is present.

49. The physician should order all of the following laboratory tests at this time EXCEPT

(A) synovial fluid analysis
(B) erythrocyte sedimentation rate
(C) C-reactive protein
(D) differential white blood cell count
(E) serum transaminase

50. Based on the data available, the most likely diagnosis is

(A) hyperuricemia with partial deficiency of hypoxanthine–guanine phosphoribosyltransferase
(B) Lesch-Nyhan syndrome
(C) osteoarthritis
(D) calcium hydroxyapatite deposition disease
(E) carpal tunnel syndrome

51. Synovial fluid analysis is done. The synovial fluid crystals are most likely composed of

(A) calcium oxalate
(B) calcium hydroxyapatite
(C) calcium carbonate
(D) sodium urate
(E) sodium oxalate

52. Biochemical studies confirm the suspected diagnosis. This patient suffers from lack of an enzyme whose product is

(A) 6-phosphogluconate
(B) citrulline
(C) inosinate
(D) oxaloacetate
(E) adenosine

53. The patient should be treated initially with

(A) adenosine replacement therapy
(B) azathioprine
(C) colchicine
(D) azidothymidine
(E) propoxyphene

54. For long-term therapy, the patient should be treated with

(A) acyclovir
(B) allopurinol
(C) amantadine
(D) acetazolamide
(E) ampicillin

55. Which of the following statements concerning primitive aortic arches and their derivatives is true?

(A) The left fourth aortic arch forms the arch of the aorta
(B) The right sixth aortic arch forms the right subclavian artery
(C) The left fifth aortic arch forms the ductus arteriosus
(D) The first aortic arch forms the common carotid artery

56. If forbidden clones are not deleted during T-cell development, a person may develop

(A) hypogammaglobulinemia
(B) a type I hypersensitivity reaction to exogenous antigens
(C) an autoimmune disease
(D) tolerance to autoantigens

57. A 60-year-old woman is brought to the hospital because of fever and confusion. One week earlier, she received chemotherapy for lymphoma. In the emergency room, she is noted to have rapid breathing; cool, clammy skin; and a blood pressure of 70/40. Complete blood count shows a white blood cell count of 200/μl. Gram stain of urine and sputum is negative. Which of the following empiric therapies would be most appropriate for this patient?

(A) Gentamicin
(B) Amikacin
(C) Chloramphenicol–gentamicin
(D) Piperacillin–gentamicin

Questions 58–60

A physician who has recommended urography for her competent, 68-year-old male patient is trying to decide whether or not to disclose the remote risk (1 in 10,000) of a fatal reaction.

58. If the physician favors nondisclosure, reasoning that it would not be in the patient's best interest to worry him with such remote risks, the physician is guided by

(A) beneficence but not nonmaleficence
(B) nonmaleficence but not beneficence
(C) both beneficence and nonmaleficence
(D) justice
(E) gratitude

59. If the physician believes that her decision should be determined by what other physicians would do in similar circumstances, she is guided by

(A) both beneficence and nonmaleficence
(B) strong paternalism
(C) weak paternalism
(D) respect for autonomy
(E) the professional practice standard

60. If the physician bases her decision on her assessment of whether or not the patient would want to learn about such remote risks, the physician is guided by

(A) respect for autonomy
(B) beneficence
(C) nonmaleficence
(D) both beneficence and nonmaleficence
(E) the professional practice standard

61. A scientist in the year 2350 is advising the NASA genetic engineering department concerning its attempts to engineer humans who can better survive the harsh climate of a planet that has high levels of ultraviolet (UV) light. The NASA engineers want to incorporate a group of genes that will allow epidermal cells to produce a light-absorbing pigment. Of the following genetic manipulations, which would be most advantageous in cells in a UV-rich environment?

(A) Removing intron DNA from the engineered genes
(B) Introducing the engineered genes in an overlapping fashion into the human genome
(C) Altering a theoretical human equivalent of the bacterial RecA protein in the cells to decrease RecA activity
(D) Producing genes with a low thymidine content

62. The photomicrograph below shows an adrenal mass that was resected from a 2-year-old child. This lesion most likely is

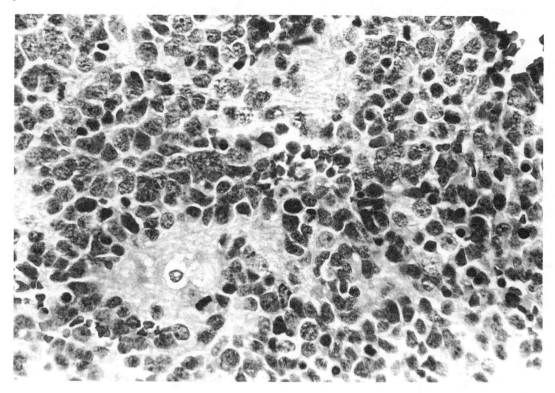

(A) Wilms' tumor

(B) a neuroblastoma

(C) a ganglioneuroma

(D) a phcochromocytoma

Questions 63–64

A 15-year-old girl presents for evaluation of short stature. She has not yet begun to menstruate. Examination reveals an intellectually normal child with short stature, webbing of the neck, a broad chest, and cubitus valgus.

63. Which of the following tests will provide the best evaluation of this patient?

(A) Amino acid analysis of urine

(B) Organic acid analysis of urine

(C) Serum long-chain fatty acids

(D) Chromosome analysis

(E) Tissue glycogen content

64. The differential diagnosis for short stature would include all of the following disorders EXCEPT

(A) Klinefelter syndrome

(B) mucopolysaccharidoses

(C) gonadal dysgenesis

(D) progeria

65. Of the following amino acids, which one is released from skeletal muscle in amounts that exceed its relative abundance in muscle protein?

(A) Aspartate
(B) Alanine
(C) Glutamate
(D) Leucine
(E) Tyrosine

66. Rapid diagnosis and determination of the causal species are essential because of the immediately life-threatening nature of which one of the following parasitic infections?

(A) Malaria
(B) Chronic Chagas disease
(C) Amebic dysentery
(D) Mucocutaneous leishmaniasis
(E) Giardiasis

Questions 67–68

A patient who weighs 50 kg is given a 20-mg/kg dose of a new drug. The plasma concentrations determined over time are illustrated in the graph below.

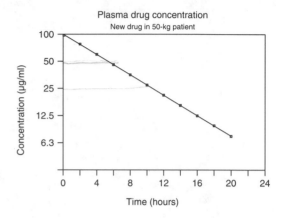

67. The drug's volume of distribution (V_d) is approximately

(A) 200 ml
(B) 1 L
(C) 2 L
(D) 10 L
(E) insufficient information to answer

68. The half-life of elimination of this drug is approximately

(A) 1 hour
(B) 2 hours
(C) 4 hours
(D) 10 hours
(E) insufficient information to answer

69. *N*-glycosylation of proteins occurs on which of the following amino acids?

(A) Asparagine
(B) Aspartate
(C) Lysine
(D) Serine
(E) Threonine

70. Tricyclic antidepressants (e.g., imipramine and amitriptyline) are useful agents for the management of endogenous depression because they

(A) reverse symptoms within days of initial administration
(B) have little effect on cardiovascular function
(C) affect dopamine receptors within the central nervous system (CNS)
(D) affect neuronal amine uptake mechanisms
(E) deplete brain serotonin levels

Questions 71–72

Cystic fibrosis is an autosomal recessive disease with an incidence of 1 per 1600 in the Caucasian population.

71. What is the frequency of the cystic fibrosis gene?

(A) 1/4
(B) 1/20
(C) 1/40
(D) 1/200
(E) 1/400

72. Of the following values, what proportion of the normal siblings of individuals with cystic fibrosis would most likely be carriers?

(A) 1/4
(B) 1/2
(C) 2/3
(D) All
(E) None

73. A 50-year-old woman with diabetes has an almost complete loss of renal function within 3 hours of a seemingly successful kidney transplant. All of the following statements concerning this type of rejection are true EXCEPT

(A) the patient had preformed antibodies to the graft
(B) the patient's rejection histologically resembles the classic Arthus reaction
(C) T cells are not directly involved
(D) administration of an immunosuppressive agent will restore kidney function

74. A 23-year-old woman with borderline personality disorder is hospitalized on a surgery ward to recover from fractures sustained in a motor vehicle accident. The patient states that her resident physician is wonderful and caring, but her primary nurse is cold and cruel. The psychologic mechanism being displayed is best termed

(A) denial
(B) projection
(C) manipulation
(D) displacement
(E) splitting

75. Baroreceptors are highly branched nerve endings that generate receptor potentials that are proportional to the rate of change in arterial blood pressure; they can also adapt to changes in arterial blood pressure over a prolonged period of time (hours to days). Which of the following statements concerning the specific properties of baroreceptors is most accurate?

(A) Baroreceptors are important for long-term regulation of blood pressure

(B) Clamping both carotid arteries after cutting both vagus nerves results in a decrease in arterial blood pressure

(C) Massaging the carotid sinus area leads to bradycardia and a decrease in arterial blood pressure

(D) A decrease in blood pressure activates baroreceptors, which, in turn, directly activate the vasomotor center

76. Lidocaine is the prototype of an amide local anesthetic and as such is

(A) free of potential central nervous system (CNS) side effects

(B) free of potential cardiac adverse effects

(C) rapidly metabolized by plasma cholinesterases

(D) a Na^+-channel blocker, especially in small, myelinated nerve fibers

(E) inappropriate for use in spinal anesthesia

77. Actin is a microfilament that is involved with all of the following activities EXCEPT

(A) endocytosis

(B) exocytosis

(C) cell locomotion

(D) mitotic spindle formation

(E) acrosome reaction

78. Mitochondria are important to the cells of eukaryotes for generating the adenosine triphosphate (ATP) necessary to carry out all energy-requiring processes. All of the following statements concerning mitochondria are true EXCEPT

(A) they contain a DNA molecule in a ring conformation

(B) mitochondrial proteins come solely from the cell nucleus

(C) the codons used by mitochondrial transfer RNA (tRNA) are not identical to those used in other mammalian genes

(D) mitochondrial proteins are encoded by gene sequences that overlap one another

79. A very painful, spreading, cutaneous edematous erythema is clinically descriptive of

(A) erysipeloid

(B) diphtheria

(C) Pontiac fever

(D) listeriosis

(E) nocardiosis

80. All of the following statements concerning gene duplication are true EXCEPT

(A) gene duplication involves unequal crossover between homologous repetitive DNA sequences during mitosis

(B) pseudogenes are nonfunctional duplications

(C) β-tubulins and β-like globins are perfect examples of duplicated gene families

(D) gene duplications are necessary to meet the cell's requirements for some RNA transcripts

81. Tay-Sachs disease occurs almost exclusively among Ashkenazi Jews, with an incidence of 1/3600. The frequency of carriers of the Tay-Sachs gene, which can be calculated by using the Hardy-Weinberg law ($p^2 + 2pq + q^2 = 1$), is which of the following?

(A) 1/4

(B) 1/30

(C) 1/60

(D) 1/600

(E) None of the above

82. Which of the endogenous substances listed is derived from the cyclooxygenase pathway of arachidonic acid metabolism?

(A) Platelet activating factor (PAF)

(B) Leukotriene D_4

(C) Eosinophil chemotactic factor (ECF)

(D) Thromboxane (TXA_2)

Questions 83–84

A 25-year-old medical student is buried by an avalanche of snow while skiing. Upon rescue, it is necessary to revive him from cardiopulmonary arrest. Although resuscitated, he remains in a coma for several hours before regaining consciousness.

83. It is known that the patient has suffered global hypoxia. The function most likely to have been lost under this condition is the ability to

(A) move facial muscles

(B) walk

(C) move arms

(D) move eyes

84. Which test of higher cortical functions would the patient most likely fail because of the hypoxic event?

(A) Remembering the name of the hospital or his physicians

(B) Reading a sentence

(C) Recognizing his cousins

(D) Adding two numbers together

85. A 65-year-old woman with degenerative joint disease secondary to rheumatoid arthritis has been admitted to the hospital for insertion of a prosthesis in her right hip (total hip arthroplasty). The physician is aware that *Staphylococcus aureus* and *Staphylococcus epidermidis* are likely to cause postoperative infection after total hip replacement. In addition, the hospital has reported a significant increase in beta-lactamase–resistant *S. aureus* isolates. Which of the following drugs is LEAST likely to be effective as prophylactic therapy in this patient?

(A) Cefazolin

(B) Methicillin

(C) Vancomycin

(D) Ampicillin

(E) Imipenem

86. A pregnant woman who is primigravida with blood type O-negative comes to the obstetrician's office for a routine visit. The patient states that her husband is AB-positive, and she is concerned about the incompatibility of the Rh factors. Her isohemagglutinin titers are normal. What would the most appropriate treatment be?

(A) Administer human anti-D globulin (RhoGAM) to the mother after the birth of the child

(B) Administer RhoGAM to the child immediately after birth

(C) Administer RhoGAM to the child if the blood is Rh-positive

(D) Do nothing at this time

87. In the figure below, the oxyhemoglobin dissociation curve is shown for a normal patient and for an anemic patient. A true statement concerning these patients is which one of the following?

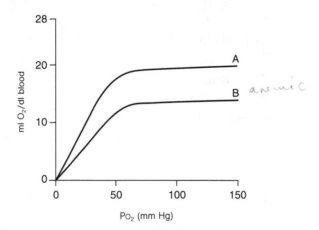

(A) Patient *A* is anemic

(B) Arterial Po_2 is likely to be similar for both subjects

(C) Venous Po_2 of the anemic subject will be greater than that of the normal subject at rest or during exercise

(D) If cardiac output is identical, oxygen delivery will be identical in subjects *A* and *B*

88. A 45-year-old woman has eaten some home-canned vegetables. Two days later she has blurred vision and difficulty swallowing. This is followed by respiratory distress and flaccid paralysis. The symptoms of her illness result from an intoxication caused by a bacterial toxin whose action involves which one of the following effects?

(A) Adenosine diphosphate (ADP)-ribosylation of elongation factor 2

(B) Blockage of release of inhibitory neurotransmitters

(C) Blockage of release of acetylcholine (ACh)

(D) Stimulation of adenylate cyclase to elevate intracellular cyclic adenosine monophosphate (cAMP) levels

(E) Hemolysis resulting from sequestration of cholesterol in membranes

89. A 22-year-old woman reports the gradual onset and relentless progression of severe pain in the lower left quadrant of her abdomen. She also reported nausea with vomiting and fever. A pelvic examination determined that there was marked tenderness both upon direct palpation and on manipulation of the cervix. A greenish-yellow discharge from the cervical os was noted, but a direct Gram stain of the discharge revealed no potential etiologic agents. Despite this finding, the patient was started on antibiotic therapy. Twenty-four hours later, laboratory culture of the discharge yielded growth of oxidase-positive, gram-negative diplococci on Thayer-Martin medium. A diagnosis of gonococcal salpingitis was made. One week post-therapy, the patient's symptoms were relieved and laboratory culture of her cervix revealed no pathogenic organisms. What is the patient's prognosis?

(A) The patient may not be cured and will require constant monitoring of her cervical flora for the next 6 months

(B) The patient may not be cured and is therefore encouraged to abstain from sexual intercourse or observe safe-sex practices for the next 6 months

(C) The patient is cured and requires no further monitoring

(D) The patient is cured but faces an increased risk of subsequent episodes of pelvic inflammatory disease, infertility, and ectopic pregnancy

90. Which of the following structures contains Hassall's corpuscles?

(A) Thyroid gland
(B) Parathyroid gland
(C) Pineal gland
(D) Thymus
(E) Spleen

91. Synthesis of glycogen from fructose in a person with essential fructosuria requires the activity of which one of the following enzymes?

(A) Transketolase
(B) Aldolase B
(C) Hexokinase
(D) Fructokinase
(E) Glucokinase

92. Renal osteodystrophy is a condition that may follow chronic renal failure. Features of this condition include osteitis fibrosa cystica admixed with osteomalacia. The pathogenesis of this condition is characterized by all of the following EXCEPT

(A) phosphate retention and hyperphosphatemia
(B) low levels of 1,25-dihydroxyvitamin D_3 (calcitriol)
(C) elevated levels of calcitonin
(D) hyperparathyroidism
(E) hypocalcemia

93. A 65-year-old woman is seen before cataract surgery. She has had no previous surgery except for a dental extraction, after which she bled for 10 days and required a 2-unit blood transfusion. One sibling died from postoperative hemorrhage during childhood, and there is a history of bleeding in a number of relatives, both male and female. Her partial thromboplastin time (PTT) is markedly prolonged, and the bleeding time is within normal limits. The most likely diagnosis is

(A) factor VIII deficiency
(B) factor XI deficiency
(C) factor XII deficiency
(D) Fletcher factor deficiency
(E) von Willebrand's disease

94. Enteric pathogens vary with respect to their ability to invade the intestinal mucosa. After infection, which one of the following enteric pathogens is most likely to invade the intestinal submucosa and then disseminate throughout the body?

(A) *Vibrio cholerae*

(B) *Salmonella typhi*

(C) *Shigella dysenteriae*

(D) Nontyphoid *Salmonella*

(E) *Campylobacter jejuni*

Questions 95–96

A 45-year-old woman is admitted to the hospital with an unremitting sore throat. She has undergone radical mastectomy for breast carcinoma and recently underwent adjuvant chemotherapy. Two weeks before, she received a seven-day course of amoxicillin–clavulanic acid (Augmentin) for a recurrent urinary tract infection. Examination of her palate reveals several patches of white, creamy, curd-like friable lesions on the tongue and other mucosal surfaces.

95. This patient most likely has which type of fungal infection?

(A) Sporotrichosis

(B) Dermatomycosis

(C) Candidiasis

(D) Cryptococcosis

96. All of the following therapies would be effective for this fungal infection EXCEPT

(A) ketoconazole

(B) oral fluconazole

(C) topical nystatin

(D) oral griseofulvin

(E) clotrimazole

Question 97

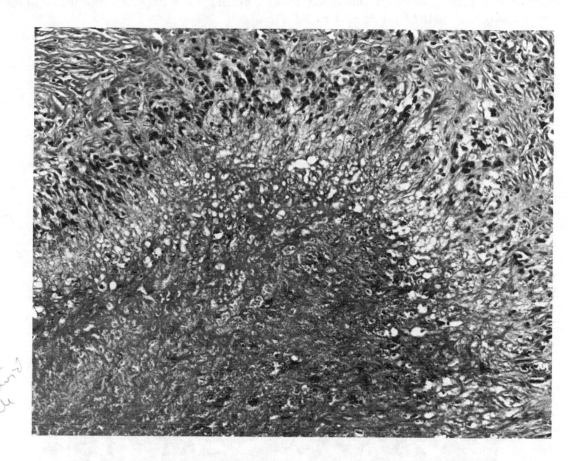

97. An elderly woman had a synovial biopsy and total knee replacement for degenerative joint disease. Sections of the synovium revealed the findings shown in the above photomicrograph, indicating a history of which one of the following conditions?

(A) Colchicine therapy for gout
(B) Repeated fractures
(C) Rheumatoid arthritis
(D) Trauma and foreign body within the joint space

98. Pictured below is a portion of large bowel resected from a middle-aged woman who had repeated bouts of crampy abdominal pain. It would be concluded from the histology that the gross appearance of the bowel would show all of the following features EXCEPT

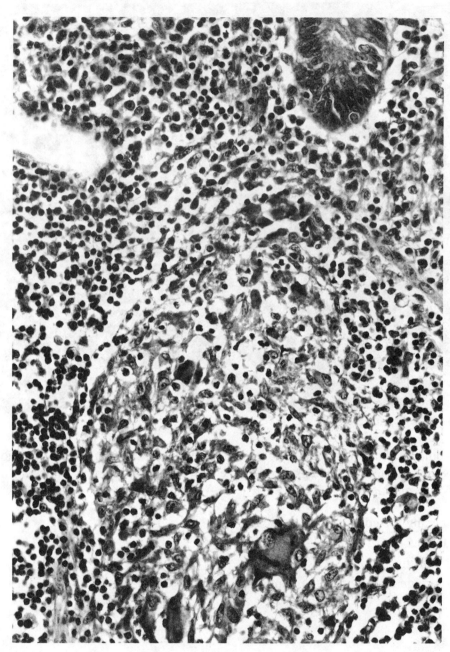

(A) segmental lesions
(B) "creeping fat"
(C) a thickened wall
(D) pseudopolyps
(E) long, snake-like lesions

99. All of the following statements about RNA are true EXCEPT

(A) RNA occurs only in a single-stranded form
(B) RNA can act to catalyze certain reactions, much like an enzyme
(C) RNA can act as primary genetic material
(D) a molecule of RNA differs from DNA in the number of hydroxyl groups present on the sugar moieties
(E) none of the above

100. Cimetidine is the prototype of a histamine receptor antagonist that

(A) causes sedation
(B) is useful for motion sickness
(C) enhances hepatic drug-metabolizing enzymes
(D) reduces gastric acid secrction
(E) is useful in the treatment of certain allergies

101. All of the following statements about the peptide bond are true EXCEPT the

(A) peptide bond is planar
(B) peptide bond has restricted rotation
(C) α-carbon atoms are in a *trans* configuration
(D) peptide bond atoms do not participate in the secondary structure of proteins
(E) peptide bond has no charge associated with it

102. Ca^{2+} is required for various processes, such as neurotransmission and muscle contraction. However, an elevated level of Ca^{2+} can be cytotoxic to cells. All of the following mechanisms are used by cells to regulate intracellular Ca^{2+} concentration EXCEPT

(A) chelation of Ca^{2+} by ethylenediamine-tetraacetic acid (EDTA)
(B) adenosine triphosphate (ATP)-independent Na^+–Ca^{2+} exchange
(C) ATP-dependent Ca^{2+} pumping
(D) sequestration of Ca^{2+} by binding proteins
(E) sequestration of Ca^{2+} in the endoplasmic reticulum

103. In a family with a disease that has an autosomal dominant inheritance pattern, seven children have been born, four of whom have the disease and three of whom do not. One parent is affected and one is not. What is the probability of the next child born having the disease?

(A) 100%
(B) 50%
(C) 25%
(D) Zero
(E) Cannot be determined

104. The inhibition observed in the Lineweaver-Burk plot below is subject to which one of the following actions? It

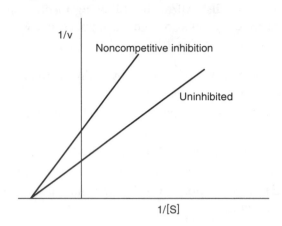

(A) can be reversed by a high concentration of substrate

(B) results from compounds that are transition-state analogs

(C) occurs through the interaction of the inhibitor at the active site

(D) results in a decrease in the V_{max} of the reaction

(E) is characterized by an increase in the K_m for the substrate

105. All of the following statements about the protein kinase C signal transduction pathway are true EXCEPT

(A) after activation, protein kinase C is degraded to protein kinase M

(B) protein kinase C phosphorylates tyrosines on proteins

(C) protein kinase C requires Ca^{2+} for full activation

(D) protein kinase C requires lipids for full activation

(E) protein kinase C is translocated to the plasma membrane

106. A patient is on a ventilator. The patient's anatomic dead space is 150 ml, and the ventilator's dead space is 250 ml. The ventilatory rate is set at 20 per minute. What should the output (tidal volume) of the ventilator be adjusted to so that alveolar minute ventilation is 4 L/min?

(A) 150 ml

(B) 250 ml

(C) 400 ml

(D) 600 ml

(E) 1000 ml

107. Each statement below concerning fenestrated capillaries is true EXCEPT

(A) fenestrations are 60 nm to 100 nm in diameter

(B) they are present in the choroid plexus

(C) they may be partially surrounded by pericytes

(D) they are present in endocrine glands

(E) they have a slit diaphragm that forms a filtration barrier in the renal glomerulus

108. Pathogenic bacteria enter the body by various routes, and entry mechanisms are critical for understanding the pathogenesis and transmissibility of each agent. Which one of the following is a correct association between a pathogen and its common entry mechanism?

(A) *Neisseria meningitidis*—sexually transmitted entry

(B) *Corynebacterium diphtheriae*—food-borne entry

(C) *Rickettsia rickettsii*—entry by contamination of wound with soil

(D) *Clostridium tetani*—inhalation entry

(E) *Borrelia burgdorferi*—arthropod vector-borne entry

Questions 109–111

A 70-year-old man is brought to the hospital, and a neurologist is called for a consultation. The residents caring for the patient tell the physician that he has spastic paralysis on one side of his body but has no sensory deficit. UMN

109. On examination, the physician finds that the patient can move neither the right side of his face nor his left extremities. He has right-sided ptosis of the eyelid, and the right eye deviates laterally. The right eye also does not respond to light or exhibit accommodation. What is the most likely site of the patient's lesion?

(A) The midbrain — *corticospinal tracts → PCA*
(B) The pons — *supplied by Basilar Artery*
(C) The medulla
(D) None of the above

110. The lesion is most likely a cerebral vascular accident, resulting in occlusion of which one of the following arteries?

(A) Basilar artery
(B) Middle cerebral artery
(C) Posterior cerebral artery *PCA*
(D) Superior cerebellar artery

111. After examining the patient, the physician is most likely to propose which of the following syndromes in his evaluation?

(A) Millard-Gubler syndrome
(B) Weber's syndrome
(C) Brown-Séquard syndrome
(D) None of the above

112. Each statement below concerning cyclic adenosine monophosphate (cAMP) is true EXCEPT

(A) cAMP levels may be increased or decreased by hormone stimulation
(B) it is the second messenger for the action of parathyroid hormone (PTH) on the kidney
(C) it activates protein kinase C by binding to the regulatory subunit and causing dissociation of the catalytic subunit
(D) it is degraded intracellularly by a family of phosphodiesterase isoenzymes
(E) it is synthesized from adenosine triphosphate (ATP)

113. Which one of the following statements about glycogen storage disease type Ia is true?

(A) Liver glycogen is decreased
(B) Renal glycogen is increased
(C) Phosphorylase A is deficient
(D) Debranching enzyme is deficient
(E) None of the above

114. Tay-Sachs disease is marked by all of the following EXCEPT

(A) it is more common among Ashkenazi Jews than other population groups
(B) it is a lysosomal storage disease
(C) it is characterized by an absence of hexosaminidase A
(D) it is characterized by an accumulation of GM_2 gangliosides
(E) it is characterized by an absence of β-galactosidase

Questions 115–118

A patient complains of chest pains that are appreciable during exercise. Electrocardiogram, stress scintigraphy, and coronary arteriography indicate that the patient has typical (exertional) angina pectoris due to atherosclerotic coronary artery disease.

115. Which of the following statements regarding coronary artery blood flow in a healthy person is true?

(A) During systole, coronary artery blood flow is uniform from subendocardial to epicardial regions of the left ventricle
(B) Myocardial oxygen extraction, not coronary artery blood flow, increases during exercise
(C) Coronary artery blood flow is directly proportional to arterial blood pressure over a range of pressures within 20–30 mm Hg of normal
(D) Coronary artery blood flow is proportional to myocardial oxygen demands
(E) Coronary artery blood flow is maximal during systole

116. Initial pharmacotherapy for the patient includes sublingual nitroglycerin at the onset of chest pain. Relaxation of vascular smooth muscle by nitroglycerin is caused by its metabolism to an intermediate that is similar in structure and activity to

(A) nitrogen dioxide
(B) nitrous oxide
(C) nitric oxide
(D) cyanide
(E) thiocyanate

117. Continued use of nitroglycerin causes profound hypotension and an increase in heart rate, which is likely to be

(A) a reflex originating from aortic and carotid baroreceptors
(B) a direct effect of nitroglycerin in cardiac pacemaker cells
(C) an atriopeptin-mediated effect originating from myocytes of the left atrium
(D) a direct effect of nitroglycerin on the central nervous system (CNS)
(E) an indirect effect of nitroglycerin via its positive chronotropic effect on the heart

118. A useful adjuvant to minimize the nitroglycerin-associated tachycardia is

(A) enalapril
(B) hexamethonium
(C) atropine
(D) isoproterenol
(E) propranolol

119. An action potential recorded from a microelectrode inserted in a nerve fiber is illustrated in the figure below. All of the following statements describe changes that take place during the action potential recorded by this electrode EXCEPT

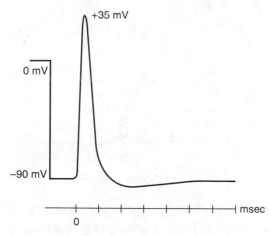

(A) at the peak of the action potential, the number of open Na^+ channels greatly exceeds the number of open K^+ channels

(B) depolarization is caused by an abrupt increase in Na^+ conductance

(C) repolarization is primarily caused by an increase in K^+ conductance

(D) repolarization is caused by activation of the Ca^{2+}–Na^+ channel

(E) chloride channel permeability does not change during an action potential

120. A 35-year-old black man presents with loss of pain sensation in the skin of the forearm and lateral border of the leg. He also exhibits loss of tendon reflexes and complains of severe stabbing pains of the legs. This condition could have been prevented by

(A) avoiding the bullet that damaged his cingulate gyrus 13 years ago

(B) early penicillin treatment

(C) avoiding exposure to varicella zoster virus infection

(D) early administration of acyclovir

121. All of the following statements concerning the major determinants of glomerular filtration rate (GFR), which are renal blood flow (RBF) and glomerular hydrostatic pressures, are correct EXCEPT

(A) constriction of the afferent arteriole decreases both RBF and GFR

(B) an increase in RBF, even with little change in glomerular pressure, increases GFR

(C) in a normal kidney, an increase in systemic arterial pressure from 100 to 150 mm Hg increases GFR severalfold

(D) constriction of the efferent arteriole decreases RBF and slightly increases GFR

122. At which of these blood neutrophil levels do patients acquire a significant risk of opportunistic infection?

(A) $<1000/\mu l$
(B) $1000–1500/\mu l$
(C) $1500–2000/\mu l$
(D) $2000–2500/\mu l$
(E) $2500–3000/\mu l$

123. A physician interested in evaluating the effects of a drug on the synthesis of RNA has decided to measure RNA production in cells after treatment with the drug by radiolabeling RNA. Which of the following radiolabeled bases should this physician use?

(A) Tritiated thymine [(^{3}H)-thymine]
(B) Tritiated guanine [(^{3}H)-guanine]
(C) Tritiated adenine [(^{3}H)-adenine]
(D) Tritiated uracil [(^{3}H)-uracil]
(E) Tritiated cytosine [(^{3}H)-cytosine]

124. Of the following statements, which best describes integral membrane proteins? They

(A) have at least one α-helical domain of approximately 20 amino acids, which spans the bilayer
(B) are stabilized within the bilayer by a combination of hydrogen bonds and electrostatic interactions
(C) may be solubilized by altering the pH or the ionic strength
(D) are frequently glycoproteins in which the carbohydrate is on the cytosolic side of the membrane
(E) may display transverse movement in the lipid bilayer

---

125. For a patient trying to prevent intercourse-related urinary tract infections, which of the following antibiotics would be the most effective and economical when administered only once after coitus?

(A) Cephalexin
(B) Nitrofurantoin
(C) Trimethoprim–sulfamethoxazole
(D) Ciprofloxacin
(E) Penicillin G

126. For which one of the following organisms do opsonic antibodies play a major role in acquired immunity to infection?

(A) *Neisseria meningitidis,* group A
(B) *Vibrio cholerae*
(C) *Clostridium botulinum*
(D) *Shigella flexneri*

127. If end diastolic volume is approximately 115 ml in the volume–pressure curve of the left ventricle below, which of the following statements is most accurate?

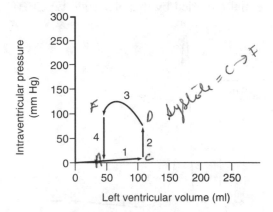

(A) The ejection fraction is approximately 30%
(B) Aortic diastolic pressure is approximately 80 mm Hg
(C) Isovolumic contraction is during the section labeled *3*
(D) Stroke volume is approximately 45 ml
(E) Left ventricular end diastolic pressure is approximately 100 mm Hg

Questions 128–130

A 45-year-old man has complained of increasing abdominal girth, fever, and malaise for the previous 4 months; he has denied having a cough. Physical examination shows a markedly enlarged spleen but no lymphadenopathy. Laboratory evaluation shows a normal chest x-ray, hemoglobin concentration of 15 g/dl, a white blood cell count of 45,000 cells/μl with no blasts seen on the blood smear, and a platelet count of 750,000/μl.

128. The most likely diagnosis is

(A) malignant lymphoma
(B) acute leukemia
(C) chronic myeloproliferative disorder
(D) pulmonary tuberculosis
(E) myelodysplastic disorder

129. The laboratory evaluation for the differential diagnosis of this problem might include all of the following tests EXCEPT

(A) measurement of leukocyte alkaline phosphatase levels
(B) chromosomal evaluation
(C) bone marrow aspiration and biopsy
(D) flow cytometric analysis
(E) determination of red blood cell mass

130. Evaluation of chromosomes shows a normal male karyotype. The leukocyte alkaline phosphatase level is low–normal, and the bone marrow is hypercellular and shows a myeloid-to-erythroid cell ratio of 10:1. Of the following conclusions, which is most appropriate?

(A) Chronic myelogenous leukemia (CML) is excluded, and the patient has a leukemoid reaction
(B) CML is excluded; therefore, the patient has an excellent prognosis and will be monitored every 6 months
(C) CML is excluded, and further workup will differentiate polycythemia vera from agnogenic myeloid metaplasia
(D) CML has not been excluded and further workup should include a molecular examination for a BCR-*abl* proto-oncogene translocation

131. Chronic Chagas disease should be considered in patients from Central and South America presenting with which set of the following signs and symptoms?

(A) Periodic fever and chills
(B) Cardiac conduction defects
(C) Multiple mucocutaneous lesions
(D) Persistent diarrhea
(E) Pneumonia

Questions 132–139

A 27-year-old woman presents with muscle weakness, including eyelid ptosis, slurred speech, and difficulty swallowing. The history shows that the woman is being treated for a gram-negative infection with gentamicin. The following tests have been ordered: thyroid function studies, serum creatine kinase, an electromyogram, and a muscle biopsy.

132. The attending physician chides the resident on the case for not ordering edrophonium, which produces a dramatic improvement in the patient's muscle strength when administered intravenously. All of the other tests that were ordered returned with normal values. The resident's working diagnosis is

(A) Duchenne muscular dystrophy (DMD)
(B) monoadenylate deaminase deficiency
(C) myasthenia gravis
(D) hyperthyroidism
(E) toxic drug myopathy

133. This patient's condition most likely results from

(A) inadequate acetylcholinesterase in the synaptic cleft
(B) production of defective acetylcholine (ACh) receptors
(C) impaired synthesis or storage of ACh in presynaptic vesicles
(D) impaired release of ACh from presynaptic terminals
(E) blockade and increased turnover of ACh receptors

134. Aminoglycoside antibotics create and exacerbate muscle weakness through

(A) inhibition of presynaptic release of ACh
(B) antagonism of the action of acetylcholinesterase
(C) potentiation of the action of acetylcholinesterase
(D) increasing the turnover of ACh receptors
(E) slowing conduction of the action potential

135. The adverse effects of the aminoglycoside antibiotics can be overcome with the intravenous administration of

(A) magnesium gluconate
(B) calcium gluconate
(C) magnesium phosphate
(D) copper sulfate
(E) creatine phosphate

136. Besides the aminoglycosides, another drug known to create muscle weakness is

(A) imipenem
(B) actinomycin
(C) tetracycline
(D) penicillamine
(E) amoxicillin

137. A more thorough physical examination of this patient would likely reveal an abnormal

(A) adrenal gland
(B) heart
(C) kidney
(D) thymus
(E) thyroid gland

138. Primary treatment of this patient's condition should begin with

(A) isoflurophate (diisopropyl phosphorofluoridate; DFP)
(B) mefenamic acid
(C) pralidoxime
(D) pyridostigmine
(E) triorthocresylphosphate

139. Long-term treatment should also include

(A) echothiophate
(B) edrophonium
(C) glucocorticoids
(D) succinylcholine
(E) vitamin and mineral supplements

140. A hospitalized patient is found to have a urinary tract infection owing to *Serratia*. A course of antimicrobial therapy with an aminoglycoside is planned. However, the patient has mild renal impairment. The best means to determine the appropriate drug dosage is

(A) body surface area
(B) serum creatinine
(C) scrum blood urea nitrogen
(D) creatinine clearance
(E) peak and trough drug levels

141. All of the following match important vasodilators with corresponding tissues EXCEPT

(A) adenosine–heart
(B) carbon dioxide–brain
(C) low oxygen–lung
(D) increased body temperature–skin

142. Surgical instruments are boiled for 10 minutes in a saline solution containing *Escherichia coli*, *Mycobacterium tuberculosis*, and *Bacillus cereus*. Which one of the following organisms is most likely to survive this procedure?

(A) *E. coli*
(B) *M. tuberculosis*
(C) *B. cereus*

143. A length–tension diagram for a single sarcomere is illustrated below. Tension that develops is maximal between points *B* and *C* because

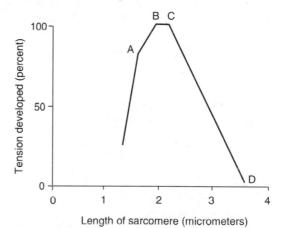

(A) there is maximal overlap between the actin filaments and the cross-bridges of the myosin filaments
(B) the actin filament has pulled all the way out to the end of the myosin filament
(C) the Z disks of the sarcomere touch the ends of the myosin filament
(D) the myosin filament is at its minimal length
(E) actin filaments are overlapping for maximal interaction with myosin

Questions 144–145

The left ventricular and aortic pressure tracings below were recorded during cardiac catheterization of a 62-year-old patient who complains of chest pain and dizziness on exertion.

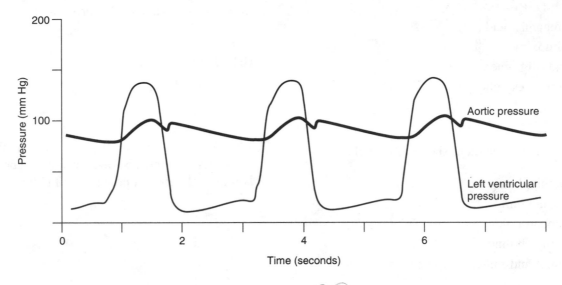

144. The left ventricular and aortic pressure tracings indicate that this patient has

(A) pulmonary stenosis
(B) aortic stenosis
(C) mitral stenosis
(D) aortic insufficiency
(E) mitral insufficiency

145. The most likely change in heart sound in this patient would be

(A) systolic murmur
(B) diastolic murmur
(C) presystolic murmur
(D) mid-diastolic murmur

146. All of the following enzymes may be targets of a new drug that inhibits cellular synthesis of DNA EXCEPT

(A) DNA-dependent DNA polymerase
(B) topoisomerase II
(C) RNA-dependent DNA polymerase
(D) RNA polymerase
(E) DNA ligase

Questions 147–148

A research laboratory has been asked to study a new viral disease, which the researchers think is caused by an arenavirus. They need a relatively simple test to determine if this is indeed true. They have found a cell line (by pure chance) in which they can culture the virus.

147. The most specific trait of Arenaviridae that would help classify the new virus as a member of this family would be

(A) an insect vector

(B) the presence of multiple genomic segments

(C) the presence of particles resembling ribosomes within the virions

(D) the presence of a viral envelope

148. What is the best method to test for the presence of this trait?

(A) Gel electrophoresis; the gel is stained with ethidium bromide

(B) Grinding up a number of the presumed insect vectors, and preparing a filtrate of this material to infect cultured human cells

(C) Addition of virion fractions to radiolabeled amino acids, adenosine triphosphate (ATP), and human messenger RNA (mRNA); then detergent gel electrophoresis

(D) Light microscopy with a simple hematoxylin–eosin stain, with visualization of viral inclusion bodies

149. The tumor pictured in the photomicrograph below arises from which one of the following types of cells?

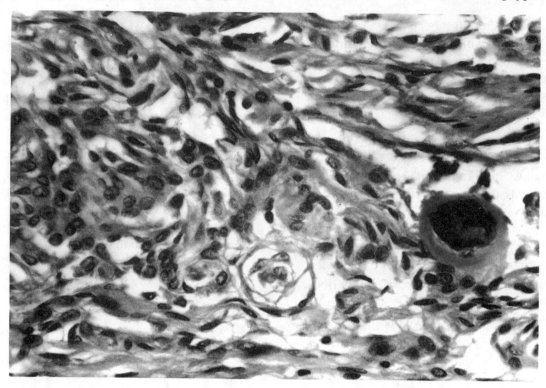

(A) Cerebellar astrocytes

(B) Leptomeningeal cells

(C) Neurons

(D) Oligodendrocytes

(E) Schwann cells

150. A 55-year-old man with a history of chronic alcoholism presents with complaints of fatigue and weakness. His laboratory values are as follows:

Hgb/Hct	11.5/34.0	
MCV	110	
MCH	38.0	
RDW	19.5	
WBC	$6.0 \times 10^9/L$	

Differential:

Polys	80%	$4.8 \times 10^9/L$
Bands	7%	$0.42 \times 10^9/L$
Lymphs	10%	$0.6 \times 10^9/L$
Monos	5%	$0.3 \times 10^9/L$

Microscopic examination of a peripheral blood smear shows poikilocytosis and hypersegmented neutrophils. This patient most likely has

(A) anemia caused by vitamin B deficiency

(B) anemia caused by iron deficiency

(C) anemia following hemorrhage

(D) sickle cell anemia

(E) thalassemia minor

151. The hepatic neoplasm pictured below has which one of the following characteristics?

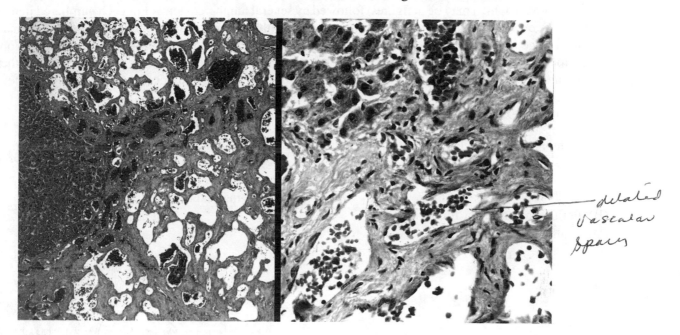

(A) An association with exposure to the carcin-
    ogen Thorotrast
(B) Highly aggressive behavior
(C) An association with thrombocytopenia
(D) Foci of hemorrhage and necrosis

DIRECTIONS: Each set of matching questions in this section consists of a list of four to twenty-six lettered options (some of which may be in figures) followed by several numbered items. For each numbered item, select the ONE lettered option that is most closely associated with it. To avoid spending too much time on matching sets with large numbers of options, it is generally advisable to begin each set by reading the list of options. Then, for each item in the set, try to generate the correct answer and locate it in the option list, rather than evaluating each option individually. Each lettered option may be selected once, more than once, or not at all.

Questions 152–155

For each organ listed below, select the region to which pain in that organ is usually referred.

(A) Inguinal and pubic regions
(B) Perineum, posterior thigh, and leg
(C) Both
(D) Neither

152. Ovary

153. Uterus

154. Epididymis

155. Testis

Questions 156–160

For each morphologic or functional description of a component of the placenta listed below, choose the appropriate lettered structure in the accompanying diagram.

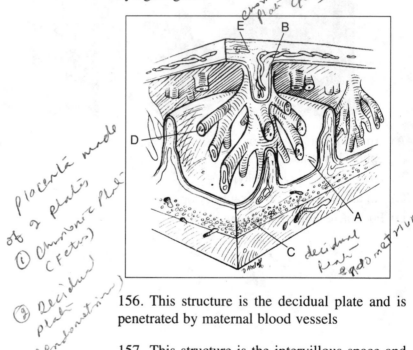

156. This structure is the decidual plate and is penetrated by maternal blood vessels

157. This structure is the intervillous space and contains maternal red blood cells

158. This structure is the chorionic plate and receives the insertion of the umbilical cord

159. This tissue column interconnects the chorionic and decidual plates

160. These structures are chorionic villi and are coated by syncytiotrophoblast

Questions 161–165

For each artery or vein comprising the vasculature of the cranium, select the lettered foramen or fissure through which it courses, shown on the illustration of the inferior aspect of the cranium below.

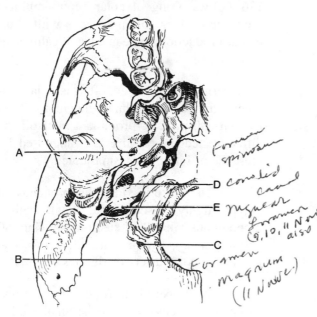

161. Middle meningeal artery

162. Internal carotid artery

163. Internal jugular vein

164. Emissary vein

165. Vertebral artery

Questions 166–170

Match each description involving thyroid hormones with the substance associated with it.

(A) Levothyroxine
(B) Thyrotropin-releasing hormone (TRH)
(C) Thyrotropin
(D) Iodine
(E) Thyroxine

166. In many forms of hyperthyroidism (Graves' disease), circulating levels of this hormone are considerably depressed

167. Propylthiouracil inhibits circulating levels of this hormone

168. This hormone is an L-pyroglutamyl-L-histidyl-L-proline amide whose intracellular signal transducing system involves phospholipase C activation

169. Deiodination of this hormone accounts for most of its ultimate biologic effects

170. A synthetic hormone useful for various forms of hypothyroidism

Questions 171–174

For each clinical state listed below, select the description of sleep architecture most closely associated with it.

(A) Sleep spindles

(B) Sleep-onset rapid eye movement (REM)

(C) Delta waves

(D) Increased percentage of REM

(E) Normal REM sleep

171. Narcolepsy

172. Major depression

173. Nocturnal penile tumescence

174. Night terrors

Questions 175–180

Lung tumors can at times have similar gross and microscopic appearances, but generally distinguishing features can be observed for the major tumor classes. Match the following descriptive features of malignant tumors with the correct neoplasm.

(A) Squamous cell carcinoma

(B) Adenocarcinoma (usual type)

(C) Adenocarcinoma (bronchioalveolar type)

(D) Large cell carcinoma

(E) Small cell (oat cell) carcinoma

(F) Carcinoid

175. Centrally located in major airways near the hilum; may have endobronchial element; large cells with optically dense cytoplasm form large irregular sheets with central necrosis; intercellular bridges; prominent host response; hypercalcemia

176. Grows along alveolar septa; multicentric foci; cuboidal or columnar cells with abundant mucus production; huge nuclei with almost no cytoplasm

177. Peripherally located; often associated with a preexisting scar; glandular, mucinous, or papillary growth pattern; prominent nucleoli; poorly differentiated tumors may be diagnosed by the presence of intracytoplasmic mucin

178. Often protrudes into the bronchus like a polyp; highly vascularized; small cells with monotonous round or fusiform nuclei; 80- to 250-nm neurosecretory granules; often grows in a pattern of clusters or ribbons of cells

179. Usually peripherally located; grows in sheets with areas of necrosis; small cells with scant cytoplasm and nucleoli that are not prominent; dense 80- to 140-nm neurosecretory granules; poor survival because of extensive metastases

180. Characterized by large nuclei, prominent nucleoli, and abundant cytoplasm; cells may be multinucleated; tumor displays well-defined cell borders; lack of mucin or keratinization often used for diagnosis

Questions 181–185

Match each description below with the appropriate organelle in the accompanying diagram.

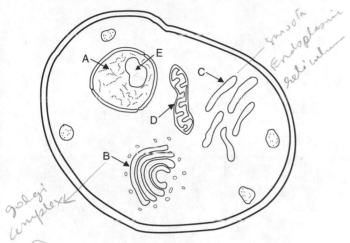

181. It is involved in sorting and targeting proteins

182. It is the site of cleavage of introns from messenger RNA (mRNA)

183. It is the site of ribosomal RNA (rRNA) synthesis

184. It is the site of steroid synthesis

185. It is the main site of adenosine triphosphate (ATP) synthesis

Questions 186–190

For each function, select the associated transport protein.

(A) Albumin
(B) Transferrin
(C) Haptoglobin
(D) Transcobalamin
(E) None of the above

186. Iron transport

187. Vitamin B$_{12}$ transport

188. Clot formation

189. Plasma osmotic pressure maintenance

190. Hemoglobin transport

Questions 191–195

Match each clinical feature with the vitamin deficiency disorder or disorders most likely to be associated with it.

(A) Pellagra
(B) Beriberi
(C) Both
(D) Neither

191. Dermatitis

192. Peripheral neuropathy

193. Cardiovascular lesions

194. Dementia

195. Diarrhea

Questions 196–200

Match each of the following conditions with the appropriate syndrome.

(A) Sheehan's syndrome
(B) Cushing's syndrome
(C) Conn's syndrome
(D) Waterhouse-Friderichsen syndrome
(E) Bartter's syndrome

196. Hyperreninemia

197. Anterior pituitary infarction

198. An overproduction of cortisol

199. Widespread petechiae, purpura, or hemorrhages

200. Aldosterone-producing adenoma

ANSWER KEY

1-D	31-A	61-D	91-C	121-C
2-A	32-C	62-B	92-C	122-A
3-C	33-C	63-D	93-B	123-D
4-A	34-C	64-A	94-B	124-A
5-B	35-B	65-B	95-C	125-E
6-C	36-D	66-A	96-D	126-A
7-A	37-D	67-D	97-C	127-B
8-D	38-A	68-C	98-D	128-C
9-E	39-E	69-A	99-A	129-D
10-B	40-C	70-D	100-D	130-D
11-E	41-A	71-C	101-D	131-B
12-B	42-A	72-C	102-A	132-C
13-B	43-D	73-D	103-B	133-E
14-D	44-C	74-E	104-D	134-A
15-C	45-B	75-C	105-B	135-B
16-C	46-A	76-D	106-D	136-D
17-A	47-C	77-D	107-E	137-D
18-C	48-E	78-B	108-E	138-D
19-C	49-E	79-A	109-A	139-C
20-C	50-A	80-A	110-C	140-E
21-A	51-D	81-B	111-B	141-C
22-C	52-C	82-D	112-C	142-C
23-D	53-C	83-C	113-B	143-A
24-D	54-B	84-A	114-E	144-B
25-A	55-A	85-D	115-D	145-A
26-D	56-C	86-D	116-C	146-C
27-C	57-D	87-B	117-A	147-C
28-A	58-C	88-C	118-E	148-C
29-B	59-E	89-D	119-D	149-B
30-B	60-A	90-D	120-B	150-A

151-C	161-A	171-B	181-B	191-A
152-A	162-D	172-D	182-A	192-B
153-C	163-E	173-E	183-E	193-B
154-B	164-C	174-C	184-C	194-A
155-A	165-B	175-A	185-D	195-A
156-C	166-C	176-C	186-B	196-E
157-A	167-E	177-B	187-D	197-A
158-E	168-B	178-F	188-E	198-B
159-B	169-E	179-E	189-A	199-D
160-D	170-A	180-D	190-C	200-C

ANSWERS AND EXPLANATIONS

1. The answer is D. (*Pathology of Barrett's esophagus*)
Barrett's esophagus is a result of protracted reflux, due to lower esophageal sphincter incompetence, with the attendant increased exposure to acid, pepsin, and bile acids. Esophageal inflammation and ulceration occur, followed by re-epithelialization and ingrowth of immature pluripotent stem cells. Rather than squamous epithelium, the new epithelium is columnar-lined with gastric or duodenal-type cells, which better tolerate prolonged acid exposure. Inflammation would only be absent in the case of postmortem ulceration and autolysis; such changes may be accompanied by "leopard spotting"—brown–black esophageal spots that form from acid digestion of hemoglobin.

2. The answer is A. (*Plasma protein binding of drugs*)
Many drugs bind to plasma proteins, which limits glomerular filtration in the kidneys because the drugs are not freely diffusible. Drug–protein interactions that are common generally occur between a wide variety of drugs and albumin or α_1-acid glycoprotein, but not immunoglobulins. Covalent interactions are rare, but when they occur it is generally with reactive antineoplastic drugs. Renal tubular secretion is generally not limited by plasma protein binding of drugs because secretion reduces free plasma drug concentration, which is quickly followed by dissociation of the drug from plasma proteins.

3–5. The answers are: 3-C, 4-A, 5-B. (*Suicide management*)
Safely removing any pill fragments from the stomach by nasogastric tube is the first step in the management of the patient described in the question because amitriptyline is an anticholinergic that retards gastrointestinal absorption, increasing the likelihood that pill fragments remain. The patient may ultimately need psychiatric hospitalization; because she is unresponsive, there is no urgency in pursuing this. An electroencephalogram would not add any useful information at this time, and seizures, if they occurred, would most likely be related to the toxicity of amitriptyline and a lowering of the seizure threshold.

Tricyclic antidepressants have antiarrhythmic effects, like quinidine. The changes on electrocardiogram, especially with increased or toxic serum levels, include a prolonged P-R interval, prolonged QRS duration, and a prolonged QT interval. In therapeutic dose ranges, tricyclics may suppress premature ventricular contraction.

Eliciting a detailed account of the events leading to the suicide attempt is important, particularly whether it was impulsive or well-planned or whether it occurred in the context of a depression. Once it has been established that suicide was in fact attempted, transfer to a psychiatric unit is imperative. In a crisis situation, the physician should avoid getting angry or overinvolved with the patient and should avoid prematurely interpreting underlying psychodynamic issues.

6. The answer is C. (*Membrane structure and function*)
The plasma membrane consists of amphipathic lipids (predominantly phospholipids and cholesterol) and amphipathic proteins. The hydrophilic portions of these molecules face the external and internal aqueous environments. The hydrophobic portions are in the internal portion of the bilayer. Phospholipids prevent free diffusion of ions and water-soluble molecules, thereby imparting selective permeability properties to the lipid bilayer. Proteins may be restricted to the external portion of the bilayer or span it entirely. In addition, the membrane is fluid, allowing lateral diffusion of even large proteins.

7. The answer is A. (*Polymerase chain reaction*)
A polymerase chain reaction is used to amplify sequences of DNA from a single copy to over 1 million copies. The template DNA is initially denatured in the presence of excess primers, which are short (15–25 base pairs) oligonucleotides homologous to sequences on the template DNA. Because the DNA is denatured and

renatured many times by multiple heating and cooling cycles, limiting amounts of primers prevents large-scale amplification of the parent strand. The temperatures at which a polymerase chain reaction is carried out are generally in the range from 55° C–95° C. Heat-resistant DNA polymerase, such as the Taq polymerase, is resistant to heat denaturation.

8. The answer is D. *(RNA structure and function)*
The primary transcript for messenger RNA (mRNA) is formed in the nucleus, where the elongation proceeds from the 5′ to the 3′ end. Most eukaryotic mRNAs are distinctive in that the 5′ ends are capped by the addition of a methylated guanylic acid residue and the 3′ ends have a polyadenylate tail of 100 to 200 adenosine nucleotides. Most precursor forms of mRNA contain intervening sequences, which are removed by a process known as splicing. The binding of steroid hormones with their receptors to specific genes results in the increased synthesis of the mRNA encoded in those genes.

9. The answer is E. *(Gastric carcinoma)*
Paget's disease of the breast is a carcinoma involving the nipple and subjacent ductal elements, and Paget's disease of the bone is an idiopathic disease characterized by a high turnover of bone. Neither form is associated with gastric carcinoma. The Leser-Trélat sign is the development of seborrheic keratosis, acanthosis nigricans, or amyloidosis in a patient with gastrointestinal malignancy. Erythema nodosum is seen occasionally with gastrointestinal malignancy.

10. The answer is B. *(Epidermis)*
The order of epidermal maturation is stratum basale, stratum spinosum, stratum granulosum, stratum lucidum, and stratum corneum. The stratum basale is the germinal layer of the epidermis. Cells migrate and differentiate from this layer at a rate equal to desquamation of keratin from the outermost layer. The stratum spinosum is superficial to the stratum basale, and its cells are in the process of growth and early keratin synthesis. The stratum granulosum is characterized by the presence of intracellular granules, which contribute to the keratinization process. The stratum lucidum is a homogeneous layer between the stratum granulosum and the stratum corneum that is present only in thick skin. The stratum corneum is the most superficial layer of the epidermis and is mainly composed of keratin.

11. The answer is E. *(Recurrent urinary tract infections)*
Longitudinal studies have shown that bacteriuria in women susceptible to urinary tract infections is preceded by colonization of the vaginal introitus with the responsible organism from the rectal flora.

12. The answer is B. *(Gaucher's disease)*
Type II Gaucher's disease is the infantile acute cerebral pattern and is characterized by a virtual absence of glucocerebrosidase, with an accumulation of large quantities of β-glucosylceramide in macrophages and hepatocytes. Type I, or the classic form, is the adult type, in which storage of glucocerebrosides is limited to the mononuclear phagocytes. Patients with type I have reduced but detectable levels of glucocerebrosidase. Both type I and type II are autosomal recessive. Niemann-Pick disease is characterized by the accumulation of sphingomyelin, which is due to a deficiency in sphingomyelinase. Tay-Sachs disease, in which ganglioside accumulates, results from lack of *N*-acetylhexosaminidase. The defective enzyme in Krabbe's disease is galactosylceramidase.

13–15. The answers are: 13-B, 14-D, 15-C. *(Histology of the epididymis)*
The micrograph shows the epididymis. The epididymis is a highly convoluted tubular organ that conveys sperm and fluid from the testis to the ductus (vas) deferens. Its luminal epithelium is a pseudostratified

columnar epithelium with numerous tall apical stereocilia. These cells secrete poorly characterized substances, which are added to the seminal fluid, and remove other poorly characterized substances from the fluids that drain from the seminiferous tubules in the testis. Apoptosis, or programmed cell death, occurs in the testis as in the thymus.

16. The answer is C. *(Pathophysiology of anthrax)*
A malignant pustule is a clinical manifestation of cutaneous anthrax. It occurs at the site of inoculation and is characterized by a black eschar at its base surrounded by an inflamed ring. Enteritis necroticans, caused by *Clostridium perfringens*, and pseudomembranous colitis, caused by *Clostridium difficile*, are diseases of the gastrointestinal tract that may be characterized by ulcerative lesions in the intestinal mucosa. Lockjaw is a lay name for tetanus; it refers to the muscle and neural spasms caused by the neurotoxin tetanospasmin. Woolsorter's disease is pulmonary anthrax—a diffuse, lethal, progressive pneumonia caused by the inhalation of spores of *Bacillus anthracis*.

17. The answer is A. *(Histopathology of seminomas)*
Seminomas comprise 30%–40% of testicular tumors and are divided into classic and spermatocytic forms. Classic seminomas, as in this case, are composed of nests of tumor cells with abundant clear cytoplasm with vesicular nuclei and angulated nucleoli *(left)*. The nests are separated by fibrous strands that contain inflammatory cells, usually lymphocytes and plasma cells (*right*). Mumps orchitis involves large numbers of giant cells; it is an inflammatory reaction, not a neoplasm, and the condition is seen in young individuals. Teratomas contain aberrant ectopic tissues (e.g., brain, cartilage, and epithelial-lined cysts), whereas choriocarcinomas have syncytiotrophoblastic giant cells and cytotrophoblasts in close apposition.

18. The answer is C. *(Platelet homeostasis)*
Examination of the peripheral blood smear is essential when evaluating a patient for thrombocytopenia. Unreported abnormalities of the red cells may offer a clue to the etiology, or occasionally one may find a discrepancy between the number of platelets seen on the smear and that found by the automated count. This occurs in pseudothrombocytopenia, where clumping of platelets in a specific anticoagulant [usually ethylenediaminetetraacetic acid (EDTA)] results in marked underestimation of the count.

19–21. The answers are: 19-C, 20-C, 21-A. *(Immunologic disorders)*
Patients with diseases that cause a deficiency in T cells are extremely prone to viral, fungal, and protozoal infections. The patient described in the question presents with severe oral thrush, which is caused by a *Candida* species, and hypocalcemia. These findings are consistent with a diagnosis of DiGeorge syndrome, which results from a defect in the embryonic development of the third and fourth pharyngeal pouches. Both the thymus and parathyroid glands fail to develop, resulting in hypocalcemia. The white blood cell count can be within normal limits, but virtually all of the circulating leukocytes are B cells and plasma cells.

DiGeorge syndrome does not appear to be genetically determined but occurs as the result of intrauterine damage. Without intervention, these patients have a poor prognosis. Transplantation of a fetal thymus not older than 14 weeks (to avoid graft-versus-host disease) has resulted in prolonged survival. Administration of antifungal agents will not really address the problem, which is a lack of T cells, and fungal infections may be a side effect of corticosteroid use.

Although both chronic mucocutaneous candidiasis and severe combined immunodeficiency result in increased susceptibility to viral, fungal, and protozoal infections, neither disease presents with hypocalcemia. Patients with chronic granulomatous disease, caused by phagocytic cell dysfunction, suffer from infections with organisms that are normally of low virulence, such as *Staphylococcus epidermidis*, and also do not present with hypocalcemia.

22. The answer is C. *(Fluid balance)*
Infusion of a hypertonic solution instantaneously adds both volume and milliosmoles to the extracellular (and total body) water space. Because the solution is hypertonic, the osmolality increases in the extracellular space (but remains unchanged in the intracellular space), thereby causing osmosis of water out of the cells and into the extracellular compartment. At equilibrium, the extracellular volume is expanded, and its osmolality is increased. In contrast, the intracellular volume is decreased, resulting in an increase in intracellular osmolality.

23. The answer is D. *(Vaccines as applied to AIDS)*
Of the vaccination procedures listed, the one most likely to be tested by the Food and Drug Administration (FDA) is the procedure that uses a human monoclonal antibody that reacts with the intact CD4 (T4) receptor. Antibodies that react with CD4 should "look like" the portion of human immunodeficiency virus (HIV) that reacts with the CD4 receptor. Therefore, the vaccinated person should make an antibody to the human monoclonal antibody, which may be protective against HIV.

24. The answer is D. *(Immunologic response)*
The necessary characteristics that a given compound must possess to be immunogenic include a high molecular weight, chemical complexity, and recognition as being foreign. Compounds with a molecular weight greater than 6000 daltons are generally immunogenic, and those with a molecular weight less than 1000 daltons generally are not. Compounds between 1000 and 6000 daltons may or may not be immunogenic, depending upon the degree of foreignness or chemical complexity.

Haptens are small, low–molecular-weight compounds that become immunogenic when coupled to a high–molecular-weight carrier, such as a conjugate of dinitrophenol and albumin. Whereas a large homopolymer of lysine would not be immunogenic because of a lack of chemical complexity, a smaller polymer containing different molecules would be immunogenic.

25. The answer is A. *(Glycolysis)*
The primary step in the regulation of glycolysis is the conversion of fructose 6-phosphate to fructose 1,6-bisphosphate. The enzyme, 1-phosphofructokinase, is an allosteric enzyme that is inhibited by adenosine triphosphate (ATP) and citrate and is activated by fructose 2,6-bisphosphate. The concentration of fructose 2,6-bisphosphate is, in turn, regulated by glucagon. Acetyl coenzyme A (acetyl CoA) is not an allosteric effector of any of the glycolytic enzymes. Glucose 6-phosphate is an inhibitor of hexokinase.

26. The answer is D. *(Renal sodium transport)*
Almost 75% of Na^+ is reabsorbed in the proximal tubular epithelium by several processes, including active transport at the basolateral surface, leading to electrogenic potential with additional passive movement; and cotransport of Na^+ at the luminal surface with glucose or amino acids. An additional 22% is reabsorbed by the active transport process in the ascending thick limb of the loop of Henle. The remaining small percentage of Na^+ that reaches the distal tubular epithelium is reabsorbed by a highly regulated aldosterone-sensitive process involving exchange with K^+

27. The answer is C. *(Papillary carcinoma)*
The photomicrograph is of a papillary carcinoma of the thyroid gland, and there is a demonstrated association of this type of tumor with previous radiation therapy to the neck. The tumor cells grow on thin fibrovascular stalks and form papillae. The cells have large overlapping nuclei; the nucleoplasm has marked chromatin, which gives the nuclei a clear, "Orphan Annie eye" appearance. Papillary carcinomas also may have stromal calcification, forming concentric laminated concretions called psammoma bodies (*top center*). These carcinomas metastasize through the lymphatics to cervical lymph nodes, but, in general, they are indolent tumors.

28. The answer is A. *(Pathogenic mechanisms of respiratory pathogens)*
Pertussis and diphtheria are caused by *Bordetella pertussis* and *Corynebacterium diphtheriae*, respectively. Both of these pathogens are extracellular bacteria, which adhere to the respiratory tract and produce exotoxins that contribute to pathogenesis. Because *B. pertussis* is gram-negative, it produces endotoxin, unlike gram-positive *C. diphtheriae.* The neurologic problems associated with the DTP (diphtheria-tetanus-pertussis) vaccine are caused by the pertussis component of the vaccine (which uses whole killed cells).

29–31. The answers are: 29-B, 30-B, 31-A. *(Geriatric depression; pharmacologic migraine headache)*
The patient described in the question is suffering from depression. Monoamine oxidase inhibitor antidepressants (e.g., phenelzine) have a safe cardiac profile (except for some initial orthostatic hypotension) and essentially no anticholinergic activity, making them a good choice in the elderly who are vulnerable to constipation, memory impairment, and urinary retention. Lithium carbonate has a prophylactic role for recurrent depression but not acute depression. The neuroleptic chlorpromazine is not indicated because the patient is exhibiting no psychotic symptoms. Benzodiazepines (e.g., clonazepam) help with anxiety, which this patient does not have, and can sedate, increase cognitive deficits, and increase depression in the elderly.

A negative neurologic examination and lack of sleep disruption from the headache make a brain tumor a less likely diagnosis. In elderly individuals, temporal arteritis is an important cause of head pain and blindness that necessitates prompt diagnosis and treatment with a corticosteroid. Computed tomography scan, cerebrospinal fluid examination, or an electroencephalogram would not aid in diagnosing temporal arteritis.

Lithium is useful for cluster headaches. Ergotamine may interrupt migraine headaches, while methysergide, propranolol, and amitriptyline have prophylactic value.

32. The answer is C. *(T-cell maturation)*   OF Thymus
Maturation of a stem cell to a resting T cell occurs earliest in the cortex. The medullary region is where the variable (V), diverse (D), and joining (J) regions of the T-cell receptor undergo rearrangement. The maturation process is independent of antigen and dependent on contact with thymic epithelial cells for purposes of proliferation and differentiation.

33. The answer is C. *(Zellweger syndrome)*
In Zellweger syndrome, the amount of cytosolic catalase is elevated, phytanic acid accumulates in central nervous system (CNS) tissues, the plasma ratio of C26:0/C22:0 fatty acids is elevated, and there is a deficiency of platelet activating factor (PAF). Zellweger syndrome results from the absence of or a grossly reduced number of peroxisomes. Peroxisomes are cellular microbodies where oxidation of a very long chain of fatty acids (C26–C40) is initiated, phytanic acid is oxidized, and plasmalogens (such as PAF) are synthesized.

34. The answer is C. *(Gonorrheal and chlamydial coinfections)*
Of all cases presenting clinically as gonorrhea, 45% have coexisting chlamydial infections. Therefore, the correct treatment for gonorrhea is the administration of both penicillin for *Neisseria gonorrhoeae* and tetracycline for *Chlamydia trachomatis.* Amoxicillin is an oral penicillin; probenecid increases its blood level by blocking its excretion.

35. The answer is B. *(Mycology)*
Cryptococcus neoformans is responsible for meningitis in this case. The india ink microscopic staining technique demonstrated the presence of yeast cells producing a capsule (the capsule appears as a clear halo), and the only encapsulated yeast among the options is *C. neoformans.* This organism is an important fungal cause of meningitis, and it often infects AIDS patients.

36. The answer is D. *(Pharmacologic action of aspirin and acetaminophen)*
Aspirin and acctaminophen are both effective antipyretic and analgesic drugs. However, acetaminophen is devoid of anti-inflammatory actions, whereas aspirin is the prototype of a group of nonsteroidal anti-inflammatory agents. Aspirin, but not acetaminophen, is associated with a risk of Reye's syndrome in pediatric patients treated for various viral diseases. Both aspirin and acetaminophen inhibit lipoxygenase activity.

37. The answer is D. *(Angiotensin-converting enzyme inhibitors)*
Captopril is the prototype of a group of angiotensin-converting enzyme (ACE) inhibitors. These agents lower blood pressure in poorly understood ways, but a critical role for inhibition of ACE (with loss of production of angiotensin II) seems apparent. ACE inhibitors do not affect renin per se, nor do they have any activity toward angiotensin II receptors.

38. The answer is A. *(Insulin-dependent diabetes mellitus type I therapy)*
Sulfonylureas and other oral hypoglycemics are contraindicated in insulin-dependent diabetes mellitus (IDDM). Insulin therapy to maintain blood glucose levels within a physiologic range is a symptomatic approach to the treatment of IDDM. Blood glucose levels are routinely monitored, and insulin is adjusted to maintain the blood glucose levels. A frequent side effect is hypoglycemia, which is best treated by ingestion of carbohydrates. Some patients who still maintain a normal response to glucagon benefit by injection of glucagon for this crisis as well. Although recombinant forms of insulin have reduced insulin insensitivity caused by an immune response, this problem still persists. Apparently the source of the hormone (animal versus human) is not the only determinant of antigenicity.

39. The answer is E. *(Allosteric enzymes)*
Allosteric enzymes have sites distinct from the active site where regulatory ligands bind and alter either the V_{max} or the K_m for the substrate. The substrate saturation curves do not obey Michaelis-Menten kinetics and frequently show sigmoidicity, which is indicative of positive cooperativity between active sites. Enzymes that obey Michaelis-Menten kinetics require an 81-fold increase in substrate concentration to achieve an increase from 10% to 90% of the V_{max}. Allosteric enzymes that display positive cooperativity require a smaller increase in substrate concentration to achieve the same increase in V_{max}. The allosteric sites may be located either on the same subunit as the catalytic site or on a separate regulatory subunit. Enzymes with these regulatory properties frequently catalyze reactions that are either rate-limiting or occupy a pivotal point in a metabolic pathway.

40. The answer is C. *(Knee)*
The medial collateral ligament prevents abduction of the leg at the knee. It extends from the medial femoral epicondyle to the shaft of the tibia. The oblique popliteal ligament resists lateral rotation during the final degrees of extension. The posterior cruciate ligament prevents posterior displacement of the tibia. The anterior cruciate ligament helps lock the knee joint on full extension.

41. The answer is A. *(Female reproductive system)*
Blood flows to the fallopian tubes through branches of the uterine vessels carried in the surrounding mesentery, which is called the mesosalpinx. The ovarian veins drain blood from the ovaries. The right ovarian vein drains into the inferior vena cava; the left ovarian vein drains into the left renal vein. Lymph from the cervix eventually drains into the internal and external iliac and obturator nodes. Visceral afferent nerves from the uterus follow two pathways: Fibers from the cervix follow the splanchnic nerves (nervi erigentes); however, the body of the uterus and uterine tubes send fibers in parallel to the sympathetic nerves.

42. The answer is A. *(Histopathology of papillomavirus)*
This cervical tissue shows the squamous epithelial changes seen with human papillomavirus (HPV) infection, an epidemic affecting primarily young women. The viral infection causes crenation of nuclei and hyperconvolution, which is accompanied by perinuclear clearing of the cytoplasm. This change has been called condylomatous or koilocytic change and is caused by HPV infection. Some subtypes of HPV predispose the cervical squamous epithelium to dysplasia, and, therefore, these patients are sometimes treated with ablative surgery.

43. The answer is D. *(Chemotherapy and biology of bacteria)*
Tetracycline inhibits protein synthesis in bacteria after it is selectively transported inside the cell by an active transport system. Tetracycline is selectively toxic not only because its transport system is peculiar to prokaryotes but also because it binds to 30S subunits of bacterial ribosomes. In bacteria (as well as in eukaryotic mitochondria), it prevents the binding of charged transfer RNA (tRNA) to the A site on the ribosomal complex, thereby inhibiting peptide bond synthesis. Thus, it is bacteriostatic, not bactericidal. Resistance can develop secondarily to altered influx or efflux of the drug in prokaryotes. It remains in the gastrointestinal tract and causes its most serious side effects there, either by direct irritation or secondary to modifications in gut flora. This can lead to life-threatening colitis. Tetracycline is hardly ever used in children because it accumulates in developing teeth and bones, causing stains and bone deformities.

44. The answer is C. *(Gluconeogenesis)*
Gluconeogenesis utilizes the enzymes in glycolysis that catalyze reversible reactions. The enzymes that catalyze irreversible steps in glycolysis are hexokinase, 1-phosphofructokinase, and pyruvate kinase. To circumvent the three irreversible reactions, the de novo synthesis of glucose requires four enzymes that are unique to gluconeogenesis: pyruvate carboxylase, phosphoenolpyruvate carboxykinase, fructose 2,6-bisphosphatase, and glucose 6-phosphatase.

45–47. The answers are: 45-B, 46-A, 47-C. *(Properties of anesthetic gases)*
Minimum alveolar concentration (MAC) is that concentration of anesthetic at 1 atm that produces immobility in 50% of patients exposed to a noxious stimulus.

If an anesthetic has a high blood:gas partition coefficient, it is very soluble in blood and is eliminated from the bloodstream into the alveolar air relatively slowly. This tends to prolong recovery time.

Relative potency of anesthetics is directly proportional to their lipid solubility. Among the commonly used agents, nitrous oxide has a very low oil:gas partition coefficient. In contrast, nitrous oxide has a rapid onset of action because of a low blood:gas partition coefficient. Nitrous oxide is neither explosive nor highly metabolized.

48. The answer is E. *(Dopamine receptor antagonism; tardive dyskinesia)*
Metoclopramide is a potent dopamine receptor antagonist that can cause tardive dyskinesia in nonpsychiatric patients. Tardive dyskinesia frequently involves the orobuccal area. Dystonia is a sustained muscle spasm that occurs as an early complication of treatment with an antidopaminergic drug. Wilson's and Huntington's diseases cause chorea, but there is no history to suggest these diseases.

49–54. The answers are: 49-E, 50-A, 51-D, 52-C, 53-C, 54-B. *(Pathophysiology and treatment of gout)*
Of the tests listed in the question, synovial fluid analysis, erythrocyte sedimentation rate, C-reactive protein, and differential white blood cell count may be useful in discriminating inflammatory versus noninflammatory musculoskeletal disorders. Synovial fluid analysis reveals clear liquid containing long, needle-shaped, negatively birefringent intracellular crystals (sodium urate). The presence of these crystals and their ingestion by macrophages are typical findings with gout.

hgprt

Neurologic workup reveals slight dysarthria and incoordination. These symptoms are sequelae of an inherited X-linked partial deficiency of hypoxanthine–guanine phosphoribosyltransferase. This enzyme converts hypoxanthine to inosinic acid. Its deficiency increases purine synthesis, which contributes to the hyperuricemia of gout. Lesch-Nyhan victims are identifiable at birth and are mentally retarded. Osteoarthritis and calcium hydroxyapatite deposition disease afflict the elderly.

Colchicine is the anti-inflammatory drug of choice for gout. Allopurinol inhibits xanthine oxidase, the enzyme that converts hypoxanthine to xanthine, and xanthine to uric acid. Thus, allopurinol decreases urate production and is efficacious for the treatment of gout.

55. The answer is A. *(Embryology of the cardiovascular system)*
Both branches of the fourth aortic arch remain intact during fetal development. In adults, the left fourth aortic arch forms the aortic arch, and the right fourth aortic arch forms the proximal segment of the right subclavian artery. During development, the first and second aortic arches all but disappear. In adults, they form the maxillary, hyoid, and stapedial arteries. The third aortic arch forms the common carotid artery. The fifth aortic arch disappears. The sixth aortic arch forms the proximal segment of the right pulmonary artery and the ductus arteriosus.

MHS

56. The answer is C. *(Etiology of autoimmune disease)*
Forbidden clones provide a supply of cells that can recognize self-antigens and will serve as cells to stimulate both humoral and cell-mediated immune responses, leading to autoimmunity. B-cell deficiency—primarily a lack of circulating B cells—is a major cause of hypogammaglobulinemia. Type I hypersensitivity (anaphylactic hypersensitivity) is mediated by humoral antibodies, which result from a normal immune response to exogenous antigens. The deletion of forbidden clones leads to tolerance to autoantigens—the opposite of autoimmunity.

57. The answer is D. *(Empiric antibacterial therapy in an immunocompromised host)*
The most likely diagnosis of this patient's condition is septic shock secondary to bacteremia. Chemotherapy for cancer is a common cause of neutropenia with subsequent fever and infection. The risk is high when the white blood cell count is less than 500/μl. In addition, cold, clammy skin is indicative of peripheral vascular shutdown. Lactic acid buildup will lead to metabolic acidosis and compensatory rapid breathing. Patients with neutropenic fever must be treated with double broad-spectrum antibacterial agents for gram-negative rods, including *Pseudomonas*. The combination of piperacillin, a broad-spectrum beta-lactam, and gentamicin, an aminoglycoside that has broad gram-negative activity, is a good choice. In addition, penicillin–aminoglycoside combinations may be synergistic because of the different mechanisms of action of these agents: Penicillins are cell wall synthesis inhibitors, and aminoglycosides inhibit protein synthesis. Single-agent therapy with gentamicin or amikacin would not be as effective for resistant organisms. Both chloramphenicol and gentamicin are protein synthesis inhibitors and would not be expected to work synergistically.

58–60. The answers are: 58-C, 59-E, 60-A. *(Medical ethics)*
If the physician's sole concern is not to harm the patient with unnecessary worry, the guiding principle is nonmaleficence. If her sole concern is to be able to benefit the patient with urography (which is impossible if the patient refuses because of concerns about the risks), the guiding principle is beneficence. Both are possible. Justice is irrelevant, and gratitude (e.g., for the patient's patronage) is, at most, marginally relevant.

If the physician decides to do what others of her profession do in like circumstances, she is acting without appeal to the independent ethical principles of beneficence and nonmaleficence. Depending on what the professional practice standard dictates, the disclosure decision might prove to be respectful of autonomy or strongly paternalistic, but the decision would still be guided by professional practice. Weak paternalism is entirely irrelevant because the patient is competent.

If the physician is guided by respect for the patient's preferences, she is acting with respect for her patient's autonomy. If the patient would want disclosure, it is possible that such disclosure could fail to benefit him or could even harm him, so neither beneficence nor maleficence is guiding the physician's thinking. Clearly, the basis for her thinking is independent of the usual practice of her profession.

61. The answer is D. *(Ultraviolet damage to DNA)*
Ultraviolet (UV) light causes cross-linking of thymidine base pairs in DNA and cross-links thymidine to cytosine (forming pyrimidine–pyrimidine dimers). In bacteria such as *Escherichia coli,* these lesions are repaired by a system of proteins called the SOS system, which includes the RecA protein, which is involved in the recombination of normal DNA and the repair of damaged DNA, and thus it would not be advantageous to decrease its activity. Also, it would be foolish to overlap the genes concerned, because one pyrimidine base pair could potentially impair all the genes involved. Removal of introns would also be disadvantageous, because introns are thought to act as buffers of inactive DNA so that a mutation can occur without disrupting the gene. Genes produced with low thymidine content, however, may be less susceptible to damage by UV radiation because fewer pyrimidine base pairs would be involved.

62. The answer is B. *(Identification of neuroblastoma)*
Neuroblastomas arise from neural crest cells of the adrenal medulla. The tumors are usually large and soft, with a red–gray cut surface. They may be calcified, with areas of hemorrhage and necrosis. The tumor cells have hyperchromatic nuclei and indistinct eosinophilic cytoplasm. The nuclei are arranged in a spoke-like pattern around a characteristic central mass of neuritic cell processes, called Homer-Wright pseudorosettes, as seen in the illustration. Like pheochromocytomas, neuroblastomas produce catecholamines, but, unlike pheochromocytomas, they do not cause systemic hypertension.

63–64. The answers are: 63-D, 64-A. *(Turner syndrome)*
The patient presented in the question is a classic example of a child with Turner syndrome (i.e., short stature, webbed neck, cubitus valgus), which is best diagnosed through chromosome analysis. The genotype of this patient is most likely to be 45,X. None of the other tests listed in the question would contribute to the diagnosis of Turner syndrome.

Short stature is not a characteristic feature of Klinefelter syndrome. Klinefelter syndrome is best defined as male hypogonadism that occurs when there are two or more X chromosomes and one or more Y chromosomes; however, the genotype 46,XXY is the most common. Short stature is a major finding in the other conditions listed in the question.

65. The answer is B. *(Amino acid catabolism)*
The amount of alanine released from skeletal muscle is greater than the amount that can be accounted for in muscle protein. The catabolism of many amino acids in muscle involves the transamination of α-amino groups from amino acids to pyruvate, producing alanine. Thus, the carbon skeleton of much of the alanine released from muscle is derived from glucose via the glycolytic pathway.

66. The answer is A. *(Malaria)*
Of the major diseases with geographic relevance, malaria is one of the few that can be rapidly life-threatening. The other diseases listed (i.e., chronic Chagas disease, amebic dysentery, mucocutaneous leishmaniasis, and giardiasis) are either chronically debilitating or subpatent in nature. Amebic dysentery and giardiasis are not life-threatening conditions, and it is not necessary to determine the causative species for treatment of either. No effective treatment exists for chronic Chagas disease, so rapid diagnosis is not essential. Although determination of the species of *Leishmania* is useful in distinguishing cutaneous and mucocutaneous leishmaniasis in terms of treatment, both are long-term infections and are not life-threatening.

67–68. The answers are: 67-D, 68-C. *(Volume of distribution; half-life of elimination)*
The volume of distribution (V_d) is approximately 10 L. V_d is defined as $V_d =$ dose/Cp, where Cp is the plasma concentration at zero time. In this case, the Cp can be estimated easily because the log plasma concentration versus time plot is linear; it is approximately 100 µg/ml. Thus,

$$V_d = \frac{(20 \text{ mg/kg}) (50 \text{ kg})}{0.1 \text{ mg/ml}}$$
$$= \quad 10,000 \text{ ml}$$
$$= \quad 10 \text{ L}$$

The half-life of elimination of this drug is approximately 4 hours. The half-life of elimination can be determined graphically from the slope of the linear plot. First, note the time when a given concentration (e.g., 50 µg/ml) was detected (5 hours). Next, determine the time when half of the original value (25 µg/ml) was detected (9 hours). Then, calculate the half-life of elimination: $9 - 5 = 4$ hours.

69. The answer is A. *(Protein post-translational modifications)*
After proteins are synthesized (translated), many are glycosylated in the lumen of the endoplasmic reticulum and the Golgi complex. Oligosaccharides are attached to proteins by *N*-glycosylation of asparagine side chains or by *O*-glycosylation of serine and threonine side chains. The transfer of oligosaccharides is mediated by an activated lipid carrier, dolichol phosphate.

70. The answer is D. *(Properties of tricyclic antidepressants)*
Tricyclic antidepressants, such as imipramine, inhibit neuronal uptake of norepinephrine, serotonin, and other central nervous system (CNS) amines. Potentiation of local concentrations of these amines may underlie the ability of these agents to reverse symptoms of depression after chronic administration over several weeks. The parent and metabolite compounds of many of these drugs can directly or indirectly affect cardiac function (including α-adrenergic receptor blockade) and, thus, may cause orthostatic hypotension and cardiac dysrhythmias. Indeed, suicide with these agents is quite common, and the cause of death is related to cardiac toxicity. The drugs do not appear to affect dopamine receptors significantly in the concentrations used clinically. Some agents are more selective for serotonin uptake (e.g., fluoxetine, which is not a tricyclic antidepressant) than for norepinephrine uptake (e.g., desipramine, which is a tricyclic antidepressant).

71–72. The answers are: 71-C, 72-C. *(Medical genetics and cystic fibrosis)*
The frequency of the cystic fibrosis gene is 1/40, the square root of the incidence. Remembering the Hardy-Weinberg law, the gene frequency is equal to the square root of the incidence (q^2). If the incidence $= q^2 = 1/1600$, then the square root of the incidence, the gene frequency (q), $= 1/40$.
   The proportion of normal siblings of individuals with cystic fibrosis who would be expected to be carriers is 2/3. Due to the recessive pattern of inheritance of cystic fibrosis, each offspring has a 1 in 4 chance of inheriting the disease. This leaves a chance that 2 of the 3 individuals will be heterozygotes, or carriers, for the cystic fibrosis gene. A simple punnet square will reveal that of the possible genotypes one can have in the offspring (of those individuals carrying a recessive disorder), 1 in 4 will have the double dose, or be homozygous for the recessive gene. Two individuals will have a single dose of the recessive gene and be carriers, and one will be normal. Because cystic fibrosis carriers are not clinically affected, there would be 3 normal individuals possible in the offspring. Two of those three will be carriers, hence the 2/3 proportion.

73. The answer is D. *(Transplant immunology; immunosuppressive agents)*
Rejection that occurs a few minutes to a few hours after transplantation is termed hyperacute rejection. It is the result of preformed circulating antibodies to the graft that were made as a result of previous transplantations, blood transfusions, or pregnancies. It usually transpires minutes after the donor kidney is anastomosed, although it can proceed over a period of a few days. The antibodies activate the complement sytem,

with ensuing swelling, interstitial hemorrhage, and thrombotic occlusion followed by outright infarction of the kidney. The only therapy is removal of the transplanted tissue.

74. The answer is E. *(Defense mechanisms)*
Borderline patients tend to view things as extremes of black and white, with little ability to perceive the gray zones. In splitting, negative feelings are split off and attributed to one person (or thing), while positive feelings are attributed to another, without the realization that people have both good and bad features. Borderline patients may also project, deny, displace, and manipulate, but the example in the question is of splitting.

75. The answer is C. *(Regulation of arterial blood pressure)*
A rise in arterial blood pressure within the carotid sinus or an increase in pressure secondary to mechanical massage leads to activation of baroreceptors, which subsequently causes inhibition of the central vasoconstrictor center with activation of the central vagal center. The net short-term effect is a decrease in blood pressure, heart rate, and cardiac output. Ultimately, baroreceptors adapt to the stimulus and are unimportant in the long-term regulation of blood pressure. Clamping of the carotid arteries (in a vagotomized animal) will decrease baroreceptor firing and remove inhibitory pathways from the central nervous system (CNS), leading to increases in pressure and heart rate.

76. The answer is D. *(Properties of lidocaine)*
Local anesthetics block Na^+ channels and decrease conductance of Na^+, thereby inhibiting depolarization and normal conduction of action potentials. Small, myelinated nerve fibers are most sensitive, and differential sensitivity explains preferential blockade for pain sensation as opposed to other sensory modalities. Lidocaine is highly lipid-soluble and may cause convulsions in the central nervous system (CNS) if sufficient amounts are delivered to the brain. By affecting Na^+ channels in cardiovascular tissue, dysrhythmia and decreased contractility may ensue. The ester anesthetics, such as procaine, are *rapidly metabolized by* substrates for plasma cholinesterases, whereas lidocaine is more slowly metabolized in the liver. Local anesthetics, such as lidocaine, are often used in spinal anesthesia to produce more widespread blockage of neurotransmission.

77. The answer is D. *(Cytoskeleton)*
In muscle cells, actin and myosin filaments cause muscle contraction by a process known as the "sliding filament hypothesis." In nonmuscle cells, actin is involved with endocytosis, exocytosis, cell locomotion, and cytokinesis. The mitotic spindle is composed of the microtubule protein tubulin, not actin.

78. The answer is B. *(Mitochondria)*
Mitochondria are organelles unlike the others within the cell. They contain a ring of DNA that codes for some of the proteins they require; the other proteins are encoded by the nuclear genes. Mitochondria also use a slightly altered genetic code than that used by other mammalian genes: Mitochondria have only 22 transfer RNA (tRNA) molecules (as opposed to 32 in the nucleus), so that 1 tRNA molecule must cover more codons. Some codons are also different (e.g., UGA, a termination codon normally, is a tryptophan codon to mitochondrial tRNA). Finally genes encoding the proteins overlap one another, perhaps reflecting the fact that the genome is so small (16,500 base pairs).

79. The answer is A. *(Presentation of cutaneous erythema)*
The etiologic agent of erysipeloid is *Erysipelothrix rhusiopathiae,* a bacterium widely distributed in the environment. Human erysipeloid is clinically described as a slowly spreading cutaneous erythema. Cutaneous edema is characteristic, and the disease is very painful. Cutaneous diphtheria is characterized by a necrotic lesion sometimes associated with insect bites; the bite apparently provides the break in the skin through which

toxigenic *Corynebacterium diphtheriae* enters the tissue. Cutaneous nocardiosis is characterized by draining sinus tracts discharging purulent exudate-containing granules. Pontiac fever and listeriosis do not have cutaneous manifestations.

80. The answer is A. *(Gene duplications)*
There are as many as 100 to 1000 gene families that contain similar sequences. β-Tubulins and β-like globins are perfect examples of duplicated gene families. There are at least two nonfunctional regions in the human β-like globin gene cluster that have sequences similar to functional β-like genes. Analysis of their DNA sequences shows that they retain their intron/exon structure, but some sequence drift has resulted in sequences that block transcription or terminate protein translation. Some gene duplications, such as those for ribosomal and transfer RNA (rRNA and tRNA), along with genes coding for histones, are necessary to meet the demands of the cell for messenger RNA (mRNA) transcripts. Although there is no accepted model for duplication, it is thought to involve unequal crossover during meiosis.

81. The answer is B. *(Hardy-Weinberg law)*
The frequency of carriers of Tay-Sachs disease can be calculated from the Hardy-Weinberg law, in which the carrier frequency is equal to 2 pq: q is calculated by taking the square root of the incidence, which gives the frequency of the gene, 1 in 60, and p is equal to $1 - q$, or $60/60 - 1/60$, which gives 59/60. As can be seen here, in most cases of rare diseases, p becomes equal to 1, and the carrier frequency then becomes 2q, or $2 \times 1/60$, which gives a carrier frequency of 1/30.

82. The answer is D. *(Lipid biochemistry and arachidonic acid metabolism)*
Leukotrienes are compounds formed as the result of the action of lipoxygenase on arachidonic acid. Platelet activating factor (PAF) is an ether phospholipid. Eosinophil chemotactic factor (ECF) is a set of peptides that produces a chemotactic gradient to attract eosinophils. Thromboxanes (TXA_2), like prostaglandins, are synthesized through the action of cyclooxygenase, a reaction that is inhibited by acetylsalicylic acid.

83–84. The answers are: 83-C, 84-A. *(Hypoxic injury)*
The first of the motor functions to become deficient during hypoxic injury to the brain would be the ability to move the arms. This is due to the fact that the most distal ends of the anterior and middle cerebral arteries anastomose in the cerebral hemispheres over the location on the motor gyrus controlling the arms. The neurons in this anastomosing zone are very sensitive to hypoxic injury.

The hippocampus is well known for its sensitivity to hypoxic injury. Because this area of the brain is involved in immediate memory recall, the patient will not remember where he is nor will he remember his physicians. He will have trouble in the future functioning independently because of this lesion. Recognition of family members would involve distant, or remote, memory, which is not involved with hippocampal functioning. The patient would also be able to perform cognitive functions, such as addition and reading.

85. The answer is D. *(Surgical prophylactic antibacterial therapy; drug resistance)*
Ampicillin is an extended-spectrum penicillin, which has greater action against some gram-negative organisms compared with penicillin G and early generation semisynthetic penicillins such as methicillin. However, ampicillin is susceptible to beta-lactamases and may not be effective when administered prophylactically against beta-lactamase–containing *Staphylococcus aureus*. Cefazolin is a prototypical first-generation cephalosporin, which has good activity against staphylococcal infections and is relatively impervious to beta-lactamases. Methicillin is prototypical of beta-lactamase–resistant penicillins. Vancomycin is a cell wall synthesis inhibitor with exclusive gram-positive antibacterial activity, owing to its large molecular size, which does not allow it to enter gram-negative bacteria through porins. Vancomycin is not susceptible to beta-lactamases. Imipenem is a beta-lactam antibiotic, which is resistant to beta-lactamases.

86. The answer is D. *(Hypersensitivity reactions)*
ABO or Rh incompatibility, the cause of erythroblastosis fetalis, is the result of blood group differences between the mother and the child. Normally, in cases of Rh-incompatible mating, human anti-D globulin (RhoGAM), an anti-Rh antibody, would be given to the mother shortly after the birth of her first Rh-positive child. This would clear the child's Rh-positive red cells from the mother's circulation before she can be immunized. In the case described in the question, the mother has blood type O negative with normal isohemagglutinin titers, so the preexisting ABO compatibility should clear her system of any "leaked" fetal blood cells. Administration of RhoGAM to an Rh-positive child will cause hemolytic anemia in that child.

87. The answer is B. *(Gas exchange)*
Anemia reduces the oxygen-carrying capacity of the blood but does not affect arterial oxygen tension. Thus, oxygen delivery is decreased and venous oxygen will have a lower partial pressure at rest and during exercise in the anemic subject. The anemic subject is patient *B* because his oxygen content is reduced for every level of Po_2.

88. The answer is C. *(Toxins; neurotransmission)*
The woman is suffering from botulism, which is caused by the neurotoxin botulin. The action of botulin involves inhibition of acetylcholine (ACh) release from peripheral nerve endings at the neuromuscular junction. Other bacterial toxins have actions described in (A), (B), (D), and (E) [i.e., diphtheria toxin, tetanus toxin, cholera toxin, and streptolysin O, respectively].

89. The answer is D. *(Gonococcal salpingitis)*
For all practical purposes, the patient is cured. However, women who suffered from gonorrhea are at risk for future complications, such as subsequent episodes of pelvic inflammatory disease, infertility, and ectopic pregnancy.

90. The answer is D. *(Hassall's corpuscles)*
Hassall's (thymic) corpuscles are found in the thymus. They are concentrically laminated structures of unknown function that appear during fetal development and increase in number with age. They are thought to be degenerated medullary epithelial cells and display varying degrees of keratinization or calcification.

91. The answer is C. *(Fructosuria; glycogen synthesis)*
Essential fructosuria results from a deficiency in fructokinase, which is found only in the liver and catalyzes the first step in the assimilation of fructose by the liver. Under normal conditions, almost all of the fructose is converted to fructose 1-phosphate and is metabolized in the liver. Hexokinase, which is present in all extrahepatic tissues, can convert fructose to fructose 6-phosphate; however, the K_m of hexokinase for fructose is sufficiently high that this reaction does not occur to any significant extent. When, as a consequence of a deficiency in fructokinase, the accumulation of fructose is high enough, it is converted to fructose 6-phosphate in extrahepatic tissues and metabolized by the glycolytic pathway. Glucokinase, which is found in the liver, is specific for glucose and cannot catalyze the phosphorylation of fructose. Aldolase B is specific for fructose 1-phosphate. Transketolase is a part of the nonoxidative phase of the pentose phosphate pathway.

92. The answer is C. *(Pathogenesis of renal osteodystrophy)*
Normally, approximately 90% of serum phosphate is not protein-bound and, thus, is filterable at the glomerulus. Of the filtered phosphate, approximately 75% is actively reabsorbed, mainly by cotransport with sodium in the proximal tubule. In chronic renal failure, hyperphosphatemia occurs as the glomerular filtration rate declines. Hyperphosphatemia produces a secondary hyperparathyroidism as excess phosphate ties up the free serum calcium, in essence leading to hypocalcemia. 1,25-Dihydroxyvitamin D_3 levels are reduced

directly by the inability of the damaged kidney to convert the 25-hydroxyvitamin D_3 produced by the liver from inactive vitamin D_3 to 1,25-dihydroxyvitamin D_3 and indirectly by the ability of high serum phosphate levels to directly inhibit renal 25-hydroxyvitamin D_3 hydroxylase activity.

93. The answer is B. *(Differential diagnosis of coagulation disorders)*
Factor XI deficiency is autosomally transmitted and can result in serious postoperative bleeding, although it may be mild enough to cause no spontaneous symptoms. Neither factor XII nor Fletcher factor deficiencies result in a bleeding disorder, and inherited factor VIII deficiency occurs only in males. Severe von Willebrand's disease could result in a positive family history and significant bleeding, but rarely is the factor VIII:C low enough to prolong the partial thromboplastin time (PTT), especially when the bleeding time is normal.

94. The answer is B. *(Enteric infections)*
Salmonella typhi is a highly invasive pathogen that is readily disseminated throughout the body. In typhoid fever, this organism invades through the intestinal mucosa and spreads through the body via the lymphatic system. In nontyphoid *Salmonella* infections, the bacteria invade the intestinal submucosa but usually do not spread into other regions of the body. *Campylobacter jejuni* and *Shigella dysenteriae* invade the intestinal mucosa but usually do not penetrate the submucosa or spread throughout the body. *Vibrio cholerae* is noninvasive.

95–96. The answers are: 95-C, 96-D. *(Etiology of fungal infections; antifungal therapy)*
The clinical signs and history are consistent with oropharyngeal candidiasis (thrush). This patient is most likely immunocompromised because of her adjuvant chemotherapy. In addition, antibacterial therapy for urinary tract infection predisposes her to develop a fungal infection because of depletion of floral bacteria. Opportunistic, endogenous *Candida* infections in the mouth are common under these conditions. Sporotrichosis is an endogenous systemic infection. Cryptococcosis is also a systemic infection. Dermatophytes usually appear on hair, nails, and skin.

Griseofulvin is effective for dermatophyte infections of nails and hair; it concentrates in the stratum corneum and outer epidermis and stops fungal growth in these tissues. Ketoconazole, fluconazole, and clotrimazole are ergosterol synthesis inhibitors, which are fungistatic or fungicidal (at high concentrations) for *Candida*. Nystatin, a polyene, binds to membrane ergosterol and affects membrane permeability and integrity. Nystatin, like the more commonly used polyene amphotericin B, is fungicidal. Nystatin is effective only in topical preparations for candidiasis, whereas amphotericin B is commonly used systemically. Clotrimazole is effective topically against candidiasis.

97. The answer is C. *(Histopathology of rheumatoid arthritis)*
The synovium pictured in the photomicrograph shows the classic features of a rheumatoid nodule in a patient with rheumatoid arthritis, a disease that affects primarily women. Rheumatoid arthritis initially affects the small joints of the hands and feet and then the larger joints of the knees and elbows. The synovium becomes infiltrated by lymphocytes and plasma cells with lymphoid follicle formation. In some cases, central fibrinoid necrosis occurs with an intense palisade of histiocytes and giant cells forming around the necrotic material, as in this case. Rheumatoid nodules occur in the skin and subcutis, particularly on extensor surfaces, but may also occur in unusual sites such as the lungs, heart, and spleen.

98. The answer is D. *(Macroscopic features of Crohn's disease)*
The photomicrograph shows chronic inflammation of the bowel, typical of Crohn's disease, or terminal ileitis. This transmural inflammation accounts for the thickened bowel wall. If the process extends into pericolic fat, thick, edematous "creeping fat" and fistulae would be seen. The presence of a small granuloma at the base of the colonic gland is helpful in confirming the diagnosis of Crohn's disease. Pseudopolyps occur in ulcerative colitis and are a means of differentiating ulcerative colitis from Crohn's disease.

99. The answer is A. *(Functions of nucleic acids)*
RNA differs from DNA by the number of hydroxyl groups present on the sugar moieties and in the kind of pyrimidine bases used; RNA has uracil substituted for thymidine. Because these differences are fairly minor, RNA can take on the same configurations as DNA; that is, it can be linear, circular, double-stranded, or single-stranded. Molecules of transfer RNA (tRNA) are a perfect example of RNA that has base-paired with itself to form double strands. RNA acts catalytically in certain messenger RNA (mRNA) splicing reactions and is the primary genetic material for a number of viruses.

100. The answer is D. *(Histamine receptor antagonists)*
Cimetidine and ranitidine are H_2-receptor blockers whose main clinical use is in the treatment of ulcers and other peptic disorders. They block the effects of histamine on gastric acid secretion. H_2 antagonists inhibit, not enhance, cytochrome P450 enzymes of the liver. H_1 antagonists (e.g., diphenhydramine, chlorpheniramine) are useful in treating allergies. They also have central effects that are useful in preventing motion sickness; however, they can also cause unwanted sedation.

101. The answer is D. *(Peptide bonds)*
The chemistry of the peptide bond imposes restrictions on higher orders of protein structure. The secondary structure of proteins is stabilized by hydrogen bonds that are formed between the amide hydrogen and carbonyl oxygen of the peptide bond. Because the atoms of the peptide bond lie in a plane, the only rotations that are permissible are around the $C\alpha$—C and the N—$C\alpha$ bonds. There is no formal charge associated with the peptide bond; the electrons of the carbonyl oxygen and the lone pair of electrons on the nitrogen atom are delocalized.

102. The answer is A. *(Calcium homeostasis)*
Ethylenediaminetetraacetic acid (EDTA) is a chelator of Ca^{2+} but is not normally found within cells and, thus, is not a mechanism by which cells regulate Ca^{2+} concentration. Two important transmembrane proteins in Ca^{2+} homeostasis are the Ca^{2+} adenosine triphosphate (ATPase) pump and the Na^+–Ca^{2+} transport chain. Ca^{2+} binds to a number of intracellular proteins, such as calsequestrin, and these proteins are found in high concentration in the endoplasmic reticulum.

103. The answer is B. *(Medical genetics)*
Every child has a 50% chance of inheriting a condition with an autosomal dominant mode of inheritance. This does not mean that in a family with eight children, four will necessarily be affected and four unaffected, although this is statistically the most likely possibility. It is also possible that all children will be affected or all will be unaffected, although these possibilities are unlikely.

104. The answer is D. *(Enzyme inhibition)*
The data in the Lineweaver-Burk plot are diagnostic of noncompetitive inhibition. The intercept on the 1/[S] axis indicates that the inhibitor has no effect on the K_m for the substrate. The increase in the 1/v intercept observed in the presence of the inhibitor indicates a decrease in the V_{max} of the reaction. Noncompetitive inhibitors interact at a site other than the active site. They usually bear no structural resemblance to either the substrate or the transition-state analogs, and their effects cannot be reversed by high concentrations of substrates. Competitive inhibitors, however, interact at the active site, are structurally related to transition-state analogs, and can be reversed by high concentrations of substrate.

105. The answer is B. *(Serine and threonine kinases)*
Protein kinase C is a member of a class of kinases that phosphorylates only serine and threonine, not tyrosines. Protein kinase C is activated by lipids and Ca^{2+}; when activation occurs, protein kinase C moves from the

cytoplasm to the plasma membrane via the process called translocation. It is degraded by a calcium-activated protease to form the lipid- and Ca^{2+}-independent protein kinase M.

106. The answer is D. *(Alveolar ventilation)*
Alveolar ventilation is the product of respiratory rate × (tidal volume − dead space). In this situation total dead space (400 ml) is the sum of the patient's anatomic dead space (150 ml) and the ventilator's dead space (250 ml). Thus, if the total output of the ventilator is adjusted to 600 ml, then 200 ml of the alveolar volume will be delivered 20 times per minute, and total minute alveolar ventilation will be 4 L/min.

107. The answer is E. *(Microcirculation)*
Fenestrated capillaries have circular pores (fenestrae), which are 60 nm to 100 nm in diameter and may be partially surrounded by pericytes. The fenestrae often are spanned by a slit diaphragm, which is filamentous and, thus, does not possess a unit membrane structure. Fenestrated capillaries are present in areas where there is a great deal of molecular exchange with blood (e.g., kidneys, small intestine, endocrine glands, choroid plexus). Although glomerular capillaries are fenestrated, they lack a slit diaphragm; a thick basement membrane forms the filtration barrier.

108. The answer is E. *(Pathogenesis of infectious microorganisms)*
Borrelia burgdorferi is spread by ticks and is the cause of Lyme disease. *Rickettsia rickettsii* also is usually spread by ticks. *Clostridium tetani* enters the body through wounds. *Neisseria meningitidis* and *Corynebacterium diphtheriae* both enter via the respiratory tract.

109–111. The answers are: 109-A, 110-C, 111-B. *(Neurologic lesions and syndromes)*
The deficits described in the question indicate destruction of cranial nerve (CN) III motor function and total autonomic function of the eye, combined with a spastic paralysis of the contralateral body, indicating upper motor neuron destruction (as opposed to flaccid paralysis, indicating lower motor neuron disease). CN III fibers leave the brain at the level of the midbrain to continue to the ipsilateral eye. CN III is responsible for moving the eye nasally and vertically in both directions; therefore, loss of CN III function results in lateral deviation of the eye. CN III also carries autonomic fibers that originate in the Edinger-Westphal nucleus and are responsible for constriction of the pupil to light and for accommodation. Riding with the oculomotor nerve are sympathetic fibers responsible for dilation of the pupil. The destruction of all of these functions together indicates a lesion of the midbrain where it intersects with the corticospinal tract.

The artery that supplies this intersection of midbrain and corticospinal tract is the posterior cerebral artery. The basilar artery supplies the pons. The middle cerebral artery supplies most of the cerebral hemisphere of either side.

Weber's syndrome is a lesion of the crus cerebri, through which the corticospinal tract passes, as well as a lesion of tissue through which the oculomotor nerve passes. Millard-Gubler syndrome is similar to Weber's syndrome, but the lesion is lower and involves the pons, causing CN VI and CN VII palsy as well as upper motor neuron paralysis of the contralateral body. Brown-Séquard syndrome is a lesion of the spinal cord, involving upper motor neuron damage and weakness of one leg, with contralateral pain and temperature sensitivity of the other.

112. The answer is C. *(Signal transduction; protein kinases)*
Protein kinase C is activated by Ca^{2+} and diacylglycerol, not by cyclic adenosine monophosphate (cAMP). Cyclic AMP is synthesized from adenosine triphosphate (ATP) in a reaction that is catalyzed by adenylate cyclase. The activity of adenylate cyclase may be either increased or decreased in response to hormone stimulation. Cyclic AMP is the second messenger for the effect of parathyroid hormone (PTH) on the kidney; cAMP also activates protein kinase A. The binding of cAMP to the regulatory subunit results in the

dissociation of the regulatory and catalytic subunits and a concomitant increase in protein kinase activity. The degradation of cAMP is mediated by a family of phosphodiesterases, which catalyze the hydrolysis to 5'-AMP.

113. The answer is B. *(Glycogen storage diseases)*

Glycogen storage disease type Ia, or von Gierke's disease, is caused by defective glucose-6-phosphatase activity and is characterized by hepatomegaly, renomegaly, and hypoglycemia. The liver shows intracytoplasmic accumulation of glycogen and a small amount of lipid along with some intranuclear glycogen. The kidney has intracytoplasmic accumulations of glycogen in the cortical tubular epithelial cells. The intestine also shows increased concentrations of glycogen.

114. The answer is E. *(Tay-Sachs disease)*

Tay-Sachs disease has a reported 1 in 30 carrier rate among Ashkenazi Jews, which is about 10 times higher than in other population groups. It is a lysosomal storage disease caused by mutations in the gene coding for hexosaminidase A, leading to a virtual absence of this enzyme. Deficiency of hexosaminidase A results in an accumulation of GM_2 gangliosides, which normally make up 1%–3% of total brain gangliosides but comprise over 90% in individuals with Tay-Sachs disease. Lack of the enzyme β-galactosidase is an autosomal recessive disorder; however, unlike Tay-Sachs disease, it results in lysosomal storage of GM_1 gangliosides.

115–118. The answers are: 115-D, 116-C, 117-A, 118-E. *(Pathophysiology and pharmacotherapy of ischemic heart disease)*

Coronary blood flow closely matches myocardial work (or oxygen consumption). Myocardial oxygen extraction is near maximal at rest and does not increase appreciably, even during exercise. Coronary blood flow is maximal during diastole, in which ventricular compression of the capillaries is minimal. In addition, there is significant heterogeneity across the ventricular wall during systole, such that subendocardial blood flow is reduced, and blood flow is shifted to the epicardial vessels. Autoregulation is normally observed in the myocardium, such that blood flow does not change over a large range of perfusion pressures.

Nitroglycerin is metabolized to nitrosothiols that are similar or identical to the endogenous endothelial-derived relaxing factor, or nitric oxide. This metabolic product of L-arginine is synthesized in the endothelium (and other cells) and diffuses to smooth muscle cells, where it activates guanylate cyclase and induces relaxation.

The most significant adverse effect of nitroglycerin is unwanted systemic hypotension. This results in a reflex tachycardia caused by decreased pressure that is sensed in peripheral baroreceptors.

A β-adrenergic receptor blocker (e.g., propranolol) is useful concomitant therapy with nitroglycerin, because it antagonizes the reflex tachycardia at the level of myocardial receptors.

119. The answer is D. *(Membrane physiology and excitation)*

The resting membrane potential is -90 mV, which is primarily due to diffusion potentials caused by K^+ (and Na^+) and the electrogenic Na^+–K^+ pump. Stimulation at time zero [e.g., as occurs with acetylcholine (ACh)] activates a Na^+ channel, thereby greatly increasing Na^+ conductance and leading to depolarization. At the peak of the action potential, the number of open Na^+ channels is 10 times greater than the number of open K^+ channels. Within a short period of time, voltage-gated Na^+ is inactivated, and a K^+ channel opens, greatly increasing the conductance to K^+ and, hence, repolarization. The Ca^{2+}–Na^+ channel (if present) is slow to be activated and normally would depolarize the membrane. Chloride channel permeability does not change during an action potential and, thus, functions passively in this process.

120. The answer is B. *(Neurologic disease)*

The patient described in the question most likely has tabes dorsalis, a disease that results from an untreated syphilis infection. The causative agent is *Treponema pallidum*, and the antibiotic of choice is penicillin. This disease results in the selective destruction of neurons in the spinal cord near the dorsal root of the spinal nerves, which causes the symptoms described in the question. Varicella zoster virus (VZV) causes shingles, a disease resulting from the activation of the virus in dorsal root ganglia of the spinal nerves, and chickenpox, a vesicular disease that usually affects children. Acyclovir is an antiviral agent that interferes with VZV as well as herpes simplex virus replication and, therefore, is not useful here.

121. The answer is C. (Glomerular filtration rate)
Blood enters the glomerulus via an afferent arteriole and leaves via an efferent arteriole. A decrease in renal blood flow (RBF) or a decrease in glomerular hydrostatic pressure tends to decrease the glomerular filtration rate (GFR). Accordingly, constriction of the afferent arteriole generally has this effect. An increase in RBF that increases hydrostatic pressure increases GFR. This effect of RBF persists even without an increase in hydrostatic pressure because of a subtle oncotic effect. Although raising systemic pressure would theoretically increase hydrostatic pressure and GFR, the effect is greatly minimized by normal autoregulation in the kidney. Thus, RBF and hydrostatic pressure are maintained by afferent arteriolar constriction in the presence of this increase over normal systemic pressures. Constriction of the efferent arteriole increases hydrostatic pressure (and GFR), but this effect is also offset by the above-mentioned decrease in RBF; thus, only a modest increase in GFR is normally observed.

122. The answer is A. (Neutropenia and infection)
Neutropenia is defined as an absolute neutrophil count of less than 1500/μl. Although there is a modest risk of acquired infection beginning at this level, patients with neutrophil counts of less than 1000/μl for any length of time are at significant risk of acquired infection and patients with counts below 500/μl are at extreme risk. The percentages of formed elements determined by peripheral blood count are of limited value; they must be multiplied by the total white cell count to arrive at absolute numbers of circulating granulocytes, monocytes, and lymphocytes. Leukocyte percentages determined by a 100-cell manual differential count have extremely broad 95% confidence intervals that may yield broad apparent shifts in absolute numbers. New cell counters with machine analysis of percentages of neutrophils, monocytes, and lymphocytes (even eosinophils and basophils) offer a better estimate of absolute number.

123. The answer is D. (DNA and RNA composition)
DNA is composed of the purines adenine and guanine and the pyrimidines thymine and cytosine. RNA is composed of the same bases with the exception that thymine is replaced by uracil. Therefore, DNA or RNA can be selectively labeled by using tritiated thymine [(^{3}H)-thymine] or tritiated uracil [(^{3}H)-uracil], respectively.

124. The answer is A. (Integral membrane proteins)
Integral membrane proteins are stabilized by hydrophobic interactions between the lipid bilayer and the amino acid side chains. Detergents are required for solubilization. Approximately 20 amino acids in an α-helical conformation are required to span the width of the bilayer. These proteins display compositional asymmetry, with the carbohydrate moieties always being on the side of the membrane away from the cytoplasm. They may display lateral, but not transverse, movement within the membrane.

125. The answer is E. (Urinary tract infection therapy)
Penicillin G is the treatment of choice. It is inexpensive, and it is a broad-spectrum antibiotic effective in the treatment of urinary tract infections. The serum levels are so low that it is unlikely to alter the natural bacterial flora of the host.

126. The answer is A. (Immunity to infection)
Opsonic antibodies are important for acquiring immunity to infection by group A *Neisseria meningitidis* because they permit recognition and destruction of *N. meningitidis* at the onset of infection. *Vibrio cholerae,*

Clostridium botulinum, and *Shigella flexneri* exert their pathogenic effects via toxins. Opsonic antibodies are not known to protect against the action of *V. cholerae*, *C. botulinum*, or *S. flexneri*.

127. The answer is B. (*Mechanics of the heart*)
At the end of the period of isovolumic contraction (2), the pressure inside the ventricle has risen to equal the pressure in the aorta at end diastole (80 mm Hg). At this point, ventricular pressures push the aortic valve open, and blood begins to pour out of the left ventricle (3) while it continues to contract. The fraction of end diastolic volume (115 ml) that was ejected was 60% because stroke volume was 115 − 45 = 70 ml. After isovolumic relaxation, left ventricular end diastolic pressure was near atmospheric pressure.

128–130. The answers are: 128-C, 129-D, 130-D. (*Genetics and pathology of chronic myeloproliferative disorder*)
An elevated platelet count and a low white blood cell count are suggestive of chronic myeloproliferative disorder. Malignant lymphoma can be eliminated as a possible diagnosis because of the lack of lymphadenopathy, and acute leukemia can be eliminated because of the lack of blasts on the blood smear. No cough and the normal chest x-ray eliminate pulmonary tuberculosis, which is often associated with myeloproliferative disorders.

Because the cytochemical stains indicate a myeloid disorder, flow cytometric analysis to determine the surface phenotype of peripheral blood and bone marrow cells is not necessary. The leukocyte alkaline phosphatase score is low in chronic myelogenous leukemia (CML) and, therefore, might be useful for differential diagnosis. Since 90% of the patients with CML have a chromosomal translocation resulting in the Philadelphia chromosome, chromosomal evaluation is appropriate. Bone marrow aspiration and biopsy distinguish CML from other chronic myeloproliferative disorders, such as polycythemia vera and agnogenic myeloid metaplasia. Determination of the red blood cell mass distinguishes between polycythemia vera and CML, because the red blood cell mass is high in the former but not in the latter.

Approximately 2% to 10% of patients with CML will not have a Philadelphia chromosome but will have a characteristic BCR-*abl* proto-oncogene translocation, which can be detected via nucleic acid hybridization methods. A leukemoid reaction can be excluded because the leukocyte alkaline phosphatase levels are not high.

131. The answer is B. (*Chagas disease*)
Patients with chronic Chagas disease present with cardiac conduction defects. The other signs and symptoms listed are classic for several diseases that are endemic in Central and South America, including malaria, visceral and cutaneous leishmaniasis, and amebiasis. Chronic Chagas disease (chronic trypanosomiasis) results from gradual tissue destruction of the heart, most likely caused by damage to myofibrils and the autonomic innervation of the heart. This results in the conduction defects and megacardia that are hallmarks of the disease. Parasitemia at this point is subpatent; parasites are difficult to detect in either the blood or tissues. Periodic fever and chills are indicative of malaria. Cutaneous and mucocutaneous lesions are seen in leishmaniasis. Persistent diarrhea and pneumonia can be the result of a number of infectious agents endemic in this region, although these symptoms are not seen in either acute or chronic Chagas disease.

132–139. The answers are: 132-C, 133-E, 134-A, 135-B, 136-D, 137-D, 138-D, 139-C. (*Neuromuscular transmission and pathophysiology and treatment of myasthenia gravis*)
Edrophonium is a short-acting acetylcholinesterase inhibitor, which increases synaptic acetylcholine (ACh) levels. An increase in muscle strength on administration of edrophonium is diagnostic of myasthenia gravis.

Myasthenia gravis is a neuromuscular disorder with muscle weakness caused by blockade of ACh receptors by autoantibodies to the ACh receptors. The antibody–receptor complex is incapable of responding to ACh and is also rapidly internalized and degraded.

Although the mechanism of action is unclear, aminoglycoside antibiotics and Ca^{2+} have opposing actions in a variety of organ systems. Thus, Ca^{2+} attenuates both the ototoxicity and nephrotoxicity of the aminoglycosides, and the aminoglycosides inhibit presynaptic release of ACh, a process known to be Ca^{2+}-dependent. Intravenous administration of a calcium salt is the preferred treatment for aminoglycoside-induced neuromuscular blockade.

Penicillamine is an effective chelator of heavy metals and is used for the treatment of copper, lead, and mercury poisoning. One of the unusual long-term side effects of penicillamine is a muscle weakness that is indistinguishable from myasthenia gravis.

About 65% of patients with myasthenia gravis have a hyperplastic thymus, and another 10% have a thymic tumor (thymoma). Surgical removal of the thymus and tumors often improves the symptoms dramatically.

Pyridostigmine is the acetylcholinesterase inhibitor most commonly used to treat myasthenia gravis. Isoflurophate (diisopropyl phosphorofluoridate; DFP) is an irreversible acetylcholinesterase inhibitor whose use is limited to ophthalmic applications; pralidoxime is the cholinesterase reactivator that is antidotal for organophosphorus poisoning; and triorthocresylphosphate, the adulterant in Jamaican ginger, was the organophosphorus poison responsible for paralysis in thousands of individuals during Prohibition.

Immunosuppression with glucocorticoids is effective in nearly all patients with myasthenia gravis. The therapy presumably works by slowing production of antibodies to the ACh receptors.

140. The answer is E. *(Pharmacokinetics of drugs)*
Nomograms (i.e., body surface area, creatinine clearance) are reliable indicators of appropriate drug dosages in only approximately 50% of patients with renal insufficiency. Actual peak and trough levels are the only way to guarantee a therapeutic level of antimicrobial agents and avoid toxicity.

141. The answer is C. *(Regulation of peripheral blood flow)*
Compared with other tissue, the lung is relatively unique in having a vasoconstrictor response to hypoxia rather than a vasodilator response. Although the mechanism remains obscure, the rationale seems to be to divert blood flow from poorly ventilated regions of the lung, thus improving the matching of ventilation and perfusion. The vascular bed in the heart, like those in many other organs, dilates to adenosine, and this vasodilator mechanism may be common in its matching of blood flow to local tissue metabolism. The brain has a very well-described and important vasodilator response to carbon dioxide.

142. The answer is C. *(Sterilization; disinfection)*
Bacterial endospores are the life-forms most resistant to heat, and they can survive boiling for several minutes. Medically important endospore-formers include members of the genera *Bacillus* and *Clostridium*. Non–spore-formers such as *Escherichia coli* and *Mycobacterium tuberculosis* are more heat-sensitive than spore-formers and are usually killed after several minutes of boiling.

143. The answer is A. *(Effect of actin and myosin filament overlap on muscle contraction)*
It is generally accepted that maximal contraction of muscle fiber will occur when the overlap between actin filaments and the cross-bridges of the myosin filaments is optimal. At point *D*, the actin filament has pulled all the way out to the end of the myosin filament without overlap, and tension is minimal. As the muscle shortens past the optimal length, *C*, actin filaments tend to overlap each other and the myosin filaments decrease in length *A*, contributing to the decline in contraction at shorter than optimal lengths.

144–145. The answers are: 144-B, 145-A. *(Cardiac dynamics)*
The gradient that occurs between the ventricular and aortic systolic pressures is diagnostic of aortic stenosis. The normal aortic valve provides a negligible resistance, and the aortic pressure is nearly identical to the ventricular pressure during the phase of rapid ventricular ejection. A similar picture is seen if right ventricular

and pulmonary pressures are measured in the presence of pulmonary valve stenosis, but the pressures are proportionately reduced because of the low resistance of the pulmonary circulation.

Semilunar valve stenosis represents an impediment to the ejection of blood from the ventricle and results in an ejection-type murmur during systole. An ejection murmur is diamond-shaped (i.e., it is a crescendo–decrescendo sound that has maximal intensity in midsystole, when the pressure gradient is largest).

146. The answer is C. *(DNA replication; retroviruses)*
RNA-dependent DNA polymerase synthesizes DNA from an RNA template and is essential for the replication of retroviruses, not cells, and is, therefore, not a potential target of the new drug. Topoisomerase II relaxes supercoiled DNA. RNA polymerase synthesizes a primer fragment for DNA-dependent DNA polymerase. DNA ligase anneals the Okazaki fragments on the lagging strand of DNA synthesis.

147–148. The answers are: 147-C, 148-C. *(Eukaryotic and viral commonalities)*
Arenaviruses are multisegmented RNA viruses with inclusion granules in the virions that contain ribosomes derived from their host cells. Although arenaviruses have envelopes, this is a trait shared by many viruses, including herpesviruses and orthomyxoviruses. Likewise, many viruses have multiple genomic segments, including orthomyxoviruses and paramyxoviruses. Only arenaviruses contain ribosomes; in fact, the Latin word ''arena'' means sand. The presence of ribosome-containing granules makes the virus look grainy under the electron microscope.

To determine if the unknown virus is an arenavirus, it is important to locate the characteristic ribosomes. To test for the presence of ribosomes in virions, it would be necessary to supply ribosomal substrates to virion fractions and test the ability of these fractions to translate cellular messenger RNA (mRNA) and radiolabeled amino acids into proteins that could be isolated on a detergent (SDS) gel. Gel electrophoresis and ethidium bromide are useful for separating and staining double stranded DNA fragments, because ethidium bromide is an intercalating dye for DNA. Light microscopy with a hematoxylin–eosin stain would be useful for viewing viruses with known inclusion-body–forming properties but not useful in determining if an unknown virus is an arenavirus.

149. The answer is B. *(Histopathology of meningiomas)*
The tumor in the photomicrograph is a meningioma, which has a marked predilection for women and arises from the pia–arachnoid cells of the leptomeninges. It is usually well circumscribed and may have a hyperostótic reaction of overlying bone associated with it. The tumor cells are arranged in whorls or nests, and they are frequently observed with concentric calcified concretions called psammoma bodies, as shown on the *right* of the photomicrograph.

150. The answer is A. *(Pathophysiology of anemia)*
The result of a diet deficient in vitamin B_{12} or folate can be macrocytic, normochromic anemia with characteristic hypersegmented neutrophils. Anemia caused by folate or vitamin B_{12} deficiency often also presents with thrombocytopenia and agranulocytopenia. Microcytic, hypochromic erythrocytes are observed in iron deficiency anemia and thalassemia minor. In addition, basophilic stippling and target cells can be seen in thalassemia minor. In sickle cell crisis, the anemia is normocytic and normochromic, as is the anemia associated with hemorrhage.

151. The answer is C. *(Microscopic features of hemangioma)*
The hepatic neoplasm pictured is a benign cavernous hemangioma. This is the most common mesenchymal tumor of the liver, and, if it reaches an enormous size, it may be associated with a bruit over the liver and thrombocytopenia owing to venous stasis and in situ thrombosis. The neoplasm is composed of dilated vascular spaces lined by flattened, cytologically bland endothelial cells (*at right*). Angiosarcomas of the liver

have highly aggressive behavior and usually have foci of hemorrhage and necrosis. They are associated with particular carcinogens, one of which is Thorotrast, a radioactive medium widely used 50 years ago.

152–155. The answers are: 152-A, 153-C, 154-B, 155-A. *(Pelvic innervation)*
Afferent nerves from the pelvic viscera travel along autonomic pathways. Afferent nerves from the ovary, testis, upper to middle ureter, uterine tubes, urinary bladder, and uterine body travel along the least splanchnic nerve to the lower thoracic segment and along the lumbar splanchnic nerves to the upper lumbar segments of the spinal cord; thus, pain is referred to the inguinal and pubic regions as well as the lateral and anterior aspects of the thigh. Afferents from the epididymis, uterine cervix, and distal ureter travel along the pelvic splanchnic nerves to the midsacral spinal segments; thus, pain is referred to the perineum, posterior thigh, and leg.

156–160. The answers are: 156-C, 157-A, 158-E, 159-B, 160-D. *(Placental anatomy)*
The placenta consists of a decidual plate (*C*) facing the endometrium and a chorionic plate (*E*) facing the fetus. The decidual plate and chorionic plate are fused at the margins of the discoid placenta. These two plates are interconnected by cytotrophoblastic cell columns (*B*). Large numbers of chorionic villi (*D*) project away from them into the intervillous space (*A*). Maternal blood vessels end on the decidual plate and pour maternal blood into the intervillous space. Maternal blood directly bathes the chorionic villi. Thus, the human placenta is said to be a hemochorial placenta.

161–165. The answers are: 161-A, 162-D, 163-E, 164-C, 165-B. *(Cranial vasculature)*
The foramen spinosum transmits the middle meningeal artery (*A*), a branch of the maxillary artery. The carotid canal (*D*) transmits the internal carotid artery, whereas the jugular foramen (*E*) contains the internal jugular vein in addition to the glossopharyngeal, vagus, and spinal accessory nerves. Each posterior condylar canal (*C*) transmits a large emissary vein. The vertebral arteries enter the cranial cavity through the foramen magnum (*B*) along with the spinal accessory nerve; the spinal cord also transmits the foramen magnum.

166–170. The answers are: 166-C, 167-E, 168-B, 169-E, 170-A. *(Regulation of thyroid hormone synthesis)*
Regulation of thyroid hormone synthesis is a complex pathway. The anterior pituitary secretion of thyroid-stimulating hormone (TSH, or thyrotropin) is controlled by the hypothalamic hormone, thyrotropin-releasing hormone (TRH). TRH is a tripeptide whose synthesis may be stimulated by such conditions as stress, trauma, or cold temperatures. TSH affects all aspects of thyroid gland physiology, including stimulation of thyroxine (T_4) secretion and to a lesser extent triiodothyronine (T_3) secretion in the presence of sufficient iodine. T_4 is activated to T_3 by peripheral deiodination. In certain forms of hyperthyroidism, high circulating levels of thyroid hormone suppress the synthesis of TSH via a direct negative feedback pathway. Propylthiouracil and other antithyroid agents are useful adjuvants to surgical or radiologic removal of the hypersecreting thyroid gland in such conditions as Graves' disease. These agents prevent thyroperoxidase oxidation in the thyroid gland and, perhaps, peripheral deiodination of T_4, resulting in a decreased circulating level and activity of T_4. Levothyroxine is a synthetic, pure compound that is used for the therapy of myxedema, cretinism, and other forms of hypothyroidism. It is available for oral use.

171–174. The answers are: 171-B, 172-D, 173-E, 174-C. *(Sleep architecture)*
In narcolepsy, sleep attacks are sleep-onset rapid eye movement (REM) periods that intrude into wakefulness. The motor paralysis component of sleep-onset REM periods that is associated with narcolepsy is called cataplexy. REM sleep normally occurs about 90 minutes after sleep onset, but in major depression it occurs after only 45 minutes. There are also increased amounts of REM throughout the night in depressed individuals. Vaginal lubrication and penile tumescence occur spontaneously during normal REM sleep. Night terrors are characterized by partial awakening in terror from stages III and IV (when delta waves occur) of slow-wave sleep (SWS).

175–180. The answers are: 175-A, 176-C, 177-B, 178-F, 179-E, 180-D. *(Gross and microscopic appearances of neoplasms)*
Grossly, the squamous cell carcinoma is a firm, white–tan mass, approximately 2 cm in diameter. Histologically, the neoplasm displays nuclei that have hyperchromatic coarse chromatin; nucleoli may or may not be observed. The tumor may be indolent, with a prominent host response consisting of inflammation and fibroblastic proliferation.

Grossly, the bronchioalveolar adenocarcinoma is white and granular and ranges from several millimeters to several centimeters in diameter. On chest x-ray, the lesion may resemble "fluffy" infiltrates of pneumonia. This tumor also follows a rather indolent course; but the multicentric foci, which appear to result from aerogenic spread, limit resectability.

Grossly, the type of adenocarcinoma usually seen often appears as a tan mass between 1 cm and 3 cm in diameter. Histologically, the tumor cell cytoplasm is pale-staining and may contain mucin vacuoles. The nuclei are round or oval, with delicate chromatin patterns and prominent nucleoli. This tumor often metastasizes early to the brain.

Grossly, carcinoid often appears as a fleshy, brown, intrabronchial polyp. Histologically, the tumor grows in a pattern of clusters or ribbons of cells. The neurosecretory granules may contain neuron-specific enolase, bombesin, serotonin, calcitonin, gastrin, adrenocorticotropic hormone (ACTH), and somatostatin, among other materials. A carcinoid often arises in the appendix and terminal ileum.

The rapidly replicating small, primitive-appearing cells of small cell (oat cell) carcinoma have finely stippled nuclei, a high nuclear:cytoplasm ratio, and nucleoli that are not prominent. The small, dense neurosecretory granules may contain markers such as neuron-specific enolase, bombesin, calcitonin, somatostatin, vasoactive intestinal polypepide (VIP), or ACTH. Long-term survival is poor because of extensive metastases to the liver, brain, bone, or adrenal glands by the time of diagnosis.

The large cell carinoma is usually 3 cm to 6 cm in diameter. It is a white–tan tumor that is partially necrotic or cavitating. In addition to the leukemoid reaction, the presence of this tumor may also be manifested by elevated serum levels of the β-chain of chorionic gonadotropin.

181–185. The answers are: 181-B, 182-A, 183-E, 184-C, 185-D. *(Cell organelle structure and function)*
The Golgi complex *(B)* is composed of flattened membranous sacs and functions in protein glycosylation, membrane recycling, and sorting and targeting of proteins. Introns are regions of DNA that are transcribed but not translated. In the nucleus *(A)*, introns are cleaved from primary RNA transcripts to produce mature messenger RNA (mRNA). Ribosomes are composed of ribosomal RNA (rRNA), which is synthesized in the nucleolus *(E)* of the cell by RNA polymerase I. Smooth endoplasmic reticulum *(C)* has various functions, including steroid synthesis; calcium homeostasis; and lipid, cholesterol, and drug metabolism. Adenosine triphosphate (ATP) is synthesized by glycolysis in the cytosol and by oxidative phosphorylation in the mitochondria *(D)*.

186–190. The answers are: 186-B, 187-D, 188-E, 189-A, 190-C. *(Transport proteins)*
The functions of transport proteins can be divided into three general classes: the control of diffusion into the tissues; the highly specific recognition of molecules; and the removal of toxins. Transferrin helps in transporting iron to storage and utilization sites in the bone marrow. The damage that free iron can cause to tissues other than the marrow is prevented when it is bound by transferrin. Transcobalamin binds vitamin B_{12} and prevents it from degrading while it is being transported to storage and utilization sites in tissues with high cellular turnover rates. Albumin is the main plasma protein responsible for the maintenance of plasma osmotic pressure. Haptoglobin is a plasma protein that binds free hemoglobin in the blood and delivers it to the liver for recycling. The degree of intravascular hemolysis is determined by measuring the levels of depleted free forms of haptoglobin in the blood.

191–195. The answers are: 191-A, 192-B, 193-B, 194-A, 195-A. *(Vitamin deficiency)*
Pellagra, a disease affecting the skin (dermatitis), the gastrointestinal tract (diarrhea), and the central nervous system (CNS) [dementia], is the result of a niacin deficiency. Because niacin can be formed from tryptophan, an essential amino acid, dietary treatment of pellagra must take into consideration daily allowances for both niacin and tryptophan. Endemic pellagra is no longer a common occurrence; however, it is a manifestation of two disorders of tryptophan metabolism, Hartnup disease, and the carcinoid syndrome. Hartnup disease is an autosomal recessive defect in which patients have a reduced ability to convert tryptophan to niacin. In the carcinoid syndrome, dietary tryptophan is metabolized in the hydroxylation pathway (a minor pathway), leaving little tryptophan for the formation of niacin. Administration of large amounts of niacin can cure the pellagra associated with these conditions.

Beriberi is a severe thiamine deficiency syndrome associated with malnutrition endemic to areas where there is a high intake of highly milled (polished) rice. Clinical characteristics of this deficiency range from cardiovascular and neurologic lesions to emotional disturbances. Cardiovascular changes include right-sided enlargement (dilatation), tachycardia, and "high-output" cardiac failure. Neuromuscular manifestations include peripheral neuropathy (neuritis), weakness, fatigue, and an impaired capacity to do work. Edema and anorexia are also characteristic. In the United States, thiamine deficiency is seen primarily in association with chronic alcoholism, which leads to Wernicke's encephalopathy, which presents with the classic triad of confusion, ataxia, and ophthalmoplegia. In thiamine deficiency, motor and sensory peripheral nerve lesions are marked by neuromuscular findings of numbness and tingling of the legs and atrophy and weakness of the muscles of the extremities compounded by the loss of reflexes. Mental depression may also accompany these findings. The dementia caused by niacin deficiency results from degeneration of the ganglion cells of the brain, accompanied by degeneration of the fibers of the spinal cord.

196–200. The answers are: 196-E, 197-A, 198-B, 199-D, 200-C. *(Endocrine syndromes)*
Bartter's syndrome is a form of secondary hyperaldosteronism in which excessive renin production occurs. The hyperreninemia results from hyperplasia of renal juxtaglomerular cells, which secrete renin primarily in response to decreased arterial blood pressure in afferent arterioles and increased renal sympathetic nerve activity.

Sheehan's syndrome, or postpartum pituitary necrosis, results from the infarction of the anterior lobe of the pituitary gland. Sheehan's syndrome usually is precipitated by obstetric hemorrhage or shock; however, it also can occur in nonpregnant women as well as in men. The infarct usually causes the destruction of 95% to 99% of the anterior lobe.

Cushing's syndrome is characterized by a prolonged overproduction of cortisol. The pituitary gland regulates the synthesis of adrenal cortisol by secreting adrenocorticotropic hormone (ACTH). The secretion of ACTH is regulated by corticotropin-releasing hormone (CRH), which is produced in the hypothalamus. Possible causes of Cushing's syndrome include ACTH-producing pituitary neoplasm, CRH-producing hypothalamic neoplasm, adrenal cortisol-producing neoplasm, and ectopic ACTH- or CRH-producing neoplasm. Cushing's syndrome can be caused iatrogenically by long-term glucocorticoid therapy.

Waterhouse-Friderichsen syndrome is most often caused by meningococcemia and is characterized by extensive cutaneous petechiae, purpura, and hemorrhages. Skin lesions appear shortly after the onset of an infectious febrile reaction, and the patient may go into circulatory collapse and die within 24 hours. In addition to lesions, extensive internal hemorrhages are present, particularly in the adrenal glands.

Conn's syndrome, or primary hyperaldosteronism, is associated with hypernatremia, hypokalemia, alkalosis, potassium wasting, and low levels of renin.

Test III

QUESTIONS

DIRECTIONS: Each of the numbered items or incomplete statements in this section is followed by answers or by completions of the statement. Select the ONE lettered answer or completion that is BEST in each case.

Questions 1–3

A 32-year-old volunteer fireman receives second-degree burns over approximately 30% of his body and third-degree burns over another 40%. Intravenous fluid and electrolyte therapy is initiated on site, and the patient is transported to the burn ward of a large metropolitan hospital. Approximately 2½ weeks after thermal injury, the patient becomes septic.

1. The most probable etiologic agent is

(A) *Serratia marcescens*
(B) *Nocardia asteroides*
(C) *Staphylococcus aureus*
(D) *Pseudomonas aeruginosa*
(E) *Streptococcus pneumoniae*

2. The patient's sepsis possibly developed because of

(A) inability of B cells to produce opsonins
(B) inhibition of chemotactic activity of mononuclear leukocyte
(C) lack of circulating segmented neutrophils in the bloodstream
(D) inhibition of the production of immunoglobulin M
(E) induction of Bruton's agammaglobulinemia by the severe thermal injury

3. The most promising chemotherapeutic agent for treatment of this patient belongs to which of the following categories?

(A) Imidazole antibiotics
(B) Immune modulators
(C) Quinolone antibiotics
(D) Thymosin fractions
(E) Amphotericin B

Questions 4–5

A 52-year-old man presents with the complaint of blood in his stools. He reports that he has experienced some changes in his bowel habits over the last 18 months and recently has become aware of the sensation that his evacuations are not complete. Proctoscopic examination reveals a large ulcerating mass in the descending colon. Biopsy results confirm the diagnosis of carcinoma of the colon, and the malignant mass is surgically removed. The patient is placed on appropriate chemotherapy and discharged 2 weeks later to be followed in the oncology clinic. Monthly blood specimens taken during the next year reveal the following carcinoembryonic antigen (CEA) levels:

	CEA (ng/ml)
Preoperative sample	50
Postoperative sample (day 1)	65
Month 1	15
Month 2	5
Months 3–9	<2.5
Month 10	10
Month 11	25
Month 12	40

4. The patient's serum CEA levels were assayed periodically because of the usefulness of CEA in

(A) localization of certain tumors in vivo
(B) diagnosing carcinoma of the colon
(C) diagnosing carcinoma of the pancreas
(D) diagnosing carcinoma of the prostate
(E) follow-up for the recurrence of certain malignancies

5. The CEA levels obtained during months 10 to 12 for this patient indicate that

(A) metastases have developed
(B) the initial diagnosis of colon cancer was incorrect
(C) surgical removal of the tumor was complete
(D) a revised diagnosis of carcinoma of the pancreas is warranted
(E) the patient is having an anamnestic response to the tumor

Questions 6–10

A 28-year-old white male presents with unexplained weight loss and lymphadenopathy of 2 months duration. He admits to using intravenous drugs and states that he has shared needles with his girlfriend, whom he has been dating for 5 years. He has also shared needles and had unprotected intercourse with one other woman. The physician suspects that the man may be infected with the human immunodeficiency virus (HIV).

6. Which of the following tests is useful in evaluating this patient for HIV infection?

(A) Enzyme-linked immunosorbent assay (ELISA) for anti-HIV antibody
(B) Complete blood count with differential
(C) Restriction fragment length polymorphism (RFLP) search for viral proteins
(D) Absolute number of CD8$^+$ lymphocytes
(E) Western blot for viral antigens

7. All of the following are opportunistic infections commonly seen in patients infected with HIV EXCEPT

(A) *Candida albicans* thrush or esophagitis
(B) Disseminated *Mycobacterium avium intracellulare*
(C) *Cryptococcus neoformans* meningitis
(D) *Pneumocystis carinii* pneumonia
(E) *Staphylococcus aureus* osteoarthritis

8. Which of the following prophylactic therapies is indicated for patients who have a T4 lymphocyte count of less than 200/μL?

(A) Acyclovir for herpes simplex esophagitis
(B) Trimethoprim–sulfamethoxazole for disseminated *M. avium intracellulare*
(C) Pentamidine for *P. carinii* pneumonia
(D) Ganciclovir for cytomegalovirus retinitis
(E) Doxorubicin for Kaposi's sarcoma

9. Which one of the following statements concerning HIV-1 is correct?

(A) The gp 120 envelope protein of the virus binds specifically to the CD8 antigen on T lymphocytes

(B) HIV-1 is a member of the lentivirus group of retroviruses and causes transformation of T lymphocytes in culture

(C) Viral reverse transcriptase causes incorporation of the viral genome into the host DNA; however, the viral DNA is not copied during cell division

(D) Viral reverse transcriptase lacks a proofreading mechanism, which results in the well-documented "microheterogeneity" of envelope proteins

(E) HIV can only be transmitted from one cell to another by direct contact of an infected lymphocyte with a healthy cell

10. All of the following are poorly understood complications of HIV infection EXCEPT

(A) Acquired immunodeficiency syndrome (AIDS)-related dementia complex

(B) Acute T4-cell leukemia or lymphoma

(C) Kaposi's sarcoma

(D) Polyclonal activation of B lymphocytes with resultant hypergammaglobulinemia

(E) Aggressive non-Hodgkin's lymphoma

Questions 11–15

A 45-year-old black history professor presents to the emergency room with shortness of breath. He has never traveled before and had just been to the doctor yesterday to prepare for his trip to central Africa. His doctor told him that his health was fine and prescribed him a prophylactic course of primaquine to prevent malaria. During the physical examination, the emergency room physician notes icterus, a jaundiced appearance to the skin, and a lack of color under the tongue. His pulse is 102, his blood pressure is 125/85, and his respiration rate is 19.

11. Which of the following diseases is indicated by the history and physical exam?

(A) Wilson's disease

(B) Polycythemia vera

(C) Disseminated intravascular coagulation

(D) Acute hemolytic anemia

(E) Hereditary spherocytosis

12. Which of the following pairs of laboratory tests would be most useful in confirming the suspected diagnosis?

(A) Unconjugated bilirubin and hemoglobin–hematocrit

(B) Bone marrow biopsy and peripheral smear

(C) Hemoglobin electrophoresis and peripheral smear

(D) Serum transaminases and abdominal computed tomography

(E) Prothrombin time and complete blood count

13. In which of the following enzyme activities is this man probably deficient?

(A) Uroporphyrinogen synthase
(B) Hexokinase
(C) Glucose 6-phosphate dehydrogenase
(D) Thymidine kinase
(E) Ribonucleotide reductase

14. Which of the following statements concerning the effect of primaquine on this man's cellular metabolism is correct?

(A) Primaquine competitively inhibited his abnormal hexokinase
(B) Primaquine reduced the metabolism of fatty acids
(C) Primaquine induced the synthesis of abnormal thymidine kinase
(D) Primaquine increased the turnover rate of hemoglobin
(E) Primaquine caused severe oxidative stress in the older erythrocytes

15. Which of the following statements accurately describes the hereditary trait causing this man's disease?

(A) It occurs frequently in Ashkenazic Jews
(B) It is most common in people from regions in which malaria is endemic because it increases a person's susceptibility to infection by *Plasmodium falciparum*
(C) It is more common in women
(D) It is rare, occurring with a frequency of less than 1% in African–American males
(E) It is sex-linked

Questions 16–19

An 8-month-old black female was brought to the emergency room with shortness of breath, icterus, and pallor under the tongue. The infant measured below the 5th percentile for her age with respect to height and weight, despite her weighing above the 80th percentile at birth. Examination of the peripheral smear indicates a hypochromic, microcytic anemia with some target cells and some teardrop-shaped erythrocytes. Unconjugated bilirubin is markedly elevated. Hemoglobin electrophoresis reveals increased fetal hemoglobin (Hb F) and double the normal amount of hemoglobin A_2 (Hb A_2); there is very little hemoglobin A (Hb A). There are no other hemoglobin bands.

16. What is the primary diagnosis for this patient?

(A) β-thalassemia major
(B) Iron deficiency
(C) Sickle cell disease
(D) Hereditary spherocytosis
(E) Methemoglobinemia

17. All of the following are common causes of this condition EXCEPT

(A) Nonsense mutation in one of the globin-chain genes
(B) Point mutation in the coding region of a globin-chain gene
(C) Point mutation in the intron of a globin-chain gene causing an abnormal splice variant
(D) Point mutation in the 5′ untranslated region of a globin-chain gene causing reduced production of a normal protein
(E) Deletion in one of the globin chains

18. Which of the following conditions is most likely to develop in this infant by adolescence?

(A) Asthma
(B) Crohn's disease
(C) Splenomegaly
(D) Chronic gastritis
(E) Iron deficiency

19. Which of the following genetically determined features makes for a more mild form of the disease?

(A) Decreased synthesis of the β-globin chain
(B) Decreased production of intrinsic factor
(C) Increased absorption of iron
(D) Increased expression of the γ-globin chain
(E) Increased expression of the α-globin chain

Questions 20–22

To answer this group of questions, refer to the following diagrammatic representation of the heart in an infant with congenital heart disease.

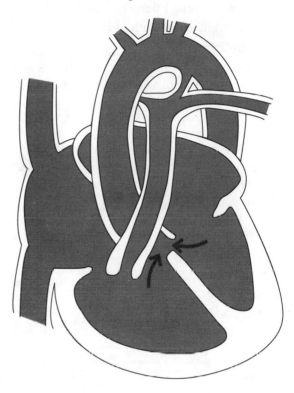

20. Which cyanotic congenital heart disease does this infant have?

(A) Truncus arteriosus
(B) Transposition of the great arteries
(C) Patent ductus arteriosus   no cyanosis (PDA)
(D) Tetralogy of Fallot
(E) Coarctation of the aorta   no. cyanosis (COA)

21. All of the following are characteristics of this heart disease EXCEPT

(A) failure of separation between the aorta and pulmonary artery
(B) ventricular septal defect
(C) right-to-left shunt with cyanosis
(D) overriding aorta
(E) obstruction of right ventricular outflow with concomitant right ventricular hypertrophy

22. Many congenital heart defects produce non-laminar, jet-stream patterns of blood flow. These turbulent jets frequently leave the infants especially susceptible to

(A) myocardial infarction
(B) rheumatic heart disease
(C) infective endocarditis
(D) valvular calcification
(E) mitral valve prolapse

Questions 23–26

A 2-year-old female is brought to her pediatrician because of progressive muscular weakness and recurrent episodes of hepatic encephalopathy with nausea and vomiting. An inherited defect in metabolism is suspected, and tests reveal low serum carnitine.

23. Which of the following correctly describes the normal function of carnitine in fatty acid metabolism?

(A) A coenzyme that is required for the dehydrogenation of acyl coenzyme A (CoA), forming a double bond between the β- and γ-carbons
(B) A coenzyme that is added to free fatty acids on the outer mitochondrial membrane
(C) A carrier protein that holds the growing acyl chain in fatty acid synthesis
(D) A carrier protein that shuttles long-chain fatty acids into the mitochondrial matrix
(E) A carrier protein that shuttles short-chain fatty acids out of the liver to adipose tissue

24. Which of the following statements concerning the β-oxidation of fatty acids is correct?

(A) Single carboxylic acids are released in successive cycles during the metabolism of fatty acids
(B) All of the energy released is stored in the form of reduced equivalents of nicotinamide–adenine dinucleotide (NADH)
(C) Phosphorylation of a fatty acid and the subsequent generation of acyl CoA are the committed steps in oxidation
(D) Fatty acids are converted into glucose by the formation of pyruvate from acetyl CoA
(E) Elevated levels of malonyl CoA activate the transfer of fatty acyl CoA into the mitochondrial matrix

25. All of the following characterizations of carnitine deficiency are correct EXCEPT

(A) Some victims of this autosomal recessive disease respond to oral carnitine therapy

(B) A diet restricted to short- and medium-chain fatty acids may prove useful

(C) Pathologic deposition of lipid is frequently seen in muscle biopsies

(D) A form of the disease confined to muscle is less severe and may involve defective transport of carnitine into the cell

(E) A deletion mutation in the gene for carnitine palmitoyltransferase would result in an entirely different phenotype

26. All of the following statements correctly pair a metabolic pathway with its appropriate subcellular location EXCEPT

(A) Oxidative phosphorylation occurs in mitochondria

(B) Fatty acid synthesis occurs in mitochondria

(C) Glycolysis occurs in the cytosol

(D) Gluconeogenesis occurs in both the cytosol and the mitochondria

(E) Ganglioside degradation occurs in lysosomes

Questions 27–31

A 30-year-old female lawyer presents to her physician's office for an increase in fatigue over the last 2 months. She has been involved in a difficult case at work and has lost five pounds. During the physical exam, the physician notes delayed capillary refill in the nailbeds and a pale appearance of the inner lining of the eyelids. A peripheral smear reveals hypochromic erythrocytes.

27. Which of the following tests would be most useful in confirming the probable diagnosis?

(A) Serum ferritin and total iron-binding capacity (TIBC)

(B) Schilling's test

(C) Glucose 6-phosphate dehydrogenase assay

(D) Hemoglobin electrophoresis

(E) Serum folate and serum cobalamin (vitamin B_{12})

28. Which of the following statements about the causes of acquired anemia is correct?

(A) Cobalamin deficiency is often secondary to chronic liver disease

(B) Methotrexate is frequently associated with hypochromic, microcytic anemias

(C) Women are more susceptible to iron-deficiency anemia because they tend to eat less red meat

(D) Folate deficiency frequently leads to neurologic disease, which may not respond to therapy

(E) Folate deficiency can develop over months in a poorly nourished person

29. Other than hematopoietic tissue, which of the following tissues is most frequently involved in folate deficiency?

(A) Liver
(B) Gastrointestinal mucosal
(C) Long bones
(D) Muscle and cartilage
(E) Central and peripheral myelin

30. Which of the following statements regarding the control of transferrin and ferritin synthesis is correct?

(A) Hepatic synthesis of transferrin and ferritin is principally regulated at the level of messenger RNA (mRNA) transcription by the presence of iron
(B) Hepatic synthesis of transferrin and ferritin is principally regulated by the level of tissue oxygenation and the presence of sufficient heme
(C) Hepatic synthesis of transferrin and ferritin is principally regulated after mRNA transcription by an iron-binding protein that is inactive in the presence of iron
(D) The rate of transferrin turnover in the serum is a function of the presence of iron
(E) The half-life of ferritin mRNA is the site of critical regulation in ferritin synthesis

31. Therapeutic intervention of megaloblastic anemias should be approached carefully because

(A) unnecessary administration of iron salts can quickly lead to iron overload and symptoms of hemochromatosis
(B) oral iron salts can increase oxygen free radical production and cause erythrocyte hemolysis
(C) cobalamin supplements will worsen the anemia in a patient with gastric mucosal atrophy
(D) excess folate cannot be excreted and is stored, leading to chronic liver damage
(E) inappropriate folate therapy in a patient with cobalamin deficiency can worsen the neurologic symptoms

32. Which of the following statements concerning fatty acid synthesis is correct?

(A) Palmitoyl coenzyme A (CoA) helps regulate the committed step in fatty acid synthesis through feedback inhibition of acetyl CoA carboxylase
(B) Hormone-dependent enzyme phosphorylation, which is important in gluconeogenesis, is not important in fatty acid synthesis
(C) Low levels of citrate increase the synthesis of malonyl CoA by reducing substrate inhibition of acetyl CoA carboxylase
(D) The growing fatty acid chain is elongated by a series of enzymes that exist as separate polypeptides in the mitochondrial matrix
(E) Niacin is the precursor for a coenzyme that is important in the addition of carboxyl groups to the growing fatty acid chain

Questions 33–37

A 40-year-old woman with refractory peptic ulcer disease presents to a gastroenterologist for a complete evaluation. She is a nonsmoker and drinks only infrequently. Endoscopy reveals ectopic ulcers in the esophagus as well as numerous ulcers in the stomach and duodenum. The physician considers a diagnosis of Zollinger-Ellison syndrome.

33. Which of the following problems characterizes the cause of peptic ulcer disease in most patients with Zollinger-Ellison syndrome?

(A) Increased vagal tone in the gastric branch
(B) Increased release of histamine
(C) Increased secretion of gastrin
(D) Increased secretion of pepsin
(E) Decreased mucous production

34. Which of the following statements correctly characterizes the secretion of acid by parietal cells?

(A) Carbonic anhydrase in the parietal cell splits carbonic acid into a bicarbonate ion, which is secreted into the blood, and a hydrogen ion
(B) Hydrogen ions are secreted passively down their gradient into the gut
(C) Cyclic adenosine monophosphate (cAMP) levels are elevated in response to either gastrin or muscarinic receptor stimulation
(D) H_2-histamine receptor activation causes elevation of intracellular calcium levels
(E) Gastrin and acetylcholine stimulate parietal cell acid production but histamine inhibits it

35. Which of the of following statements correctly pairs a commonly prescribed ulcer medication with its mechanism of action?

(A) Atropine blocks acetylcholine release by the vagus nerve
(B) Ranitidine and cimetidine competitively block the gastrin receptor
(C) Colloidal bismuth inhibits gastrin release
(D) Omeprazole irreversibly inhibits the hydrogen–potassium adenosine triphosphatase
(E) Sucralfate competitively inhibits carbonic anhydrase

36. An extensive laboratory evaluation reveals hypercalcemia, and the patient recalls having had "kidney stones" last year. Which of the following diseases does this patient probably have?

(A) Ataxia-telangiectasia
(B) Neurofibromatosis
(C) Hemochromatosis
(D) Niemann-Pick disease
(E) Multiple endocrine neoplasia type I (MEN I)

37. What other abnormality would this patient be likely to develop during her lifetime?

(A) Immunodeficiency
(B) Hypoglycemia
(C) Adrenal insufficiency
(D) Bronchogenic carcinomas
(E) Panhypopituitarism

Questions 38–41

A 75-year-old woman with a 35-year history of noninsulin-dependent (type II) diabetes mellitus is admitted to the hospital for mental status changes. The physician considers a diagnosis of chronic renal failure and investigates the possibility of dialysis.

38. All of the following are common characteristics of chronic renal failure EXCEPT

(A) hypokalemia
(B) elevated triglycerides
(C) uremic fetor
(D) normochromic, normocytic anemia
(E) proteinuria

39. All of the following kidney lesions are regularly seen in diabetic patients EXCEPT

(A) interstitial nephritis
(B) diffuse glomerulosclerosis
(C) amyloid deposits in hypercellular glomeruli
(D) Kimmelstiel-Wilson lesions
(E) hyaline arteriosclerosis

40. Which of the following statements correctly characterizes the role of the kidney in acid–base homeostasis?

(A) Cells of the proximal tubule are the only cells in the body with the complete enzymatic machinery for urea biosynthesis, an important route for excreting acid
(B) Carbonic anhydrase, located on the brush border of tubule cells, splits carbonic acid into a bicarbonate anion and a hydrogen ion; the hydrogen ion is pumped into the cell
(C) Bicarbonate is actively synthesized from pyruvate in the distal tubule cells
(D) Tubule cells actively secrete bicarbonate anion as a potassium salt
(E) The tubule cells secrete ammonia as one of the mechanisms to excrete excess acid

41. An arterial blood gas reveals a pH of 7.26, and her anion gap is 12. Which of the following statements correctly describes her metabolic acidosis due to renal failure?

(A) A large anion gap is indicative of better compensation
(B) The metabolic acidosis is caused by an excess production of ammonia in the tubule cells
(C) The large anion gap indicates that her plasma bicarbonate is elevated
(D) This patient has probably already passed the hyperchloremic phase of her acidosis
(E) Long-standing metabolic acidosis is not related to renal osteodystrophy

Questions 42–45

A neurologist postulates that the extent of physical disability following a cerebrovascular accident (CVA) is related to personality type. Five hundred such patients were classified according to the severity of their physical deficit (mild or severe) and simultaneously assigned to one of four personality groups (1 = most prone to depression and 4 = least prone to depression), based on a personality assessment questionnaire developed by the investigator. The table below depicts the number of subjects in each category.

Personality Type	Severity of Condition		
	Severe	Mild	Totals
1	60	40	100
2	60	40	100
3	132	68	200
4	48	52	100
Totals	300	200	500

42. This study is an example of a

(A) prospective cohort study
(B) case–control study
(C) cross-sectional study
(D) experimental study
(E) randomized controlled clinical trial

43. What is the most appropriate statistical test for determining whether a significant association exists between the extent of physical disability and personality type?

(A) Analysis of variance
(B) Independent sample (pooled) t test
(C) Paired t test
(D) Chi-square test
(E) Correlation/regression analysis

44. The neurologist computes a test statistic of 9.00; the tabulated critical value for $\alpha = .05$ is 7.81. What is the most appropriate conclusion that can be drawn from this result?

(A) Reject H_O at the 5% level of significance; conclude that the severity of the disability is related to personality type
(B) Reject H_O at the 5% level of significance; conclude that no association exists between the extent of disability and personality type
(C) Do not reject H_O at the 5% level of significance; conclude that there is no association between the severity of the physical deficit and personality type
(D) Do not reject H_O at the 5% level of significance; conclude that there is an association between the extent of the disability and personality type
(E) None of the above

45. In a similar study, the investigators report that there is a statistically significant association between the severity of the physical deficit observed after a CVA and personality type ($P < .001$). What is the most appropriate interpretation of this finding?

(A) There is a strong, clinically important association between personality type and the degree of physical disability after a CVA
(B) Those patients who are most prone to depression are least likely to make a full recovery after suffering a CVA
(C) All competing explanations for the observed association have been eliminated (i.e., all potential sources of bias have been controlled)
(D) It is unlikely that a sample giving rise to an association as large as that observed would have been drawn at random from a population in which no association exists between the two study variables

Questions 46–49

A 29-year-old man with no prior medical history is transported to the hospital after being involved in a serious motor vehicle accident. The bleeding has been slowed by the paramedics, but the man has lost a substantial amount of blood. His blood pressure on arrival at the hospital is 72/30. Right heart catheterization with a Swan-Ganz catheter is performed. The physician begins volume replenishment with units of packed red blood cells and plasma.

46. Which of the following pharmacologic agents would be most useful in supporting this man's cardiovascular system?

(A) Albuterol
(B) Propranolol
(C) Furosemide
(D) Dobutamine
(E) Tubocurarine

47. Which of the following tissues is most likely to sustain damage following hypovolemic shock?

(A) Brain
(B) Liver
(C) Intestines
(D) Peripheral muscle
(E) Heart

48. All of the following cause shock accompanied by an increased peripheral vascular resistance EXCEPT

(A) sepsis
(B) pericardial tamponade
(C) pulmonary embolus
(D) large myocardial infarction
(E) gastrointestinal blood loss

49. The physician estimates that the patient's systemic circulation was compromised for a total of 4 hours. In the intensive care unit 36 hours later, his serum potassium level is 5.7, increased from 4.8 when he was admitted (normal = 3.4–5.0). Which of the following tests would be most useful in confirming the origin of this man's new problem?

(A) Antinuclear antibody screen
(B) Blood urea nitrogen and serum creatinine
(C) Antistreptolysin O (ASO) titer
(D) Complete blood count
(E) Digoxin level

Questions 50–53

An 8-year-old girl is taken to her pediatrician's office because of blood in her urine and "puffiness." Her mother indicates that the child has also been lethargic for the past 2 or 3 days. The girl has no history of cardiac or renal disease. The mother reveals that her child had a sore throat that kept her from 2 days of school about 12 days ago. The girl's blood pressure is 140/100.

50. Which of the following diseases is suggested by the history and physical findings?

(A) Systemic lupus erythematosus
(B) Acute tubular necrosis
(C) Acute glomerulonephritis
(D) Juvenile onset (insulin-dependent) diabetes mellitus
(E) Hyperaldosteronism

51. A complete laboratory evaluation would probably reveal all of the following EXCEPT

(A) Elevated serum creatinine
(B) Proteinuria
(C) Cellular and granular casts in the urine
(D) Hyponatremia
(E) Increased serum complement factor C3

52. Which of the following would you expect to see on renal biopsy?

(A) Complement and immunoglobulin deposits in clumps along the mesangium and basement membrane
(B) Occlusion of tubular lumen by casts with large gaps in luminal epithelia
(C) Linear or ribbon pattern of immunoglobulins directed against the glomerular basement membrane
(D) Hypertrophy of the macula densa
(E) Proliferation of mesangial cells *lupus*

53. Which of the following factors was most likely involved in the pathogenesis of this child's problem?

(A) Bacterial lipopolysaccharide *(by gram –ive)*
(B) IgG directed against glomerular basement membrane
(C) Antinuclear antibodies
(D) Immune complex formation stimulated by an unknown bacterial antigen
(E) Excess renin production

Questions 54–58

A 35-year-old woman presents to the emergency room with severe, stabbing abdominal pain that is constant and radiating from the epigastrium to the back and chest. She is nauseated and says that her abdomen feels bloated as well as painful, and the pain is worse lying down. During the physical exam, the physician notes tachycardia, a low-grade fever, an absence of bowel sounds, guarding, and an exquisitely tender abdomen. The remainder of the physical exam is noncontributory. Further questioning reveals that the patient drank excessive amounts of alcohol last night; she has no prior medical or family history for cardiac disease. A plain radiograph of the abdomen shows no air under the diaphragm.

54. Which of the following processes is most likely in this patient?

(A) Perforated duodenal ulcer
(B) Myocardial infarction
(C) Abdominal aortic aneurysm
(D) Acute pancreatitis
(E) Renal colic

55. Which one of the following sets of tests is most useful in ascertaining a diagnosis?

(A) Serum lipase and amylase
(B) Bilirubin, alkaline phosphatase, and γ-glutamyl transpeptidase (GGTP)
(C) Routine and microscopic urinalysis
(D) Upper gastrointestinal radiographic imaging with barium contrast
(E) Electrocardiogram and creatine kinase level

56. A more complete physical exam on admission reveals muscle spasms, including a positive Chvostek's sign (i.e., facial muscle spasm), and a lengthened QT interval. Which of the following is most likely to be causing these new findings?

(A) Hyperkalemia
(B) Vitamin B$_{12}$ deficiency
(C) Cocaine abuse
(D) Severe hemolysis
(E) Hypocalcemia

57. A social worker's report indicates that this woman has been seen by other physicians in the same hospital quite frequently, and the social worker thinks that she may be an alcoholic. Considering this information, which of the following therapies will probably be required to alleviate the neuromuscular symptoms described in the preceding question?

(A) 5% dextrose in normal saline
(B) Packed red blood cells
(C) Magnesium replacement
(D) Furosemide
(E) Vitamin B$_{12}$

58. All of the following are criteria for diagnosing alcoholism EXCEPT

(A) Alcohol-related relationship problems leading to separation or divorce
(B) Loss of memory while using alcohol (blackouts)
(C) Loss of a job due to alcohol-related problems
(D) Alcohol-related disease including delirium tremens, hepatitis, or cardiomyopathy
(E) Two or more arrests related to alcohol

59. Which of the following statements concerning α_1-antitrypsin deficiency is correct?

(A) Liver disease is always preceded by lung disease
(B) The deficiency may be a common but unrecognized cause of many cases of neonatal hepatitis
(C) Direct restriction fragment length polymorphism (RFLP) analysis of the gene is the only means of definitive diagnosis
(D) Of individuals who are homozygous for the deficiency, panacinar emphysema develops in about 33% of persons surviving into adulthood
(E) There is no interaction between smoking and the protein deficiency

60. Which of the following is appropriate pharmacologic management of routine delirium tremens (i.e., alcohol withdrawal)?

(A) Haloperidol therapy for up to 3 weeks
(B) Phenytoin (Dilantin) tapered over 10 days
(C) Chlordiazepoxide (Librium) tapered over 5 days
(D) Morphine for up to 1 month
(E) Nortriptyline for up to 6 months

Questions 61–65

An 11-year-old boy with a history of episodic dyspnea associated with wheezing has the following spirometric tracings in the pulmonary function laboratory:

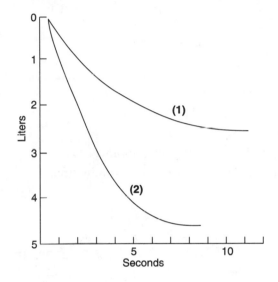

61. Which of the following is the most likely description of curves (*1*) and (*2*)?

(A) Before (*1*) and after (*2*) inhalation of methacholine
(B) Before (*1*) and after (*2*) inhalation of metaproterenol
(C) Before (*1*) and after (*2*) inhalation of cromolyn sodium
(D) Before (*1*) and after (*2*) inhalation of beclomethasone
(E) Curves (*1*) and (*2*) arise from normal variation of forced expiratory maneuvers within a subject

62. A possible pharmacotherapeutic approach to control this boy's symptoms may include which one of the following agents?

(A) Antihistamine
(B) Propranolol
(C) Ibuprofen
(D) Theophylline
(E) Bethanechol

63. Inhalation of an irritant that stimulates nonmyelinated C fibers near epithelial cells lining the airway lumen produces reflex bronchoconstriction via the

(A) sympathetic nerve endings
(B) hypoglossal nerve
(C) phrenic nerve
(D) vagus nerve
(E) intercostal nerve

64. All of the following are potential stimuli that may precipitate an acute episode of bronchospasm EXCEPT

(A) potassium metabisulfite
(B) ozone
(C) parainfluenza virus
(D) exercise
(E) acetaminophen

65. If an allergic component contributes to the boy's disorder, which one of the following cells plays a critical role in initiating the early response to inhaled antigen?

(A) Mast cells
(B) Bronchial epithelial cells
(C) Eosinophils
(D) Polymorphonuclear cells
(E) Endothelial cells

Questions 66–67

A 68-year-old woman suddenly develops a fever of 38.2° C and a severe headache one evening. The following morning she also experiences a stiff neck and uncharacteristic drowsiness. At the emergency room, her temperature is 38.8° C, and there is pain and resistance on flexion of her neck. The patient is noted to be mentally competent although lethargic. A cerebral spinal fluid sample is obtained by lumbar puncture.

66. On the basis of the history and physical examination of this patient, what is the most probable diagnosis?

(A) Viral meningitis
(B) Fungal meningitis
(C) Bacterial meningitis
(D) Viral encephalitis
(E) Brain abscess

67. On the basis of the patient's age, the probable etiologic agent is

(A) *Staphylococcus aureus*
(B) *Haemophilus influenzae*
(C) *Streptococcus pneumoniae*
(D) *Neisseria meningitidis*
(E) none of the above

Questions 68–70

A 48-year-old homeless man appears ataxic and confused in the emergency room. He is unshaven, mildly jaundiced, and has a bleeding scalp wound over the right frontotemporal area.

68. The physician should first

(A) ask the nurse to shower him, using antilice treatment
(B) suture his head wound
(C) order skull films
(D) obtain a serum ethanol level
(E) perform a neurologic examination

69. The patient suddenly falls into unconsciousness. The most emergent condition to assess would be

(A) subdural hematoma
(B) epidural hematoma
(C) delirium tremens
(D) hepatic encephalopathy
(E) AIDS

70. Appropriate treatment of delirium tremens includes all of the following EXCEPT

(A) monitor for generalized seizures
(B) treat with intravenous fluids
(C) monitor vital signs for autonomic arousal
(D) treat with chlordiazepoxide
(E) treat with disulfiram (Antabuse)

Questions 71–74

A previously healthy 60-year-old man collapsed while playing with his grandchildren. Although he quickly regained consciousness and became fully alert, his family called an ambulance. The emergency medical team found no abnormalities on the electrocardiogram or on physical examination. However, the patient was admitted to the coronary care unit of the local hospital. During the evening, the patient was noted to have a fast rhythm with a wide complex on his monitor followed by hypotension and loss of consciousness.

71. After electrical cardioversion with 200 watt-seconds of direct current, possible therapy may include

(A) intravenous propranolol
(B) digitalis
(C) intravenous lidocaine
(D) intravenous diltiazem
(E) epinephrine

72. Blood is drawn from the patient serially over the next 8–48 hours, and serum enzyme studies are consistent with a diagnosis of myocardial infarction. The most likely change noted was

(A) a decrease in aspartate aminotransferase
(B) an elevation in creatine kinase muscle brain isoenzyme (CK-MB)
(C) an increase in lactate dehydrogenase
(D) a decrease in pseudocholinesterase
(E) a decrease in alkaline phosphatase

73. A radionuclide scan (with technetium 99m pyrophosphate) performed in the hospital 48 hours after the initial incident indicates significant damage to the anterior wall of the left ventricle. Subsequent coronary artery angiography most likely shows occlusion of the

(A) right coronary artery
(B) left circumflex artery
(C) coronary sinuses
(D) left anterior descending coronary artery
(E) atrioventricular nodal artery

74. After being discharged from the hospital after successful coronary artery bypass surgery, the patient is placed on low-dose aspirin therapy. The rationale for selecting this therapy includes

(A) lowering the patient's body metabolism
(B) decreasing anxiety
(C) inhibiting endothelial cell prostacyclin metabolism
(D) inhibiting platelet thromboxane A_2 synthesis
(E) decreasing circulating leukotriene D_4

75. Which one of the following fatty acids found in a normal diet is metabolized by the α-hydroxylase pathway?

(A) Linoleic acid
(B) Phytanic acid
(C) Arachidonic acid
(D) Palmitic acid
(E) Decenoic acid

76. Low levels of cellular 3-hydroxy-3-methyl-glutaryl coenzyme A (HMG CoA) reductase activity in humans is most likely to result from

(A) a vegetarian diet
(B) the administration of a bile acid–sequestering resin
(C) familial hypercholesterolemia
(D) a long-term high cholesterol diet

Questions 77–78

A 35-year-old man contracts something resembling the flu, receives no treatment, and is sick for a few days. Three and one-half weeks later, he develops "a feeling of pins and needles" in his fingers and toes. Three days after that he has trouble speaking and eating, and he keeps cutting the right side of his face while shaving because "it is numb." The next day, upon waking, he has trouble with his gait. He goes to the hospital, and he tells the physician that he has never been ill before in his life. He is barely able to lift his arms to a horizontal position, and he cannot walk well. All of his tendon reflexes are absent.

77. Which one of the following diseases is the patient most likely to have?

(A) Myasthenia gravis
(B) Polio
(C) Guillain-Barré syndrome
(D) Raynaud's phenomenon

78. This disease is thought to be caused by

(A) destruction of anterior horn cells due to picornavirus infection
(B) autoantibodies to the acetylcholine (ACh) receptors
(C) damage to spinal nerves
(D) peripheral arteriosclerosis

Questions 79–83

The figure below shows flow–volume curves after inhalation to total lung capacity (TLC) and a forced expiratory maneuver to residual volume (RV) from a normal person and a patient. Absolute volume of gas within the thorax was determined independently in a body plethysmograph. The patient was a middle-aged man with a history of chronic cough with expectoration and complaints of shortness of breath and an increasing inability to exercise. In addition, a chest x-ray revealed an enlarged heart and congested lung fields with increased markings attributable to old infections.

79. From the following flow–volume curve, which of the following statements is correct regarding the patient?

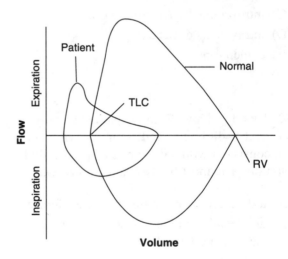

(A) TLC is greatly reduced
(B) RV is reduced
(C) Vital capacity is greatly increased
(D) Flow rate over most of expiration is less than predicted
(E) Elastic recoil of lung is likely to be greater than predicted

80. An arterial blood gas is drawn from the patient and his arterial P_{CO_2} is 50 mm Hg (normal = 40 mm Hg) and P_{O_2} is 55 mm Hg (normal is >90 mm Hg). Which of the following factors is most likely to have contributed to his CO_2 retention?

(A) A low physiological shunt
(B) An increased minute ventilation
(C) A decreased work of breathing
(D) A large increase in physiologic dead space
(E) Diminished ventilatory drive (in relation to their arterial blood gas values)

81. On examination, during inspiration, neck vein distention is noted, and an early diastolic gallop and holosystolic murmur are detected. These symptoms are likely due to

(A) atrial fibrillation
(B) tricuspid regurgitation
(C) a decrease in atrial pressure
(D) atrioventricular blockade
(E) aortic insufficiency

82. A histopathologic hallmark of the disease in this patient is

(A) caseating necrosis
(B) noncaseating granuloma
(C) hypertrophy of mucous glands
(D) thickening of the interstitium of the alveolar wall
(E) destruction of respiratory bronchioles

83. All of the following are potential contributory factors to a patient with chronic bronchitis EXCEPT

(A) smoking
(B) overproduction of α_1-antitrypsin
(C) rhinovirus infection
(D) exposure to sulfur dioxide
(E) exposure to toluene diisocyanate

Questions 84–86

A 28-year-old woman with a family history of skin cancer presented with a rapidly growing (3 to 6 months) asymptomatic lesion on her right scapular area. The lesion was brown with a bluish-red *or Black* (violaceous) color, and its border was palpably elevated.

84. The lesion described is likely to be a

(A) hemangioma
(B) pigmented basal cell carcinoma
(C) pigmented dermatofibroma
(D) melanoma
(E) subungual hematoma

85. Although a full excisional biopsy and regional lymph node excision indicate a good prognosis, several months later significant hepatic dysfunction is noted. All of the following are important biochemical changes that may have taken place within the lesion EXCEPT for the synthesis of

(A) collagenase
(B) lysosomal hydrolase
(C) plasminogen activator
(D) endothelial cell tumor adhesion-like molecules
(E) fibronectin

86. After failure to respond to high dosage chemotherapy, the woman is enrolled in an experimental adoptive immunotherapy protocol. Which of the following cytokines will be used to treat her lymphocytes, ex vivo, in an attempt to generate lymphokine-activated killer (LAK) cells?

(A) Interleukin-1
(B) Interleukin-2
(C) Interleukin-6
(D) Interferon-γ
(E) Tumor necrosis factor

87. Topoisomerase enzymes are important in the replication of DNA because they

(A) anneal Okazaki fragments
(B) relax supercoiled DNA
(C) degrade histone proteins
(D) "proofread" newly synthesized DNA
(E) synthesize the RNA primer fragment

Questions 88–90

A teenager who is below average in both weight and height is seen for complaints of vomiting of bile-stained material, abdominal distention, and pain. Further questioning reveals a periodic history of respiratory infections. Cystic fibrosis is suspected, and the diagnosis confirmed when pilocarpine iontophoresis produces an abnormally high sweat chloride concentration (> 60 mEq/L).

88. The mode of inheritance for cystic fibrosis is autosomal recessive. If the parents of the child described above are both disease-free carriers, then the chance that a sibling also has this disorder is

(A) 1/4
(B) 2/4
(C) 3/4
(D) 4/4

89. The patient is noted to have pancreatic achylia (absence of secretion of pancreatic digestive enzymes). As a result of the achylia, deficiency in absorption of which of the following vitamins may result in prolonged prothrombin times?

(A) Vitamin A
(B) Vitamin B_6
(C) Vitamin C
(D) Vitamin D
(E) Vitamin K

90. A history of frequent respiratory infections is noted in the patient. A recent sputum analysis indicates the presence of *Staphylococcus aureus*, *Haemophilus influenzae*, and *Pseudomonas aeruginosa*. Although the value of antibiotic therapy in cystic fibrosis remains unclear, a conventional approach to such therapy based on sputum culture might include

(A) gentamicin and ceftazidime
(B) nalidixic acid and kanamycin
(C) nitrofurantoin
(D) pentamidine
(E) rifampin and isoniazid

91. In the United States, the most common tumor in males is found in which one of the following organs?

(A) Kidney
(B) Colon
(C) Prostate gland
(D) Liver
(E) Testis

Questions 92–93

A patient is noted to have paroxysmal episodes of hypertension, tremor, weakness, and sweating. Urinary catecholamines and their metabolites are elevated, and a computed tomography (CT) scan of the abdomen detects a mass within the adrenal gland.

92. The tumor most likely involves which one of the following cells?

(A) Zona glomerulosa
(B) Zona fasciculata
(C) Zona reticularis
(D) Chromaffin cells of the medulla

93. If the tumor is deemed inoperable, pharmacotherapy of the above disorder may include which one of the following drugs?

(A) Clonidine
(B) Propranolol
(C) Methyldopa
(D) Phenoxybenzamine

94. Correct statements concerning toxic exposure to organophosphates include which one of the following?

(A) Aminophylline is the agent of first choice in reversing the respiratory symptoms
(B) Atropine and pralidoxime are useful antidotes
(C) Exposure must be inhalational since organophosphates are not well absorbed through the skin
(D) Immediate injection of epinephrine is a useful antidote

95. In general, tolerance to self-antigens exists, even if the antigens are not expressed in the thymus. For example, antigens on the pancreatic islet cells produce insulin. Which of the following statements is a reasonable explanation for this?

(A) Pancreatic antigens are shed and are transported to the thymus via the circulation; at the thymus, they are associated with the major histocompatibility complex (MHC) and induce positive selection of immature T cells
(B) Immature $CD4^+CD8^+$ thymic T cells are transported to the pancreas, where they undergo negative selection; they then return to the thymus for final maturation
(C) Mature T cells circulate to the pancreas, recognize pancreatic antigen in context of self MHC, which stimulates them via the T-cell receptor; however, no interleukin-1 is produced, so T cells are inactivated
(D) T-cell progenitors in the bone marrow circulate to the pancreas before being transported to the thymus; they undergo negative selection at the pancreas and then proceed to the thymus where T-cell differentiation occurs

96. Which of the following structural motifs is important for the transcriptional activation produced by some steroid-bound hormone receptors?

(A) zinc fingers
(B) EF hands
(C) β-pleated sheets
(D) immunoglobulin folds
(E) gly-X-Y repeats

DIRECTIONS: Each of the numbered items or incomplete statements in this section is negatively phrased, as indicated by a capitalized word such as NOT, LEAST, or EXCEPT. Select the ONE lettered answer or completion that is BEST in each case.

97. The retroviruses have many unique biologic and biochemical features. All of the following are properties of the retroviruses EXCEPT

(A) they are genetically diploid
(B) the particles contain an RNA-dependent DNA polymerase
(C) they require integration into the host genome for proper replication
(D) the RNA has minus polarity
(E) the retroviral group antigens are highly reactive between strains

98. All of the following complications are common in patients with chronic hemolytic anemias EXCEPT

(A) cardiac arrhythmias
(B) emphysema
(C) congestive heart failure
(D) severe infection by encapsulated organisms
(E) chronic liver failure

99. All of the following statements about immunoglobulin classes are correctly paired with a characteristic feature EXCEPT

(A) immunoglobulin A (IgA) is found in mucosal secretions from the breast, gut, and respiratory tract
(B) immunoglobulin G (IgG) crosses the placenta
(C) immunoglobulin M (IgM), frequently found as a pentamer, efficiently activates the complement cascade
(D) immunoglobulin D (IgD) antibodies against IgG are present in high titers in many patients with rheumatoid arthritis
(E) immunoglobulin E (IgE) mediates type I hypersensitivity by activating mast cells and basophils

100. All of the following statements concerning hemoglobin genes and thalassemia are correct EXCEPT

(A) normal individuals inherit four copies of the α-chain, two from each parent
(B) most α-thalassemias involve deletions of α-chain genes due to a nonhomologous crossover
(C) α-thalassemias vary in severity depending on the number of defective α-chain genes
(D) α-thalassemias are sex-linked because the α-chain genes are located on the X-chromosome
(E) α-chain abnormalities can generally be confirmed by the use of restriction endonucleases

101. All of the following statements about multiple endocrine neoplasia (MEN) type IIb are correct EXCEPT

(A) pheochromocytoma and the accompanying sympathomimetic signs are a common presentation
(B) the disorder is hereditary, and the gene has been mapped to chromosome 10
(C) some research suggests that the neoplastic clones may have arisen from abnormal neural crest cells
(D) neuromas of the conjunctival, labial, and buccal mucosa are not unusual
(E) Zollinger-Ellison syndrome is present in about 20% of cases

102. All of the following are characteristics of nephrotic syndrome EXCEPT

(A) proteinuria
(B) hematuria
(C) generalized edema
(D) hyperlipidemia
(E) focal segmental glomerulosclerosis

103. All of the following may result from chronic alcohol abuse EXCEPT

(A) cerebellar degeneration and ataxia
(B) esophagitis and Mallory-Weiss tears
(C) testicular atrophy or amenorrhea
(D) mild-to-moderate hypertension and elevated serum triglycerides
(E) bronchogenic carcinoma

104. Acute pancreatitis is associated with all of the following EXCEPT

(A) alcohol ingestion
(B) biliary tract disease
(C) elevated serum triglycerides
(D) α_1-antitrypsin deficiency
(E) major abdominal surgery or trauma

105. All of the following statements describe the biologic properties of immunoglobulin E (IgE) EXCEPT

(A) it has the shortest half-life of all classes of immunoglobulins
(B) low levels of circulating IgE are due in part to the high-affinity binding of the Fc portion to mast cells and basophils
(C) it can cause agglutination of particulate antigens
(D) it is elevated in cases of certain parasitic infections

106. A patient hospitalized for multiple fractures was placed on a prophylactic antibiotic. Two days prior to discharge, diarrhea developed, requiring intravenous rehydration. The antibiotic was changed to a broad-spectrum cephalosporin, but diarrhea continued and the patient's condition deteriorated. All of the following actions are appropriate EXCEPT

(A) sigmoidoscopic examination
(B) proper isolation of the patient
(C) Gram stain of feces for white blood cells
(D) a request for *Clostridium difficile* toxin test
(E) changing the antibiotic to clindamycin

107. Agnogenic myeloid metaplasia with myelofibrosis is characterized by all of the following features EXCEPT

(A) hypocellular bone marrow
(B) normal levels of leukocyte alkaline phosphatase
(C) teardrop-shaped erythrocytes
(D) hepatomegaly
(E) splenomegaly

108. All of the following characteristics of warfarin are accurate EXCEPT

(A) it is useful in pregnant women because it does not cross the placenta
(B) it affects hepatic synthesis of clotting factors present in blood
(C) it is effective after oral administration
(D) it is primarily used in chronic therapy
(E) therapy can be reversed by administration of vitamin K

109. Each of the following enzymes is essential for protecting red blood cells from the hydrogen peroxide generated in vivo EXCEPT

(A) glutathione peroxidase
(B) 6-phosphogluconate dehydrogenase
(C) catalase
(D) transketolase
(E) glutathione reductase

110. All of the following statements concerning the Arthus reaction are true EXCEPT

(A) it usually requires large amounts of antibody and antigen
(B) it results in localized rupture of vessel walls followed by tissue necrosis
(C) neutrophils and platelets are present at the site of the reaction
(D) it is the most common type III reaction seen in humans

111. Zidovudine (ZDV) [formerly known as azidothymidine (AZT)] has all of the following properties EXCEPT

(A) ZDV reduces the chances of progression to AIDS in asymptomatic HIV-infected subjects
(B) ZDV improves the clinical symptoms of immunologic function, survival period, and quality of life of advanced AIDS patients
(C) ZDV is very toxic to bone marrow
(D) ZDV is effective only in the treatment of patients with advanced AIDS
(E) prolonged treatment with ZDV (1–3 years) results in resistance to this drug

112. All of the following mediators released during mast cell activation cause an increase of vascular permeability EXCEPT

(A) histamine
(B) eosinophil chemotactic factor (ECF)
(C) serotonin
(D) slow-reacting substance of anaphylaxis

113. Major risk factors for the development of chronic obstructive pulmonary disease (COPD) include all of the following EXCEPT

(A) smoking
(B) air pollution
(C) occupational exposure to irritant gases and particles
(D) α_1-antitrypsin deficiency
(E) intravenous drug abuse

114. Characteristics of Duchenne muscular dystrophy (DMD) include all of the following EXCEPT

(A) decreased amounts of dystrophin in affected muscles
(B) hypertrophy of affected muscle groups
(C) autosomal dominant inheritance via mutated chromosome 20
(D) one-third of the cases resulting from spontaneous mutation
(E) sarcomere hypercontraction and contraction band formation

115. A young child develops pharyngitis, a fever, and a rash. β-Hemolytic, gram-positive cocci in chains are isolated from the throat and are found to be catalase-negative. All of the following statements about the virulence factors of this pathogen are true EXCEPT

(A) hemolysis results from production of extra-cellular hemolysins
(B) the organism produces membrane-bound protein (M protein), which has antiphago-cytic properties
(C) the organism produces lipoteichoic acid, which is necessary for attachment to mucosa
(D) the organism is not encapsulated
(E) the rash is produced by a toxin distinct from the hemolysins

116. Cushing's syndrome is a complex array of symptoms that are due to excess glucocorticoid levels. All of the following statements about Cushing's syndrome are correct EXCEPT

(A) the disease may be associated with an ade-noma of the pituitary corticotropes
(B) the disease may be secondary to abnormal hypothalamic function with excessive re-lease of corticotropin releasing factor (CRF)
(C) the disease may be due to ectopic adrenocor-ticotropic hormone (ACTH) synthesis
(D) some aspects of the syndrome may be due to long-term therapy with glucocorticoids
(E) increased long bone length is common in pa-tients prior to puberty

117. All of the following statements about pro-tein synthesis are true EXCEPT

(A) the activated form of an amino acid is called aminoacyl transfer RNA (tRNA)
(B) the addition of aminoacyl tRNA to the grow-ing peptide chain and subsequent transloca-tion is an energy-requiring process
(C) the formation of the peptide bond is catalyzed by peptidyltransferase
(D) synthesis occurs in the mitochondria as well as in the cytoplasm of cells
(E) synthesis can occur in the absence of RNA

118. Each statement below concerning osteo-clasts is true EXCEPT that they

(A) are found in Howship's lacuna
(B) resorb bone
(C) are stimulated by calcitonin
(D) are multinucleated
(E) help remodel bone

119. Asymptomatic bacteriuria is noted in a 35-year-old pregnant woman in her second trimester. Five years ago, during her first pregnancy, she presented with acute pyelonephritis, which re-quired hospitalization and parenteral antibacterial therapy. Since then, recurrent sexual intercourse–related urinary tract infections have been pre-vented by a single dose of nitrofurantoin after coitus. All of the following agents would be con-traindicated for this patient during the remainder of her pregnancy for prevention of acute pyelone-phritis EXCEPT

(A) trimethoprim/sulfamethoxazole
(B) minocycline
(C) amoxicillin
(D) gentamicin

120. Thymomas are associated with all of the following diseases EXCEPT

(A) myasthenia gravis

(B) systemic lupus erythematosus

(C) hypogammaglobulinemia

(D) Graves' disease

(E) neutrophil agranulocytosis

(F) polymyositis

121. All of the following statements concerning the human immunodeficiency virus (HIV) are true EXCEPT that

(A) the virus can infect T cells, macrophages, and any other cell type with a CD4 receptor

(B) viral infection can spread between cells without the involvement of free virus

(C) the viral infection process involves endocytosis of the HIV particle into the cell

(D) replication of the viral nucleic acid occurs in the nucleus

122. For antibiotic therapy, it is useful to understand both the action of the prescribed antibiotic and the pathogenesis of the bacteria responsible for a patient's infection. For example, the aminoglycoside antibiotic gentamicin does not enter mammalian cells and, therefore, is ineffective against intracellular pathogens. Considering only this information, gentamicin is effective against all of the following infections EXCEPT

(A) *Haemophilus influenzae* type B epiglottitis

(B) *Pseudomonas aeruginosa* burn infections

(C) *Klebsiella pneumoniae* respiratory infections

(D) *Escherichia coli* urinary tract infections

(E) *Chlamydia trachomatis* infections

DIRECTIONS: Each set of matching questions in this section consists of a list of four to twenty-six lettered options (some of which may be in figures) followed by several numbered items. For each numbered item, select the ONE lettered option that is most closely associated with it. To avoid spending too much time on matching sets with large numbers of options, it is generally advisable to begin each set by reading the list of options. Then, for each item in the set, try to generate the correct answer and locate it in the option list, rather than evaluating each option individually. Each lettered option may be selected once, more than once, or not at all.

Questions 123–127

For each area of the brain listed below, select the most appropriate test for functional evaluation. (The patient's language function is assumed to be normal.)

(A) Recall of four items after 5 minutes

(B) Repetition of digits, forward and reversed

(C) Interpretation of proverbs

(D) Serial 7's subtraction

(E) Copying simple shapes and objects

123. Visual cortex; visual association areas of parietal lobe; motor areas of frontal lobe

124. Pontine and midbrain reticular activating system (RAS)

125. Prefrontal cortex

126. Left hippocampus and temporal lobe

127. RAS; left parietal lobe; hippocampus and other cortical and subcortical memory areas

Questions 128–131

Match each of the following measurements with the corresponding letter on the diagram of a typical pulmonary function trace, which is shown below.

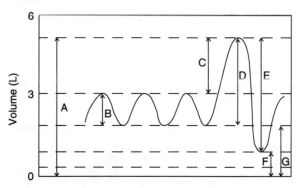

128. Residual volume

129. Tidal volume

130. Vital capacity

131. Functional residual capacity

Questions 132–136

Match each treatment technique with the school of family therapy most associated with that technique.

(A) Behavioral–psychoeducational approaches
(B) Structural–strategic approaches
(C) Intergenerational–experiential approaches
(D) Sociobiological approaches

132. Clarification of transgenerational relationship patterns

133. Clarification of relationship patterns within the nuclear family

134. Training in social learning theory

135. Cognitive reframing

136. Elaboration of the family's identity

Questions 137–139

Match each description below with the most appropriate abdominal fascia.

(A) Camper's fascia
(B) Scarpa's fascia
(C) Both
(D) Neither

137. Prominent over the abdominal wall

138. Supports sutures

139. Called Colles' fascia in the perineum

Questions 140–144

A 15-year-old boy develops insulin-dependent diabetes mellitus (IDDM). His parents want to know the risk of their other children developing diabetes. The pedigree below was developed for the family. Match each of the affected son's siblings in the pedigree to the best estimate of risk.

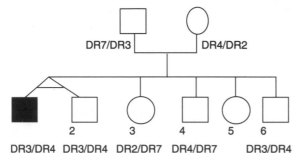

DR3/DR4   DR3/DR4   DR2/DR7   DR4/DR7   DR3/DR4

(A) 2%
(B) 5%
(C) 20%
(D) 50%
(E) 100%

50% 140. The proband's monozygous twin (II-2)

141. The proband's sister with human leukocyte antigen (HLA) DR2/DR7 (II-3)

142. The proband's brother with HLA DR4/DR7 (II-4)

5% 143. The proband's sister for whom no HLA typing is available (II-5)

144. The proband's brother with HLA DR3/DR4 (II-6)

Questions 145–149

Match each of the following clinical or pathological descriptions with the appropriate heavy metal.

(A) Arsenic
(B) Lead
(C) Tin
(D) Cadmium
(E) Mercury

145. Intense exposure to the vapor causes acute interstitial pneumonitis

146. Inorganic form commonly used in insecticides and rodenticides; gas is produced in smelting and refining of metals and causes severe hemolysis and hematuria

147. Produced epidemic levels of disease in preschool children; with chronic exposure, it causes cognitive impairment, language dysfunction, and, when severe, mental retardation

148. Chronic exposure to vapors leads to neurologic symptoms including insomnia, excitability, and memory loss

149. Uncouples oxidation and phosphorylation in glycolysis by forming an unstable acyl intermediate

Questions 150–154

Match each of the following descriptions of cell signalling with the hormones or cells identified in the figure.

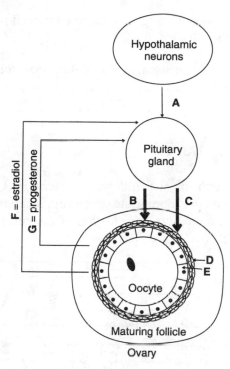

150. Responds to luteinizing hormone (LH) with increased synthesis of androstenedione and testosterone, which are used as substrates for estradiol synthesis

151. Increases pituitary responsiveness to gonadotropin-releasing hormone (GnRH) during the follicular phase in preparation for the LH surge

152. Elicits the correct response only when secreted in a pulsatile manner; precocious sexual development can be arrested by constant infusion of a synthetic analogue

153. Causes ovulation at midcycle

154. Estradiol and inhibin act together to decrease the pituitary gland's synthesis of this hormone

Questions 155–158

For each characteristic of lung carcinoma listed below, select the corresponding tumor.

(A) Adenocarcinoma
(B) Squamous cell carcinoma
(C) Small cell carcinoma
(D) Bronchioloalveolar adenocarcinoma

155. Associated with the *ras* oncogene amplification and mutation

156. Presence of neurosecretory granules

157. Similar to jaagsiekte disease in sheep

158. Association with the *myc* oncogene amplification and mutation

Questions 159–163

Match the following biochemical activities or nutritional information with the appropriate vitamin.

(A) Vitamin A
(B) B vitamins
(C) Vitamin C
(D) Vitamin D
(E) Vitamin E
(F) Vitamin K

159. Source of a methyl group in the synthesis of methionine from homocysteine

160. Lipid-soluble antioxidant whose use in Parkinson's disease is being studied

161. Water-soluble reducing agent in the hydroxylation of amino acids

162. Precursor of visual pigments; derivatives are used to treat cystic acne

163. Precursor for the electron transport moiety in flavin nucleotides

Questions 164–168

A deranged former employee snuck into the hospital nursery and clipped the identification bracelets from five newborn boys. To correct the situation, blood typing has been done on the infants and their parents. Match the following parents to the correct infant.

(A) Infant A: O, MN, Rh$^+$
(B) Infant B: A, MN, Rh$^-$
(C) Infant C: A, M, Rh$^+$
(D) Infant D: AB, N, Rh$^+$
(E) Infant E: B, MN, Rh$^+$

	Mother Blood Group			Father Blood Group		
Family	**ABO**	**MN**	**Rh**	**ABO**	**MN**	**Rh**
164.	B	N	Rh$^-$	A	MN	Rh$^-$
165.	B	N	Rh$^+$	AB	N	Rh$^-$
166.	AB	MN	Rh$^+$	O	MN	Rh$^+$
167.	O	M	Rh$^+$	A	M	Rh$^+$
168.	A	M	Rh$^+$	A	N	Rh$^+$

Questions 169–172

Match each description with the psychosocial stage of cancer it best characterizes.

(A) Diagnosis
(B) Treatment
(C) Remission *– decrease in pain + symptom*
(D) Recurrence
(E) Terminal phase

169. Period of short-term focus, when palliation of pain and patient support are paramount

170. Period during which denial may prevent proper management

171. Anxious waiting may cause emotional pain during this phase

172. Malaise, nausea, and vomiting may foster noncompliance

Questions 173–177

Match each of the following descriptions or events with the appropriate structure or location in the diagrammatic representation of the cell pictured below.

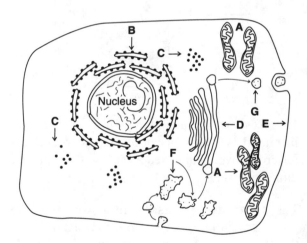

173. O-linked glycosylation as well as acylation and sorting of many proteins

174. Translation of hexokinase

175. Ultimate destination for cytosolically synthesized proteins with special amino-terminal sequence signals

176. Ultimate destination for proteins with mannose 6-phosphate signals

177. Translation of proteins with signal sequences

Questions 178–182

Match each of the following diseases that affect the brain with its most characteristic neuropathologic finding.

(A) Lewy bodies
(B) Hippocampal neurofibrillary tangles
(C) Argentophilic intraneuronal inclusions
(D) Prions
(E) Multinucleated giant cells

178. Alzheimer's dementia

179. AIDS

180. Parkinson's disease

181. Creutzfeldt-Jakob disease

182. Pick's disease

Questions 183–187

Using the following diagrammatic representation of nucleic pre-messenger RNA, match the following descriptions with the correct lettered structure.

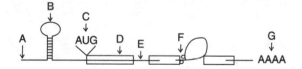

183. Site of translation initiation once the message has entered the cytoplasm

184. Site of autocatalytic activity of some RNA molecules; small nuclear ribonucleoproteins (snRNPs) can bind here

185. Site of specially modified base (N7-methylguanylate)

186. Secondary structural motif which has different functions in different messages, for example preventing message breakdown or hiding initiation sequences

187. Post-transcriptional modification of variable length; the length is probably related to the message's half-life

Questions 188–192

Match each of the following descriptions of neurochemistry with the enzyme that is most likely to be associated with it.

(A) Tyrosine hydroxylase
(B) Monoamine oxidase (MAO)
(C) Choline acetyltransferase
(D) Tryptophan-5-hydroxylase
(E) Catechol-O-methyltransferase

188. Decreased in Alzheimer's dementia

189. Rate-limiting step for catecholamine synthesis

190. Located on the mitochondrial membrane

191. Levels increase with increasing age

192. Found in neurons of the dorsal raphe nuclei

Questions 193–195

Match each phrase describing a feature of inflammatory heart disease with the disease it characterizes.

(A) Acute rheumatic fever

(B) Chronic rheumatic heart disease

(C) Acute bacterial endocarditis

(D) Subacute bacterial endocarditis

(E) Libman-Sacks endocarditis

193. Fusion of the commissures

194. Infection by group A β-hemolytic streptococci

195. Infection by α-hemolytic (viridans) streptococci

Questions 196–200

Match each of the following hormones with its function in the pregnant woman and fetus.

(A) Human chorionic gonadotropin (hCG)

(B) Human chorionic somatomammotropin (hCS)

(C) Progesterone

(D) Estrogens (estradiol, estriol)

(E) Prolactin

(F) Relaxin

196. The principal substrate for cortisol and aldosterone production by the fetal adrenal gland

197. Stimulates continuous growth of the uterine myometrium

198. Stimulates corpus luteum production of progesterone and estradiol

199. Suppresses pituitary luteinizing hormone (LH) secretion; stimulates milk production

200. Stimulates development of ductal tissue in the breast

ANSWER KEY

1-D	30-C	59-B	88-A	117-E
2-B	31-E	60-C	89-E	118-C
3-C	32-A	61-B	90-A	119-C
4-E	33-C	62-D	91-C	120-D
5-A	34-A	63-D	92-D	121-C
6-A	35-D	64-E	93-D	122-E
7-E	36-E	65-A	94-B	123-E
8-C	37-B	66-C	95-C	124-B
9-D	38-A	67-C	96-A	125-C
10-B	39-C	68-E	97-D	126-A
11-D	40-E	69-B	98-B	127-D
12-A	41-D	70-E	99-D	128-F
13-C	42-C	71-C	100-D	129-B
14-E	43-D	72-B	101-E	130-E
15-B	44-A	73-D	102-B	131-G
16-A	45-D	74-D	103-E	132-C
17-E	46-D	75-B	104-D	133-B
18-C	47-C	76-D	105-C	134-A
19-D	48-A	77-C	106-E	135-B
20-D	49-B	78-C	107-D	136-C
21-A	50-C	79-D	108-A	137-C
22-C	51-E	80-E	109-D	138-B
23-D	52-A	81-B	110-D	139-B
24-C	53-D	82-C	111-D	140-D
25-E	54-D	83-B	112-B	141-A
26-B	55-A	84-D	113-E	142-B
27-A	56-E	85-D	114-C	143-B
28-E	57-C	86-B	115-D	144-C
29-B	58-B	87-B	116-E	145-E

146-A	157-D	168-A	179-E	190-B
147-B	158-C	169-E	180-A	191-B
148-E	159-B	170-A	181-D	192-D
149-A	160-E	171-C	182-C	193-B
150-D	161-C	172-B	183-C	194-A
151-F	162-A	173-D	184-F	195-D
152-A	163-B	174-C	185-A	196-C
153-B	164-B	175-A	186-B	197-D
154-C	165-D	176-F	187-G	198-A
155-A	166-E	177-B	188-C	199-E
156-C	167-C	178-B	189-A	200-D

ANSWERS AND EXPLANATIONS

1–3. The answers are: 1-D, 2-B, 3-C. *(Sepsis following severe burn)*
Pseudomonas aeruginosa is a major cause of sepsis in burn patients. The bacterium is ubiquitous in the environment and is a member of the indigenous flora of some people. Once it gains entry through the physical barrier of the skin, *P. aeruginosa* causes significant tissue damage. It is capable of invading the epithelium of blood vessels, leading to repeated seeding of the bloodstream. *Serratia marcescens* is a leading cause of sepsis and urinary tract infections in patients with indwelling catheters. *Nocardia asteroides* is seen primarily in patients receiving long-term antirejection therapy. *Staphylococcus aureus* causes localized skin infections and deep abscesses associated with foreign bodies. *Streptococcus pneumoniae* causes pneumonia in patients with underlying diseases affecting antibody production and cell-mediated immunity; patients with splenectomy are particularly at risk.

Patients with burns over more than 20% of their body demonstrate a lack of chemotactic activity of mononuclear leukocytes 15 to 45 days after the thermal injury. Inhibition of activity corresponds to the appearance of a chemotactic inhibitor in the serum. An inability to produce opsonin antibodies and a decrease in the production of immunoglobulin M (IgM) are associated with splenectomy. A decrease in the number of circulating segmented neutrophils occurs during bone marrow failure. Bruton's agammaglobulinemia is a sex-linked genetic dysfunction.

Pseudomonas aeruginosa and other pseudomonads frequently display multiple drug resistance. The mortality rate in pseudomonas septicemia approaches 80%. A new group of antibiotics, the quinolones, have shown good in vitro activity against *P. aeruginosa;* the number of cases of disease successfully treated with the quinolones is increasing. Imidazole antibiotics and amphotericin B are antifungal agents; the imidazoles are now considered alternatives to amphotericin B therapy in some mycoses. Immune modulators, such as thymosin and interferon, have shown potential in treating infections controlled by the cell-mediated immune system.

4–5. The answers are: 4-E, 5-A. *(Carcinoembryonic antigen analysis)*
Carcinoembryonic antigen (CEA) is associated with carcinoma of the colon and pancreas; however, because CEA also occurs in nonmalignant conditions (e.g., as a result of cigarette smoking), it is not considered to be diagnostic of, but merely suggestive of, a cancerous condition. Assays for CEA show their greatest promise in monitoring for the recurrence of certain malignancies after surgery or chemotherapy.

The presence of CEA in the serum is correlated with the tumor burden of the host. The higher the level of CEA, the greater is the patient's tumor mass. Following surgical excision of the tumor, the CEA level should drop very low, perhaps even to indiscernible levels. If the CEA level increases again, it suggests that the tumor has metastasized and appropriate therapeutic or surgical intervention is indicated. The patient presented in the questions is gravely ill. Surgical removal of the tumor was incomplete, and metastases have developed, as indicated by the rise in CEA in months 10 to 12. The chemotherapeutic regimen should be reevaluated, and the patient should be thoroughly examined for possible radiologic and surgical treatment.

6–10. The answers are: 6-A, 7-E, 8-C, 9-D, 10-B. *(HIV, AIDS)*
An enzyme-linked immunosorbent assay (ELISA) for anti-HIV antibody is the mainstay in screening for HIV. ELISA is relatively sensitive (as any screening should be), but its low specificity requires confirmation with a Western blot for the anti-HIV antibody. A Western blot for viral proteins is not effective. Although viral proteins do circulate in the serum of infected individuals, the concentration of antigen is not detectable. The absolute number of CD4+ lymphocytes is used to monitor the progress of HIV-infected patients but is not particularly useful as a screening tool. In most cases, any substantial loss of T4 cells occurs many years after infection. Polymerase chain reaction (PCR) techniques, which allow extremely sensitive detection of a small fragment of viral (or any) DNA sequence, are currently being investigated as a potential tool in screening for

HIV infection. A complete blood count with standard differential is not useful in the diagnosis of HIV infection because decreases in the number of white blood cells differentiated by routine light microscopy occur only late in the disease. Furthermore, elevations in the white cell count can be indicative of a host of inflammatory processes, which may or may not be related to HIV.

Opportunistic infections, by definition, do not normally occur in immunocompetent individuals. Therefore, *Staphylococcus aureus* osteoarthritis, which is an extremely severe and relatively common infection in anyone who has suffered traumatic injury to a joint, is not opportunistic. *Pneumocystis carinii* is the most common opportunistic infection in AIDS patients, and it is seen in more than 80% of HIV-infected individuals at some point during the course of their disease. *Candida albicans* thrush or esophagitis, disseminated *Mycobacterium avium intracellulare*, and *Cryptococcus neoformans* meningitis are familiar sources of morbidity and mortality in people suffering from AIDS.

Patients who have had a previous infection with *Pneumocystis* pneumonia or those who have the low number of CD4+ cells cited above are placed on prophylactic regimens of aerosolized pentamidine. *P. carinii* infection is a common presentation for a new case of AIDS, and this opportunistic parasite is a significant source of AIDS morbidity and mortality. Trimethoprim–sulfamethoxazole (Bactrim) is an effective therapy for *P. carinii* infection as well as a mainstay in some opportunistic infections of the gut. Ganciclovir is required as lifelong maintenance therapy once an AIDS patient has been infected with cytomegalovirus. However, ganciclovir prophylaxis is not recommended. Acyclovir therapy is only indicated in active herpes simplex infections. Doxorubicin therapy has resulted in transient improvement in active Kaposi's sarcoma; however, all chemotherapies are immunosuppressive and therefore of questionable value in HIV-infected patients. Treatment of active Kaposi's sarcoma is only indicated for cosmetic or functional reasons; prophylactic therapy for Kaposi's sarcoma is never indicated.

The HIV-1 virus is a cytopathic member of the lentiviruses; it lyses T lymphocytes in culture whereas its sister virus human T-cell lymphotrophic virus (HTLV) transforms them into an immortal cell line. The two viruses are related by the enzyme reverse transcriptase, which uses the viral RNA genome to synthesize linear DNA. The DNA is incorporated into the cellular genome via recombination and forms a template for normal mammalian replication processes. Once incorporated, the viral DNA is replicated and given to all of the cell's progeny. New strategies for intervention are focused on more effective chronic therapy for infected people and vaccination for uninfected people. Lysis of an infected cell results in a prolific release of viral progeny that are capable of infecting a large number of uninfected T4-helper cells. Direct contact is not required, and research efforts toward binding these free particles with soluble CD4 antigen may prove fruitful. The envelope proteins, including gp 120, are important in the binding, entry, and uncoating of the virus. The gp 120 envelope protein is involved in the recognition of the CD4 antigen. Efforts to develop an effective vaccine have been elusive because the envelope antigens are subject to frequent mutation. This high rate of mutation is probably the result of selection pressure, which favors a viral transcriptase prone to frequent error. Most other DNA-synthesizing enzymes (including all of the DNA synthases in healthy mammalian cells) have extensive proofreading mechanisms, which HIV reverse transcriptase lacks.

Fully developed AIDS is associated with lysis and death of CD4+ lymphocytes, the T4-helper cells. The disease is staged, and therapy is indexed by the absolute number of circulating T4 cells. No T4 leukemias or lymphomas have been reported to date. A closely related virus, the HTLV-1, does cause T-cell leukemias and lymphomas; however, this virus is a transforming virus not a cytopathic virus like HIV. AIDS-related dementia is probably associated with HIV infection of microglia, which are monocytes in the central nervous system. The dementia clinically manifests in 70% of AIDS patients, and neuropathologic lesions are present in 80%–90% of autopsies in AIDS victims. Kaposi's sarcoma is another regular feature of AIDS whose cause remains enigmatic. The polyclonal activation of B lymphocytes and non-Hodgkins (B-cell) lymphomas may be different manifestations of a common problem, but further research is needed to clarify the pathologic process of these two problems familiar to many AIDS patients.

11–15. The answers are: 11-D, 12-A, 13-C, 14-E, 15-B. (*Glucose 6-phosphate dehydrogenase deficiency, hemolytic anemia*)

Pallor under the tongue, delayed capillary refill in the nailbeds, and, in Caucasian people, general lack of color are indicative of anemia. The acute onset, obvious signs of jaundice, the patient's race, and the recent prescription of primaquine indicate acute hemolytic anemia resulting from glucose 6-phosphate dehydrogenase deficiency. The patient's tachycardia and tachypnea are a reflection of the sympathetic activation produced by inadequate tissue oxygenation. Such sympathetic activation is not unusual, and some patients with more chronic hemolytic anemias develop prominent high-output S3 flow murmurs as a result of chronic hypoxia. Wilson's disease is a complex of symptoms (primarily liver and pancreatic failure) related to the inappropriate storage of copper; jaundice (but not hemolysis) develops over time in a patient with Wilson's disease. Polycythemia vera is the neoplastic growth of hematopoietic stem cells, which gives rise to an unregulated excess of the cellular components of blood; platelets, erythrocytes, and lymphocytes can be elevated individually or in combination. Disseminated intravascular coagulation occurs when the clotting cascade is inappropriately activated and platelets (not erythrocytes) are depleted to a dangerous low. Hereditary spherocytosis does cause hemolytic anemia, but the disease is not generally triggered but rather is present early in adulthood. The anemia is a chronic, lifelong anemia secondary to a defect in the plasma membrane of the erythrocytes. The name spherocytosis reflects the odd appearance of the erythrocytes in the peripheral smears from these patients.

Unconjugated bilirubin is an accurate indicator of hemolysis; erythrocyte lysis releases heme proteins into the blood, where they are degraded to bilirubin. During an episode of acute hemolysis, the capacity of the liver to conjugate bilirubin with glucuronate is soon exceeded and unconjugated bilirubin rises dramatically. The hemoglobin–hematocrit test is useful in differentiating hemolysis as a cause for elevated unconjugated bilirubin from other disease states (e.g., acute liver failure). If the results of the hemoglobin–hematocrit test are low, elevated unconjugated bilirubin is a relatively specific indicator of hemolysis. A bone marrow biopsy is rarely indicated as an initial test in the evaluation of a probable anemia. Hemoglobin electrophoresis, whereas it is extremely useful in diagnosing hemoglobinopathies, is very expensive and rarely indicated until a hemoglobinopathy is almost certain. Although the peripheral smear should certainly be ordered in the evaluation of any problem involving the blood, it is not reasonable for it to be paired with a bone marrow biopsy or hemoglobin electrophoresis. The correct pair of tests would more specifically rule in hemolysis. Serum transaminases are reliable indicators of damage to hepatocytes; however, in this patient, there is sufficient evidence to indicate that his jaundice and icterus are not related to primary liver failure. Prothrombin time is useful for evaluating a suspected coagulopathy not an anemia. A complete blood count would be useful in this patient, but, again, it was not reasonably paired with another useful test.

Uroporphyrinogen synthase is an enzyme involved in the erythrocyte's synthesis of heme rings. Defects in this enzyme result in ineffective erythropoiesis not hemolysis. Hexokinase is the enzyme that phosphorylates glucose in most of the cells of the body, thus trapping glucose with negative charge and beginning the glycolytic process. A substantial defect in hexokinase manifests itself in infancy. Thymidine kinase is involved in the synthesis of nucleotides. It is especially significant because acyclovir, an antiviral medication commonly used for herpes infections, specifically targets the viral but not the mammalian form of the enzyme. Ribonucleotide reductase is also involved in nucleotide biosynthesis. A tolerable deficiency in either of these enzymes is imaginable, especially as a side effect of a potential chemotherapeutic; however, the resultant anemia would probably not be acute in onset, and it would reflect ineffective erythropoiesis not hemolysis.

Glucose 6-phosphate dehydrogenase is an enzyme in the pentose phosphate pathway, which is also known as the hexose monophosphate shunt. This pathway is essential in both erythrocytes and the liver as an important source of the reduced form of nicotinamide–adenine dinucleotide phosphate (NADPH). This reducing equivalent is absolutely essential for maintaining an adequate supply of reduced glutathione, which in turn is used by the various enzyme systems that catalyze the removal of oxygen free radicals (e.g.,

oxygen
free radicals

superoxide dismutase, catalase). Oxygen free radicals are continuously generated by most cells of the body as an ordinary part of metabolism and cell signalling. Normally, the NADPH generated by the hexose monophosphate shunt sufficiently maintains a quantity of reduced glutathione so that these free radicals are easily neutralized. However, the extra stress of primaquine metabolism (which generates additional free radicals) taxed this patient's inadequate system beyond its limits. Older erythrocytes are more easily damaged by the oxygen free radicals because their membranes have already been subjected to more damage. Furthermore, the enzymes in the pathway seem to lose their efficiency over time. None of the other answers provide a reasonable explanation for an acute hemolytic crisis.

The gene that encodes glucose 6-phosphate dehydrogenase is located on the X chromosome. Therefore, males have only one copy, and a defective gene always leads to a phenotypic expression. X-chromosome inactivation (i.e., Barr body formation) in the cells of normal women results in insufficient activity in some erythrocytes. However, random processes generally leave heterozygous women with an adequately large pool of normal erythrocytes so that their phenotype is normal. Thus, glucose 6-phosphate dehydrogenase deficiency is sex-linked, and this hereditary trait occurs in 15% of African–American males. Research indicates that the trait may make erythrocytes less susceptible to infection by *Plasmodium falciparum* and thus has been selected in areas with endemic malaria. The hereditary trait cannot be more common in women because it is sex-linked. Crohn's disease, an inflammatory bowel disease, is one of the several hereditary conditions that is more commonly seen in the population of Ashkenazic Jews.

16–19. The answers are: 16-A, 17-E, 18-C, 19-D. (*β-thalassemia genetics and pathology*)
Hemoglobin A (Hb A) is the normal hemoglobin tetramer with a subunit stoichiometry of $\alpha_2\beta_2$ and most individuals have a hemoglobin composition with 97% Hb A. Hemoglobin A_2 has a subunit stoichiometry of $\alpha_2\delta_2$ and normally accounts for less than 3% of total hemoglobin. Normal adults usually have less than 1% of their total hemoglobin comprised of the fetal form (i.e., Hb F), which has the subtypes $\alpha_2\gamma_2$. Infants with β-thalassemia major usually present after the sixth month, when the hemoglobin promoters gradually switch from γ subunit production (for Hb F) to β subunit production (for Hb A). White people of Mediterranean descent have the highest carrier frequency, and the heterozygous state is also relatively common in people from central Africa, Asia, and parts of India. Jaundiced skin, icterus, elevated unconjugated bilirubin, and pallor under the tongue are a relatively specific indication of hemolytic anemia. The infant's failure to thrive indicates a chronic course that is now emerging. The peripheral smear indicates a hypochromic anemia but specifically lacks evidence of spherocytosis or sickle cell anemia. In addition, sickle cell disease is rare in a female infant because it is sex-linked. Spherocytosis has a much more chronic course that often emerges in the second or third decade of life. Iron deficiency is a possibility, but ineffective erythropoiesis is not the only problem; iron deficiency does not cause hemolysis. The unconjugated bilirubin and teardrop cells indicate active destruction as well as ineffective erythropoiesis; therefore, iron deficiency is not a sufficient explanation. The inherited form of methemoglobinemia causes an anemia that is much less severe than the one described and would probably not be noted except as an incidental finding on routine evaluation.

The thalassemias are diseases in which there is a quantitative problem in hemoglobin subunit synthesis: One of the protein subunits is not produced in sufficient quantity to correctly pair with the other. β-thalassemia major, in which two defective β-subunit genes are inherited, is almost never due to a major deletion or major gene rearrangement event. This is clinically significant because standard restriction fragment length polymorphism (RFLP) testing is very sensitive to such major changes in the gene structure. Because α-thalassemia is almost always caused by major structural changes to the gene, a patient with suspected α-thalassemia can generally be diagnosed with standard RFLP. Diagnosis of β-thalassemia can require more sophisticated linkage analysis to identify the polymorphisms that are transmitted with the thalassemia trait. Each of the listed abnormalities in the β-globin gene can give rise to the disease. A nonsense mutation is usually caused by a point mutation leading to an inappropriate stop codon; thus a nonsense mutation in a globin-chain gene and a point mutation in the coding region of a globin-chain gene are essentially the same. The β-globin gene has a number of introns, so abnormal splice variants are also a common cause. Defective sequences in the promoter, enhancer, or *trans*-acting elements can cause insufficient quantities of a qualitatively intact subunit. Each of these molecular causes gives rise to the same cellular problem: insufficient β subunit. Erythrocyte maturation takes longer, and the ineffective development leads to an excess production of α subunits. Aggregates of the α subunits lead to Heinz body formation. The spleen sequesters these abnormal cells, if they have not already lysed in the capillary beds because of their lack of deformability. Thus, the anemia is a result of ineffective erythropoiesis, hemolysis, and sequestration.

The chronic sequestering of large numbers of red cells causes splenomegaly sometime during the first decade of life. As with sickle cell patients, splenectomy relieves some of the sequestering and allows the abnormal erythrocytes to continue circulating even if their oxygen-carrying capacity is limited. Thus, the surgery is generally indicated as a palliative measure. However, because the spleen is a major site of antigen presentation, these patients are then chronically susceptible to infections caused by encapsulated bacteria, particularly *Haemophilus influenzae* and *Streptococcus pneumoniae*. Iron overload generally results from multiple transfusions, and metal chelating therapy is generally indicated if transfusions are used frequently. There is no evidence to support a relationship between the thalassemias and inflammatory bowel disease, asthma, or chronic gastritis.

Some patients with chronic hemolytic anemias have milder clinical courses; most of these patients have an elevated amount of Hb F, the fetal hemoglobin whose oxygen carrying capacity is not ideal but is much better than Hb A_2. This seems to be a result of an enhanced expression of the γ subunit; the explanation for this enhanced expression is not known, but there does seem to be variability of γ expression even in the normal population. Decreased synthesis of the β-globin chain is the cause, not the palliation, of β-thalassemia. Decreased production of intrinsic factor leads to a deficiency of vitamin B_{12} or cobalamin, which can cause megaloblastic anemia as a result of ineffective nucleotide biosynthesis. Some research has actually justified supplementation of folate and cobalamin to provide substrate to bolster the struggling hematopoietic marrow. Increased absorption of iron will not help and, as noted above, iron overload is generally a problem. The α chain is automatically up-regulated as part of the body's somewhat futile attempt to produce more hemoglobin and relieve the lack of tissue oxygenation.

20–22. The answers are: 20-D, 21-A, 22-C. *(Tetralogy of Fallot)*
Congenital heart disease occurs in 1% of births and is usefully classified into two categories: cyanotic and noncyanotic. An infant with a cyanotic heart disease generally begins to show signs of oxygen desaturation within hours to days after birth, depending on the severity of the lesion. The cyanosis results from poor oxygenation in the blood and peripheral tissues. Generally speaking, cyanosis indicates a lesion that causes a substantial right-to-left shunt or a lesion in which the lungs are left out of the circulation. Patent ductus arteriosus and coarctation of the aorta are typically noncyanotic lesions at birth, although a patent ductus can lead to cyanosis later. Truncus arteriosus is a cyanotic lesion in which the aorta and pulmonary artery have fused into one large vessel that overrides both chambers; typically there is also a ventricular septal defect to accommodate the combined outflow. The diagram clearly shows two different outflow vessels. Transposition of the great arteries is a cyanotic lesion in which the right ventricle sends its output to the system and the left ventricle sends its output to the lungs. Because the return flows are not switched in the common variety of transposition, the result of transposition is two entirely separate circulations (unless the ductus arteriosus remains patent). The systemic circulation is never oxygenated, and the pulmonary circulation is never deoxygenated.

Tetralogy of Fallot is defined by an aorta that overrides a ventricular septal defect, some degree of pulmonary stenosis with right ventricular hypertrophy, and right-to-left shunt. The lesion is usually cyanotic, but if the amount of pulmonic stenosis is mild, then the resulting pulmonic perfusion may be sufficient. As the pulmonic stenosis increases, the right-to-left shunt becomes significant, and the cyanosis develops. Truncus arteriosus is the result of a failure in differentiation between the aorta and pulmonary artery.

The abnormal flow patterns associated with most congenital heart defects cause local jet streams; that is local regions of fluid with high-velocity turbulent flow. Unlike the laminar flow that normally predominates, jet streams can be directed at the tissue (especially on the valves), resulting in tiny lesions to the delicate endocardium. The intact endocardium is resistant to most organisms, but the damaged endocardium provides a rough surface that is ideal for bacterial or viral attachment. Infectious endocarditis is an important source of morbidity and mortality in infants with congenital heart disease. Because it involves coronary artery disease in over 90% of cases, myocardial infarction is highly unusual in men younger than 20 and women younger than 30 years, even when the patients have a positive family history for cardiac disease. Mitral valve prolapse is a common finding, occurring in about 7% of adults between the ages of 20 and 40 years. Mitral valve prolapse is unusual in children and is not increased in infants with congenital heart defects, unless they also have connective tissue diseases. In most adult cases, mitral valve prolapse is asymptomatic except for their increased incidence of valvular endocarditis. By definition, rheumatic heart disease always follows a streptococcal infection (usually of the pharynx), and it is thought that the pathophysiology is related to immune dysregulation (not structural abnormalities in the heart). Valvular calcification is generally related to endocardial damage, but calcification is a process of long-term inflammation and calcium deposition.

23–26. The answers are: 23-D, 24-C, 25-E, 26-B. *(Carnitine deficiency, fatty acid oxidation, compartmentalization of metabolism)*
Carnitine deficiency is a relatively rare hereditary disorder with two forms: The form illustrated in this question is systemic, whereas the other variant is confined only to muscle and tends to manifest itself in older people after they exercise strenuously. Carnitine is important for transporting long-chain fatty acids into the mitochondria where β-oxidation occurs. Flavin adenine dinucleotide (FAD) is the coenzyme that is required for the formation of carbon–carbon double bonds in virtually all metabolic pathways. Free fatty acids are acetylated with acetyl coenzyme A (CoA) on the outer surface of mitochondria; then, carnitine is exchanged for acetyl CoA, and the carnitine-complexed fatty acid is moved into the mitochondria. A different enzyme catalyzes the second exchange, this time freeing the carnitine by replacing it with acetyl CoA. Acyl carrier protein is the pantothenate derivative that holds the growing fatty acid during synthesis. Very low density lipoprotein (VLDL) is the carrier for fatty acids being exported by the liver to adipose tissue.

The discovery that oxidation occurs in cycles that release two carbon units in the form of acetyl CoA was a major advance in understanding fatty acid metabolism. The hydrolysis of pyrophosphate following formation of acyl CoA commits a fatty acid to degradation in the oxidative pathway. Adenosine triphosphate (ATP) molecules are not directly synthesized in the oxidative sequence; rather, energy is stored in reduced equivalents of both NADH and FADH$_2$. Because malonyl CoA is a substrate for fatty acid synthesis, high levels of malonyl CoA inhibit the fatty acid oxidation pathway to prevent a futile cycle of synthesis and oxidation. Understanding that fatty acid degradation cannot result in glucose is absolutely fundamental in understanding how the various metabolic pathways are integrated by the body. Because the body cannot make pyruvate (the building block for glucose) from any of the products of fatty acid or ketone breakdown, the β-oxidative pathway can produce only reducing equivalents and acetyl CoA units.

Oral carnitine replacement therapy should always be tried, but patients are not uniformly responsive. Because short- and medium-chain fatty acids do not require carnitine for their transport into mitochondria, a diet that excludes long-chain fatty acids may provide a great deal of relief. However, designing such a diet is far from trivial, and most patients find it difficult to comply. In the nonsystemic form, muscle biopsies are frequently taken to determine the cause of muscular weakness. The reasons for the lipid accumulation remain obscure. Because carnitine is a carrier that is attached and then immediately cleaved following fatty acid transfer, a deficiency in the enzymes for attachment or for cleavage would mimic a substrate carnitine deficiency almost identically. There are two separate enzymes (one for attachment and one for cleavage) named carnitine palmitoyltransferase I and II, respectively.

In order to allow for integration of different metabolic pathways, some key substrates are found in several different pathways. For some reactions, the energy state of the cell regulates the direction that a substrate like acetyl CoA follows. In other pathways, the entrance of a substrate is mainly regulated by substrate availability; in these cases, if a substrate is available to the enzymatic machinery, it is utilized. Thus, pathway compartmentalization within the cell keeps substrates from being available to the wrong pathway and helps prevent futile cycles of synthesis and degradation. Oxidative phosphorylation and fatty acid oxidation occur in the mitochondria; glycolysis and fatty acid synthesis occur in the cytosol. The pathways for gluconeogenesis and urea synthesis have enzymes in both the cytosol and mitochondria. Gangliosides and other complex lipid–carbohydrate molecules are degraded in the acidic lysosome. Several lysosomal storage disorders have been described in which particular lysosomal enzyme activities are deficient, which results in buildup of substrate.

27–31. The answers are: 27-A, 28-E, 29-B, 30-C, 31-E. (*Differential diagnosis of acquired anemia*)
Nutritional deficiencies, drugs, and several gastrointestinal disorders can give rise to acquired anemias. The principal classification of anemias is based upon the size and color of the circulating red blood cells. Megaloblastic anemias are generally hyperchromic and macrocytic. In the bone marrow, the maturation of the cytoplasm proceeds at a normal rate, whereas cell division is slow, and thus the cells are especially large. The slow cell division is a result of inefficient DNA synthesis. Deficiencies in either folate or cobalamin are a common cause of megaloblastic anemia; both of these nutrients serve essential roles in nucleotide biosynthesis. However, this woman's anemia is not megaloblastic. Schilling's test reveals the exact cause of cobalamin deficiency in a patient with low levels of serum cobalamin by determining the body's secretion of intrinsic factor and measuring the ileum's ability to absorb the intrinsic factor–cobalamin complex. Iron deficiency is a common cause of new onset hypochromic, microcytic anemias, and total iron-binding capacity (TIBC) and serum ferritin provide confirmation. TIBC is a measure of transferrin (the serum's iron transfer protein), which is increased in patients who are iron deficient because the body attempts to trap all available iron for hematopoiesis. Ferritin, the body's storage form of iron, is usually decreased in patients who are iron deficient and is increased in patients who are iron overloaded. Glucose 6-phosphate dehydrogenase deficiency is generally restricted to people of Asian, African, or Mediterranean descent, and the acute anemia is almost always traceable to a new prescription or infection. In addition, the anemia is hemolytic and is thus accompanied by signs of acute hemolysis (e.g., jaundice, icterus, elevated unconjugated bilirubin). A hemoglobinopathy becoming clinically significant this late in life is unusual; in addition, hemoglobinopathies are not common in white people.

Cobalamin deficiency is probably the most serious cause of anemia, because cobalamin deficiency can also result in irreversible damage to the nervous system. The neurologic complications begin with demyelination and can eventually include damage to the cerebral cortex. Cobalamin deficiency also has a more insidious onset due to the low daily requirement and the relatively large stores of cobalamin in the liver. Thus, patients can cease to absorb new cobalamin and not show symptoms for years. In some cases, the anemia may not present until after the neurologic complications because the anemia emerged too slowly to become symptomatic. Pernicious anemia is the most common cause of cobalamin deficiency. In pernicious anemia, atrophy of the gastric mucosa leads to decreased secretion of intrinsic factor (IF). Because IF is required for ileal absorption of cobalamin, the cobalamin deficiency that results from gastric atrophy can be quite severe. Both ileal resection and Crohn's disease can interfere with sufficient absorption of the cobalamin–IF complex and cause a similar deficiency. Although neither cobalamin nor folate deficiency is directly associated with chronic liver damage, folate deficiency is relatively common in alcoholics who may have associated cirrhosis. The liver's store of folate is relatively small in relation to the daily requirement of folate. Since most alcoholics are malnourished, the stores can be depleted rather quickly (i.e., in months) resulting in a relatively sudden onset of symptomatic folate deficiency. In contrast, cobalamin stores are relatively large in relation to the daily requirement, and a malnourished person is able to use the stored reserve of cobalamin for 1 to 2 years. Women are more susceptible to iron deficiency because they menstruate, which drains their iron stores each month. Even a short period of poor nutrition can result in relatively quick depletion of iron stores, especially in a woman with insufficient starting reserves.

Folate and cobalamin are required in large quantities for any cells that are undergoing rapid division. Therefore, the same cells that are susceptible to damage by chemotherapeutic drugs are most susceptible to damage from folate and cobalamin deficiency: hematopoietic stem cells, the gastrointestinal mucosa, and, to a lesser extent, the skin and hair. Hepatocytes divide only infrequently, and the cells of muscle and cartilage rarely divide. Although long bones are constantly undergoing remodeling, this process does not require a substantial amount of rapid cell division. Damage to myelin in cobalamin deficiency is thought to be directly related to cobalamin's role in methionine synthesis. Methionine is important in the methylation of myelin basic protein and choline-containing phospholipids.

The iron-binding protein of liver illustrates a classic case of coordinated protein synthesis; levels of transferrin and ferritin are regulated in opposite fashions by a single mechanism that is post-transcriptional [i.e., following the synthesis of messenger RNA (mRNA)]. Transferrin mRNA is normally degraded rapidly, but in the presence of the activated (i.e., iron free) iron-binding protein, a $3'$ stem–loop structure is stabilized, and the mRNA is no longer susceptible to degradation. Ferritin, the storage form of iron, has a $5'$ stem–loop structure that is recognized by the activated iron-binding protein. When the activated protein is bound to the stem–loop, initiation of ferritin translation is prevented. Therefore, when there is no iron to inactivate the iron-binding protein, the transferrin message is stabilized, and transferrin synthesis increases, while ferritin translation is blocked. When iron binds to the protein and inactivates it, ferritin translation begins proportional to the amount of message, and the transferrin message is rapidly degraded prior to translation.

Both folate and vitamin B_{12} are water soluble and, therefore, easily excreted if they are present in excess. Iron overload is a process that generally takes years, because the body can store a large amount of iron. Thus a short course of oral iron salts could not generate an iron overload. Furthermore, the symptoms of hemochromatosis require long-standing iron overload. Oxygen free radical toxicity is a source of hemolysis in glucose 6-phosphate dehydrogenase deficiency. Although iron overload is probably associated with an increase in free radical production, this process takes years, as stated above. Folate replacement should not be initiated until it has been clearly ascertained that a vitamin B_{12} deficiency does not coexist. The reason is twofold. First, folate replacement may reverse the anemia associated with a vitamin B_{12} deficiency, even if folate was not deficient in the beginning. This apparent recovery may allow neurologic complications to develop because the anemia will no longer serve a warning function. Secondly, if neurologic abnormalities have emerged, folate replacement may actually worsen the neurologic damage. The reason for this paradoxical turn for the worse is unclear.

32. The answer is A. *(Fatty acid synthesis)*
Feedback inhibition of pathways is common throughout cellular metabolism. The ultimate product inhibits the committed step so that when sufficient product is available, the enzymatic sequence is completely stopped. This prevents energy from being lost by moving a substrate partly through the pathway. Enzyme phosphorylation, in response to elevation of cyclic adenosine monophosphate (cAMP), is also an important part of a variety of catabolic and anabolic pathways. Elevated levels of citrate indicate a high-energy status within the cell and, therefore, activate acetyl coenzyme A (CoA) carboxylase to increase fatty acid production. The enzymes that catalyze fatty acid synthesis exist as independent domains on one large polypeptide. This provides for the most efficient shuttling of substrate from one reaction to the next, and obviates the need for diffusion and random collision with the next enzyme. The acyl carrier protein (ACP) is a pantothenic acid derivative that is covalently bound to the growing chain. Biotin is the main carrier of carboxyl groups in nearly every reaction that requires transfer of activated bicarbonate anions. Niacin is important in the biosynthesis of nicotinamide–adenine dinucleotide (NADH), which is essential for reactions that oxidize hydroxyl groups into carbonyl groups.

33–37. The answers are: 33-C, 34-A, 35-D, 36-E, 37-B. *(Peptic ulcer disease and multiple endocrine neoplasia)*
Zollinger-Ellison syndrome was initially described in a person with refractory, erosive peptic ulcer disease. Most cases involve a pancreatic islet cell tumor that secretes gastrin, which is the most potent physiologic

stimulator of parietal cell acid production. Aggressive medical treatment is sometimes not sufficient to block the copious production of acid in these patients, and usually the gastrin-secreting tumor must be extracted surgically or treated medically. Increased vagal tone results in increased acid production, but vagal hyperactivity is rarely sufficient to account for acid production of this magnitude. Increased release of histamine also leads to hyperactivity of the parietal cells. However, histamine is produced by mast cells located near the parietal cells, and mast cell tumors are not a common cause of Zollinger-Ellison syndrome. Pepsin is the proteolytic enzyme whose activation is pH dependent; hypersecretion of pepsin is uncommon and, in any case, would not lead to the refractory ulcers in this patient. Decreased mucosal production is probably involved in many cases of peptic ulcer disease, most notably those induced by stress or nonsteroidal anti-inflammatory drugs (NSAIDs). Locally produced prostaglandins are important in regulating the production of mucus by the cells lining the stomach, and stress as well as NSAIDs can inhibit prostaglandin production. However, peptic ulcer disease of this magnitude, particularly a condition that includes esophageal ulcers, could not be caused by insufficient mucous production.

The production of acid by parietal cells is regulated by the interplay of three main substances: histamine, gastrin, and acetylcholine, all of which can stimulate acid production. Parietal cells have receptors for all three signals, and each of the three signals can regulate release of the other signals independent of the parietal cell receptors. H_2-histamine receptor activation causes an elevation of cyclic adenosine monophosphate (cAMP) and the subsequent activation of cAMP-dependent protein kinases. Acetylcholine from the vagus nerve mediates its actions via muscarinic-type receptors. These muscarinic receptors, as well as their gastrin receptor analogues, mediate their signals through an elevation of free intracellular calcium. Acid production is a two-step process; in the first step, carbonic anhydrase splits the carbonic acid molecule into a bicarbonate anion and a hydrogen ion. In the second step, the movement of the bicarbonate anion into the blood causes the measurable and physiologically normal "alkaline tide" during meals (i.e., when the arterial pH increases slightly), and the hydrogen ion is pumped against a million-fold concentration gradient into the stomach by the hydrogen–potassium adenosine triphosphatase.

The H_2-histamine receptor blockers (e.g., ranitidine and cimetidine) are the mainstay of peptic ulcer disease treatment. They competitively block the receptors and powerfully downregulate parietal cell acid production, thus providing adequate therapy for most patients with peptic ulcer disease. Sucralfate and omeprazole are relatively new drugs whose efficacy is being demonstrated as their use continues to grow. Sucralfate specifically targets the ulcer bed and coats it for up to 12 hours; it shows very little affinity for normal mucosa, and it is not absorbed systemically. Omeprazole is absorbed systemically, although it is not associated with any substantial systemic toxicities. The irreversible mechanism of action of omeprazole makes it especially useful in the treatment of refractory cases due to Zollinger-Ellison syndrome. Colloidal bismuth is another coating agent whose mechanism of action may also involve antibiotic effects against the organism *Helicobacter pylori*, which can be identified in a substantial majority of patients with chronic peptic ulcer disease. There is evidence to indicate that *H. pylori* may destroy the mucosal lining, and, therefore, make patients susceptible to gastritis as well as to peptic ulcer disease. Atropine blocks the muscarinic receptors on the parietal cells, but it is not as efficacious as the histamine receptor blockers. Furthermore, oral or intravenous atropine is associated with a myriad of systemic side effects and is, therefore, not commonly used for chronic medical conditions. There are no clinically useful gastrin receptor blockers available for prescription in the United States.

Multiple endocrine neoplasia type I (MEN I) is a hereditary disorder whose pattern of inheritance has not been clearly defined; the gene has tentatively been mapped to chromosome 11. The syndrome consists of tumor involvement in a variable number of organ systems and is usually accompanied by a family history of endocrine abnormalities. According to the classic definition, MEN I causes tumors in the parathyroid, the pituitary, and the islet cells of the pancreas. Parathyroid tumors give rise to hypercalcemia, which, when untreated, can lead to calcium oxalate stones in the urinary tract. A variety of pituitary and islet cell tumors have been described. About 66% of patients actually have tumors in two cell types, whereas only 20% of patients have tumors in all three cell types. Various other tumors of the endocrine system, including carcinoid tumors, have also been described. The syndrome can manifest at any age and has no apparent gender preference. Although it is relatively rare, MEN is important because of the severity of the presenting symptoms, its hereditary transmission, and its responsiveness to therapy. Hemochromatosis is a hereditary iron-storage disorder whose cause remains enigmatic; liver and pancreatic disease are responsible for most of the classic signs. Patients with hemochromatosis are frequently diabetic and hypogonadal due to pancreatic insufficiency and dysregulated steroid production, respectively. Ataxia-telangiectasia is an autosomal recessive disorder whose clinical features include early-onset ataxia, oculocutaneous capillary growths (i.e., telangiectasia), and immunodeficiency. Endocrine manifestations include diabetes mellitus and adrenal hypoplasia. Niemann-Pick disease is an autosomal recessive lysosomal storage disorder, in which a sphingomyelinase deficiency causes the buildup of sphingomyelin and cholesterol. Most infants with this disorder come to clinical attention with mental retardation, ataxia, and seizures. Liver damage is common, but these infants usually do not live long enough to have clinically relevant endocrinopathies. Neurofibromatosis is a relatively common disorder inherited in an autosomal dominant fashion, although as many as 50% of cases can be new mutations. There are several forms of neurofibromatosis; von Recklinghausen's disease, the most common type, has three major characteristics: multiple neural tumors, numerous pigmented skin lesions, and pigmented iris hamartomas.

In addition to gastrinomas, other pancreatic islet cell tumors are common in MEN I; insulinomas can cause patients to present with profound hypoglycemia. Immunodeficiency is not a common characteristic of MEN, and, although the syndrome is hereditary, MEN does not seem to involve immune system dysfunction. Adrenal hyperplasia due to pituitary adenomas that secrete adrenocorticotropic hormone is common in patients with this syndrome, but adrenal insufficiency is unrelated. Carcinoid tumors of the lung, although unusual, have been described in patients with this disease. The tumor cells secrete serotonin and histamine, causing a variety of symptoms. Their embryonic origin has not been clearly defined, but the neoplastic cells are not bronchogenic and are much less malignant than are true bronchogenic cancer cells. Panhypopituitarism is not a common finding in patients with MEN; pituitary tumors in these patients are generally not malignant enough to erode all normal pituitary tissue.

38–41. The answers are: 38-A, 39-C, 40-E, 41-D. *(Metabolic acidosis and chronic renal failure)*
End-stage renal disease is the cause of death in up to 30% of patients with noninsulin-dependent diabetes mellitus. Chronic renal failure is characterized by increased glomerular filtration rate, proteinuria, and the systemic symptoms of urinary protein loss. Because the kidneys have a tremendous reserve for maintaining potassium balance, neither hypokalemia nor hyperkalemia is common in patients with renal failure. However, when potassium balance is lost, hyperkalemia is more common, generally resulting from acidosis, oliguria, or excess potassium ingestion. Proteinuria is one of the earliest findings in many types of kidney disease; the compromised glomeruli have leaky basement membranes, and albumin, as well as other small proteins, is lost from the serum. The liver increases production of all serum proteins in response to the loss. The mechanism causing triglyceride elevation is complex and poorly understood, but it is thought that the liver's production of lipoproteins is inappropriately increased in addition to the necessary increase in albumin production. Red blood cell production is dependent on the kidneys' synthesis of the growth factor erythropoietin. Although the reserve production of erythropoietin is substantial, most patients with end-stage disease have a clinically significant anemia. In the past, normochromic, normocytic anemia used to be a much more serious problem in patients with renal failure. With the development of recombinant erythropoietin, this problem is easily treatable. Patients with renal failure have a pungent odor in their sweat and on their breath called uremic fetor as a result of their elevated serum urea and creatinine.

Kimmelstiel-Wilson bodies are the hallmark of nodular glomerulosclerosis; the glomerular nodules are the remains of normal tissue destroyed by fibrin and lipid deposition. Kimmelstiel-Wilson bodies are fairly specific to diabetic nephropathy. Interstitial nephritis generally results from ischemia and inflammation. Atrophy of tubules and the chronic presence of inflammatory cells are seen in biopsy, and this lesion is common to many different kidney diseases. Vascular pathology is the hallmark of diabetic disease, and the kidneys usually reflect this with hyalinization of the small arteries and arterioles. Diffuse glomerulosclerosis is the description given to the thickened mesangium and associated destruction of most normal tissue in the glomerular tufts; it is not specific to diabetes, and, in most patients, it probably represents the progression from nodular glomerulosclerosis. Amyloid deposition in the glomeruli and interstitium of the kidneys is characteristic of primary amyloidosis, a heritable condition associated with deposits of protein throughout the body, most notably in the heart, brain, blood vessels, and kidneys. The specific test for amyloid involves a congo red stain of the tissue; under polarized light, the protein deposits display apple-green birefringence.

Ammonia is one of the nontitratable acids in the urine and is a major route of acid excretion. Ammonia is synthesized in the cells of the kidney tubules and freely diffuses into the tubule fluid. Any free hydrogen ions are bound by the ammonia, making the charged ammonium ion, which does not diffuse back into the cells. Ammoniagenesis is tightly regulated by the kidney and is the major factor in the kidney's ability to handle large acid loads. The complete enzymatic pathway for urea synthesis is found only in hepatocytes. Urea synthesis plays no significant role in acid–base homeostasis; excretion of urea is the major route for disposal of nitrogenous wastes. Bicarbonate recycling by the tubule cells involves a complex set of transport processes. Carbonic anhydrase on the brush border of the proximal tubule cells synthesizes carbon dioxide and water from bicarbonate and hydrogen ion in the tubule fluid. The carbon dioxide diffuses into the cell, where another carbonic anhydrase synthesizes the bicarbonate anion from the incoming molecule and hydroxyl anion. The bicarbonate is transported with sodium into the bloodstream, whereas the hydrogen ion is secreted into the tubule fluid, resulting in a net reabsorption of bicarbonate. Pyruvate is a substrate for gluconeogenesis in the liver, and potassium is secreted in exchange for sodium reabsorption in the distal tubules.

In the initial phases of metabolic acidosis, the anion gap is small because the deficiency in serum bicarbonate is replaced by chloride anion. This phase is called hyperchloremic acidosis and reflects the initial stage in which some level of compensation is maintained. As the active transport of bicarbonate by the kidneys continues to drop, unmeasured anions like phosphate and sulfate begin to fill the gap. Because they are unmeasured, the apparent "gap" between the measured cations (i.e., sodium and potassium) and the measured anions (i.e., bicarbonate and chloride) starts to increase. The source of the phosphate that fills the anion gap is most likely the bone. Thus, hydrolysis of calcium salts in the bone provides the anions to compensate for the failure of the kidneys to synthesize ammonia and reabsorb bicarbonate. It is thought that metabolic acidosis plays a significant role in the pathophysiology, which leads to renal osteodystrophy. The synthesis of ammonia in the kidney tubules is important in acid secretion, and, as discussed above, it is seriously compromised in patients with renal failure.

42–45. The answers are: 42-C, 43-D, 44-A, 45-D. *(Cross-sectional study of severity of disability in cerebrovascular accident and personality type)*
The patients participating in this study were simultaneously classified according to the severity of their disability and their personality type. Therefore, this is an example of a cross-sectional study.

When the data are in the form of counts (i.e., the number of people in each combination of categories), the chi-square test is used to test for the presence of a significant association between the two study variables. Both the paired and pooled t tests, as well as the analysis of variance, use continuous, not frequency, data to test for the equality of means. Correlation analysis estimates the magnitude of the association between two quantitative variables, whereas regression analysis is used to derive an equation for predicting the value of one variable based on values of the other.

The calculated test statistic exceeds the tabulated critical value; therefore, the P value is less than $\alpha = .05$. The null hypothesis (H_O) is rejected at the 5% level of significance, indicating there is a statistically significant association between the severity of the physical deficit and personality type.

A statistically significant result indicates that it is unlikely (here, a less than .1% chance) that an association equal to or greater than that observed could be obtained from a sample drawn from a population in which no association exists between the two study variables. Statistical significance, however, does not provide an estimate of the strength of the association, nor does it imply the existence of a cause-and-effect relationship. Because a cross-sectional design was used, this study is particularly vulnerable to antecedent–consequence uncertainty. No statistical test can overcome flaws in the study design that lead to a biased comparison.

46–49. The answers are: 46-D, 47-C, 48-A, 49-B. *(Management of shock)*

Dobutamine is the agent of choice for a hypovolemic crisis. Other adrenergic-activating agents have two drawbacks. Many (e.g., epinephrine) are not β-receptor specific and, therefore, cause vasoconstriction, which is undesired because in these patients vasoconstriction is already severe and may be causing intestinal or renal damage. Other β-specific agents (e.g., isoproterenol) are chronotropic as well as inotropic. Because increased chronotropism carries a greater risk of ischemia, and because increased inotropism is a more efficient way to increase cardiac output, the selectively inotropic agent dobutamine is best suited. As an added benefit, dobutamine also activates an unusual class of dopaminergic receptors in the kidneys, causing vasodilation at a time when the kidneys may be suffering clinically significant ischemia. Albuterol is a relatively selective agonist of the β_2 class of adrenergic receptors and is commonly prescribed to relieve the acute bronchoconstrictive symptoms during episodes of asthma and chronic obstructive pulmonary disease. Because the cardiac receptors are principally representatives of the β_1 subtype, albuterol would not offer any substantial cardiac effects. Propranolol is a nonselective β-adrenergic receptor antagonist used as a class II antiarrhythmic as well as an antianginal agent. It decreases cardiac output and is not indicated for the management of shock. Furosemide is a loop diuretic that can induce rapid and large increases in urine output and would be strictly contraindicated in this patient. Tubocurarine blocks neurotransmission at nicotinic cholinergic synapses and is used to provide muscular paralysis prior to intubation. It may be necessary to intubate patients during a hypovolemic crisis, but tubocurarine does not support the man's cardiovascular system.

The brain and heart have tightly regulated local circulations that prevent ischemic damage as long as some cardiac output is maintained; therefore, the severe vasoconstriction induced by hypovolemic shock is usually not felt by the brain or heart until cardiac arrest. Peripheral muscle is usually not metabolically active in these patients and, therefore, has very low oxygen requirements. Blood flow to the liver is not completely closed off during a vasoconstrictive crisis in most patients, but the splanchnic vessels demonstrate profound vasoconstriction in response to hypovolemia and the resultant sympathetic outflow. Thus, many patients who have survived a near-fatal episode of shock may recover only to need major surgery to remove infarcted bowel.

Gram-negative sepsis induced by the body's reaction to lipopolysaccharide endotoxin is almost always manifested by widespread vasodilation and a resultant loss of blood pressure. The locally present lipopolysaccharides have a vasodilatory effect, which is resistant to the nonetheless massive sympathetic outflow (which accompanies all forms of shock). None of the other causes of shock (pericardial tamponade, pulmonary embolus, large myocardial infarction, and gastrointestinal blood loss) has a locally mediated vasodilatory effect, which must be overcome. Pericardial tamponade and a large myocardial infarction both dramatically reduce cardiac output; the former by constraining ventricular filling and the latter by interfering with ventricular contraction and, in many cases, impulse conduction. A large pulmonary embolus blocks flow through the pulmonary circulation and increases in pulmonary resistance, which is normally quite low. The net result is similar to the intracardiac causes (e.g., substantially diminished cardiac output). Gastrointestinal blood loss results in the same hypovolemic shock that affects a patient with traumatic blood loss.

In addition to the intestines, the kidneys are especially sensitive to hypovolemic shock that lasts 30 minutes to 1 hour. Acute tubular necrosis is the most common kidney lesion seen in patients recovering from hypovolemic shock, and hyperkalemia quickly ensues (primarily the result of oliguria). In the absence of a substantial external potassium load, most patients will only experience modest potassium accumulation, with rises in serum potassium of about 0.4 mM in a 24-hour period. As with all causes of kidney failure, serum blood urea nitrogen (BUN) and creatinine are markedly elevated (creatinine as high as 8–12; normal =

0.8–1.5). An antinuclear antibody screen is useful in diagnosing systemic lupus erythematosus. A positive antistreptolysin O (ASO) titer is generally adequate evidence to demonstrate a recent streptococcal infection and is especially useful in diagnosing acute rheumatic fever as well as post-streptococcal glomerulonephritis. A complete blood count provides information that may be important in diagnosing infection, anemia, or neoplasia. A digoxin level is important if digoxin toxicity is suspected. However, digoxin is most commonly prescribed to support patients with congestive heart failure, which is an unlikely condition in this 29-year-old man. Furthermore, digoxin toxicity is usually manifested in cardiac conduction disturbances and arrhythmias, not in renal failure.

50–53. The answers are: 50-C, 51-E, 52-A, 53-D. *(Post-streptococcal glomerulonephritis)*
Post-streptococcal glomerulonephritis is a relatively common complication of pharyngitis in children 6 to 10 years of age. Most cases are caused by group A β-hemolytic streptococci with specific types of M antigen. The child's puffiness is due to dramatically decreased glomerular filtration and the resultant oliguria with salt and water retention. As with all cases of nephritis, there is significant hematuria and proteinuria. The loss of protein combined with the salt and water retention produces the characteristic edema, and the increased blood volume is sufficient to explain her modest hypertension. Although systemic lupus erythematosus can be associated with glomerulonephritis, renal symptoms characteristic of the nephrotic syndrome are more common in the early stages; and, it would be unusual for an 8-year-old to present with lupus. Acute tubular necrosis can be associated with water retention, edema, and high blood pressure, but hematuria is not common in these patients. Furthermore, most cases of acute tubular necrosis are preceded by an identifiable ingestion of some acutely nephrotoxic agent or ischemic damage secondary to shock. Juvenile-onset diabetes frequently presents with renal symptoms, but these changes are usually nephrotic rather than nephritic in nature (i.e., lack of hematuria and more substantial proteinuria). The onset of diabetes is generally more gradual, and significant edema would probably evolve over a longer period of time. Finally, all cases of diabetes manifest with polyuria, and salt and fluid retention are rarely seen prior to the onset of chronic renal failure late in the disease. Isolated hyperaldosteronism is rare and would not be associated with hematuria.

Positive antistreptolysin O (ASO) titers and substantially decreased serum complement C3 levels are the hallmarks of the inflammatory damage involved in post-streptococcal glomerulonephritis. Although the specific antigenic component has not been identified, immune complexes with complement can be found deposited throughout the glomerular tufts. Inappropriate fixation of complement is thought to be the factor responsible for the destruction of renal function. In acute glomerulonephritis, hyponatremia is the result of salt and water retention secondary to decreased glomerular filtration. Proteins, cells, and cell casts are found in the urine as a result of damage to the basement membrane and its subsequent leakiness. Elevated serum creatinine, as in all cases of renal failure, is the result of decreased glomerular filtration.

As suggested above, clumps of antigen–antibody complexes with associated complement can be seen with electron microscopy and immunofluorescence in renal biopsies of patients with post-streptococcal glomerulonephritis. Thus, the damage falls within the realm of class III hypersensitivity reactions. Occlusion of tubular lumens with cellular casts and gaps in the luminal epithelia indicates acute tubular necrosis. Proliferation of mesangial cells can be seen in any of a number of systemic diseases but the most common example is systemic lupus erythematosus. The linear pattern of immunofluorescence is pathognomonic for Goodpasture's syndrome, in which antibodies targeted against basement membrane antigens are found in the lungs and kidneys. The difference between the pathology in Goodpasture's and post-streptococcal glomerulonephritis is substantial. In this case, the antigens are most likely extrarenal, and the immune complexes are formed prior to filtration. The glomerulus is, therefore, the unfortunate bystander during complement cascade activation, whereas in Goodpasture's syndrome the glomerular antigens are the target of immune attack. Hypertrophy of the macula densa is not a lesion commonly found in any disease.

The bacterial antigen stimulating confusion between self and nonself continues to elude scientists. The etiology of post-streptococcal glomerulonephritis seems to be similar to rheumatic fever, in which a streptococcal antigen stimulates inappropriate identification and destruction of tissue in the heart. The difference is that renal antigens are not targeted in post-streptococcal glomerulonephritis but, as described above, the kidney is the unfortunate bystander during complement cascade activation when the antibody–antigen complexes are trapped in the glomeruli. Streptococci are gram-positive and, therefore, do not have gram-negative bacterial lipopolysaccharide. Immunoglobulin G directed against basement membrane antigens is important in Goodpasture's syndrome, as described above. Antinuclear antibodies, possibly important in the cause of drug-induced lupus and systemic lupus erythematosus, are not implicated in post-streptococcal glomerulonephritis. Excess renin production is unusual and, as indicated earlier, would not cause hematuria.

54–58. The answers are: 54-D, 55-A, 56-E, 57-C, 58-B. *(Pancreatitis, hypocalcemia, alcoholism)*
The description of abdominal pain with guarding and hypoactive bowel sounds is classic for pancreatitis. Other causes of an acutely painful abdomen need to be considered, however. The absence of free air under the diaphragm eliminates visceral perforation from the differential diagnosis in this patient with an acutely painful abdomen. Myocardial infarction is very unlikely in a 35-year-old woman with a negative family history for cardiac disease; furthermore, most patients do not describe the pain of infarction as stabbing but rather crushing. Similarly, an aortic aneurysm is generally a disease of older adults and is the result of chronic hypertension and atherosclerosis, which are unlikely in this woman of 35 years. The pain of renal colic is much different than what this patient described. Located primarily in the flank, it radiates to the groin in classic cases and is almost always described as a pain that comes severely in 10- to 20-minute waves. Renal colic is not usually worsened by lying supine.

A serum lipase test is more sensitive and specific than a serum amylase test, in most laboratories, and, where available, it is the test of choice. Serum amylase tests are more routinely available in smaller labs, and they are sufficiently sensitive to establish the diagnosis in most cases. Bilirubin, alkaline phosphatase, and γ-glutamyl transpeptidase (GGTP) are the most sensitive markers of obstructive liver disease (e.g., acute cholecystitis, acute cholelithiasis). This patient has no specific indications of obstructive liver processes. A urinalysis does not add any useful information to the diagnosis of acute pancreatic disease, although it is routinely ordered in patients thought to have acute liver disease. An upper gastrointestinal series with barium contrast is useful for assessing peptic ulcer disease but is highly contraindicated if the physician has any reason to suspect visceral perforation. An electrocardiogram with the muscle–brain fraction of creatine kinase is useful in ruling out a myocardial infarction.

A positive Chvostek's sign is highly specific to hypocalcemia-induced tetany, although it is not as sensitive. The lengthened QT interval in a patient with Chvostek's sign confirms the presence of hypocalcemia, even without a laboratory evaluation. The physician should be looking for these signs specifically because hypocalcemia is a routine complication of pancreatitis. The cause of hypocalcemia in these patients is generally the result of a number of factors. In most patients, the pancreatitis is accompanied by the formation of calcium soap salts in the pancreas secondary to the inappropriate release of pancreatic digestive enzymes within the tissue; normal mechanisms frequently serve to maintain calcium homeostasis. But in patients with alcoholism, chronic malnutrition has generally left them magnesium deficient. This becomes important in answering the next question. Hyperkalemia is not a routine result of pancreatitis, and the electrocardiogram findings for hyperkalemia include peaked T waves not QT prolongation. Vitamin B_{12} deficiency would manifest in neurologic signs and megaloblastic anemia; such a deficiency is not uncommon in the alcoholic patient. However, vitamin B_{12} deficiency is not associated with electrocardiogram findings. In addition, Chvostek's sign is specific to hypocalcemia, and the neurologic manifestations of vitamin B_{12} deficiency are mainly associated with demyelination (e.g., proprioceptive loss, loss of distal light touch and vibration). Cocaine abuse needs to be considered in this woman, but lengthening of the QT interval is not likely in a patient with significant levels of serum cocaine. Severe hemolysis is not a routine finding in the patient with pancreatitis, and neither of the symptoms given indicates hemolysis.

Alcoholic pancreatitis contributes substantially to the morbidity and mortality of alcoholism, and alcohol ingestion is a common cause of acute pancreatitis. A secondary diagnosis of hypocalcemia in alcoholism is often related to magnesium deficiency, which results from chronic malnutrition. Magnesium is important in the parathyroid gland's release of parathyroid hormone (PTH) as well as its action on target tissues. Synthesis of PTH is not impaired because magnesium replacement is usually followed by rapid correction of calcium homeostasis. If PTH synthesis were impaired due to magnesium deficiency, there would be a delay following replacement therapy during which PTH synthesis would occur. Because there is no delay in correcting PTH (and calcium) values once magnesium is replaced, it is fairly certain that only the PTH release process is affected by low serum magnesium. It is clear that magnesium is also involved in the signalling cascade secondary to PTH-receptor activation, because PTH administration in a magnesium-deficient patient is not sufficient to restore calcium homeostasis. In fact, calcium gluconate is usually unable to correct the problem. Furosemide causes diuresis by acting at the distal loop of Henle and is not useful for any of the patient's symptoms. Thiazide diuretics, however, are important adjuncts to calcium gluconate in other causes of hypocalcemia. There is no evidence implicating hypovolemia or anemia in this woman, so neither dextrose–saline nor packed red cells are indicated. Vitamin B_{12} may be necessary in this malnourished woman, but it will not have any impact on her hypocalcemia.

Making a diagnosis of alcoholism is the responsibility of all physicians, since alcohol represents one of the most important causes of morbidity and mortality in the United States. Blackouts are frequently described by individuals who have drunk alcohol excessively on one or two occasions and are not sufficient reason to diagnose alcoholism in the absence of one of the other criteria listed. Each of the other problems (i.e., relationship problems, work problems, disease, arrests all related to alcohol) is a *Diagnostic and Statistical Manual IV (DSM-IV)* criterion for diagnosing alcoholism. The key unifying factor in all four of these problems is that a socially significant, undesirable repercussion of the drinking behavior had no effect in changing subsequent drinking.

59. The answer is B. (*α_1-Antitrypsin deficiency*)

α_1-Antitrypsin deficiency may first present as acute hepatitis with impressive jaundice, elevated serum transaminases, and compromised blood clotting (especially in children). However, the phenotypic expression of this genotype is variable, even in persons who are homozygous for the deficiency. Some patients with heterozygous genotypes, and even individuals with homozygous mutations, may experience emphysema and symptoms of chronic obstructive pulmonary disease before liver disease, especially if they smoked. All homozygous individuals who live into adulthood will have panacinar emphysema by their early forties. Although restriction fragment length polymorphisms (RFLPs) are useful in providing information for genetic counseling of the patient, the definitive diagnosis can be made by directly assaying the serum for protein activity. The pathophysiology seems to involve a deficiency of the protein's normal inhibitory effect on the serine proteases released by the neutrophils residing in the lung and liver. Because both tissues have antigen-presenting cells that are regularly active, there is a small population of neutrophils normally releasing proteases, nucleases, and elastases. In unaffected individuals, the antitrypsin protein irreversibly inhibits the destructive effects of elastases and proteases, thus checking the level of local tissue inflammation. In affected individuals, this small amount of inflammation grows unchecked, causing significant tissue destruction and the recruitment of more inflammatory effector cells. Since it is known that individuals who smoke have an increased number of neutrophils and macrophages in their lung tissue, smoking results in a significantly greater amount of damage than it would in an unaffected individual.

60. The answer is C. (*Alcohol withdrawal*)

Physical dependence on alcohol implies that withdrawal of the depressant results in clinically significant physical and behavioral changes. Benzodiazepines are appropriate as a substitute for the depressive effects of alcohol while the acute physical symptoms are still active (approximately 5–7 days). Chlordiazepoxide, a commonly prescribed benzodiazepine, is a good choice based upon its intermediate half-life and long history of use. The drug should be prescribed at a sedative dose and tapered over a 5-day period, so that the physician avoids exchanging one addiction for another. Phenytoin should not be routinely prescribed because seizures are an uncommon complication, and, in the few cases involving seizures, the episode had passed before adequate phenytoin levels were achieved. If the alcoholism coincides with clinically significant depression, nortriptyline may be appropriate in conjunction with appropriate counseling. However, nortriptyline is an antidepressant and is not directed at the delirium tremens. Haloperidol, a commonly prescribed antipsychotic, is not appropriate therapy for delirium tremens. Since morphine, a therapeutically useful narcotic analgesic, can be just as addictive as alcohol, it is certainly contraindicated.

61–65. The answers are: 61-B, 62-D, 63-D, 64-E, 65-A. *(Asthma diagnosis and treatment)*
Asthma is a potential underlying cause of episodic dyspnea associated with wheezing in an 11-year-old boy. Although it is often difficult to establish a diagnosis of asthma in the laboratory, a reduction in forced expiratory volumes (*curve 1*) that is reversible after the inhalation of a bronchodilator such as metaproterenol (*curve 2*) is consistent with a diagnosis of hyperreactive airway disease. Although variability in spirometric testing is common, a forced expiratory volume in 1 sec (FEV_1) of less than 1 L/min is of concern even in a patient of this age. Methacholine is a useful provocative agent that will reduce FEV_1 at a lower dose in an asthmatic patient than in normal subjects. Although cromolyn sodium and beclomethasone are useful agents in the therapy of asthma, neither agent is likely to produce acute reversal of airway obstruction.

Theophylline is one of a number of methylxanthines that is useful for the chronic therapy of asthma. Although it can increase intracellular levels of cyclic adenosine monophosphate (cAMP) via phosphodiesterase inhibition and relax bronchial smooth muscle, theophylline appears to affect symptoms of asthma via other mechanisms, including affecting adenosine receptors or intracellular calcium homeostasis. Propranolol is a β-adrenergic receptor antagonist that is contraindicated in patients with asthma because it may exacerbate their symptoms. Although local concentrations of histamine contribute to the pathogenesis of asthma, antihistamines do not have an accepted role in the therapy of asthma except to manage associated rhinitis. Bethanechol is a moderately long-acting parasympathomimetic and, as such, is contraindicated in asthmatics. Ibuprofen and other nonsteroidal antiinflammatory agents (which inhibit cyclooxygenase) may also produce an airway narrowing effect (perhaps by shuttling arachidonic acid via the bronchoconstricting lipoxygenase pathway) and are often contraindicated in a subset (e.g., aspirin-hypersensitive) of asthmatics.

Stimulation of irritant receptors leads to reflex bronchoconstriction via a vagal reflex. Indeed, normal resting tone is set by the parasympathetic nervous system, and some aspects of hyperreactive airway disease are thought to involve a relatively high influence of vagal tone at the expense of sympathetic efferent bronchodilator activity. The intercostal and phrenic nerves are important nerves to the accessory respiratory muscle and the diaphragm, respectively.

Asthma is a collective term for a variety of disorders of unknown etiology leading to hyperreactive airways. Although common pathogenic factors remain ill-defined, it is quite clear that a large subset of patients may undergo symptoms of airway narrowing and unstable lung function after exposure to food preservatives (e.g., sulfites), air pollutants (e.g., ozone), pathogens (e.g., parainfluenza virus), exercise, cold temperatures, and emotional stress. Nonsteroidal antiinflammatory agents, such as aspirin, also may produce similar symptoms in many patients, but acetaminophen does not produce asthma-like manifestations in a significant number of patients.

Allergic asthma is the causative factor in 25% to 35% of all cases and is a contributing factor to approximately an additional 30% of all cases. Interaction of antigen with mast-cell–bound IgE receptors results in elaboration of a number of soluble mediators that cause bronchospasm, airway edema, and the ultimate recruitment of eosinophils and neutrophils to the airspace.

66–67. The answers are: 66-C, 67-C. *(Bacterial meningitis)*
The findings of fever, headache, nuchal rigidity, and lethargy with an acute onset and the lack of dramatic neurologic manifestations suggest acute bacterial meningitis. Viral meningitis causes much of the same symptomatology, but the onset typically is more insidious and the patient usually is less acutely ill. Patients with viral encephalitis display the same general symptomatology as those with viral meningitis, but encephalitis is differentiated by dramatic neurologic manifestations and a much poorer prognosis. Fungal meningitis is more chronic and frequently is seen with other systemic signs of mycotic disease. Brain abscess usually is seen with other foci of infection, and the patient typically has deficits that reflect the location of the lesion.

Streptococcus pneumoniae is the most common cause of bacterial meningitis among the elderly. *Haemophilus influenzae* type B is the most common cause of bacterial meningitis overall. Its incidence is highest in infants 6 to 12 months old and decreases with age; the incidence of meningitis caused by *H. influenzae* is low in adults. Meningococcal meningitis occurs primarily among young adults, and *Neisseria meningitidis* serogroups A, B, C, and Y cause most cases. *Staphylococcus aureus* occasionally causes meningitis but is a common cause of brain abscess.

68–70. The answers are: 68-E, 69-B, 70-E. *(Acute neurologic management; alcohol withdrawal)*
The most important action to take with the ataxic and confused homeless man is to determine what, if any, brain injuries he may have sustained. The scalp wound can be handled initially with a bandage before suturing. If a fracture is suspected, skull films can be obtained after an acute neurologic condition has been ruled out. A serum ethanol level is indicated, and though important, it is not a priority. Hygiene is relevant but not urgent.

Although all of the problems listed in the question must be considered in the differential diagnosis of this patient, the epidural hematoma is the most emergent potential problem listed. An epidural hematoma classically presents as an initial brief period of unconsciousness followed by a lucid period that is followed by unconsciousness. If a sufficient tear of the middle meningeal artery has occurred, death can ensue rapidly. The encephalopathies, including delirium, could progress to coma, but hepatic encephalopathy is not the most urgent choice listed.

Disulfiram (Antabuse) is used as a deterrent to further drinking; it is not a treatment for alcohol withdrawal. Hydration is important to prevent cardiovascular collapse. Benzodiazepines are cross-tolerant with barbiturates and ethanol and permit controlled withdrawal from ethanol. Changes in vital signs, including increased blood pressure, heart rate, and temperature, accompany ethanol withdrawal and should be monitored.

71–74. The answers are: 71-C, 72-B, 73-D, 74-D. *(Myocardial infarction; physiology and treatment)*
A fast rhythm with a wide complex is usually consistent with a ventricular tachycardia. It is highly likely that the 60-year-old man described in the question suffered a myocardial infarction associated with ventricular tachycardia. The treatment of choice for ventricular tachycardia associated with myocardial ischemia is lidocaine. Lidocaine is typical of a group of antiarrhythmic agents that block sodium ion channels that are the current-carrying processes responsible for depolarization in fast fibers of the heart (ventricular and atrial). It suppresses these channels in the infarct area in cells with abnormal resting membrane potential. Although the mechanism underlying this selectivity is poorly understood, it is thought that abnormal tissue ion channels tend to be in inactivated states, which would increase the binding and efficacy of use-dependent agents, or that damaged myocardial tissue tends to accumulate agents such as lidocaine to a greater extent. Agents such as diltiazem, propranolol, or digitalis affect electrical propagation and conduction in sinoatrial and atrioventricular nodal tissue, where parasympathetic input predominates, and calcium is the current carrying ion. Although propranolol has been shown to have some utility in reducing subsequent damage after myocardial infarction, it is contraindicated in patients with hypotension and potential poor left ventricular function. Epinephrine increases oxygen demands on the heart by directly stimulating beta receptors as well as increasing afterload, and, in this case, it appears to be contraindicated.

Creatine kinase (CK) is an enzyme that catalyzes the transfer of high energy phosphates and is found largely in tissues that use large amounts of energy. The two most common isoforms are CK-MM (muscle) and CK-BB (brain). There is an isoform that contains both M and B subunits (CK-MB), which is found only in the myocardium. In the heart, CK is approximately 85% CK-MB. An increase in both total CK and CK-MB (secondary to myocardial injury) has proven to be highly sensitive and specific for the diagnosis of myocardial infarction. Lactate dehydrogenase (LDH) is often elevated 48–72 hours after injury.

Significant injury to the anterior wall of the left ventricle may be due to occlusion (>70%) of the left anterior descending coronary artery. Alternatively, occlusion to a lesser degree of the left mainstem coronary artery may also produce the above condition. The left circumflex artery may affect the anterior wall but is more likely to involve inferior or posterior parts of the heart.

Low-dose aspirin has become an important component of pharmacotherapeutic approaches to reducing the risk of recurrent myocardial infarction. The desired effect is to irreversibly inhibit platelet cyclooxygenase (thereby reducing platelet-derived thromboxane A_2), while allowing for resynthesis of endothelial cell cyclooxygenase and maintaining a useful production of prostacyclin. Aspirin does not affect lipoxygenase activity and, therefore, it does not decrease circulating levels of any of the leukotrienes. Aspirin does not reduce normal body temperature.

75. The answer is B. *(Fatty acid metabolism; nutrition)*
Because of a methyl group on the third carbon, phytanic acid cannot be metabolized through β-oxidation. Phytanic acid is converted to pristanic acid in peroxisomes by the decarboxylation of the hydroxylated intermediate. Pristanic acid can then be used as a substrate for β-oxidation, as can linoleic acid, arachidonic acid, palmitic acid, and decenoic acid. Phytanic acid is toxic if it is not metabolized.

76. The answer is D. *(Cholesterol biosynthesis)*
The rate-limiting and regulated step of cholesterol biosynthesis is the formation of mevalonate from 3-hydroxy-3-methylglutaryl coenzyme A (HMG CoA) catalyzed by HMG CoA reductase. This enzyme is inhibited by dietary cholesterol and endogenously synthesized cholesterol. A vegetarian diet, a diet low in cholesterol, and the administration of a bile acid–sequestering resin all result in a reduced intake of cholesterol, which will not inhibit HMG CoA reductase activity. Familial hypercholesterolemia is a result of a deficiency of low-density lipoprotein (LDL) receptors.

77–78. The answers are: 77-C, 78-C. *(Neurologic disease topography)*
Guillain-Barré syndrome presents with peripheral sensory defects as well as motor defects, which progress from distal areas of the body to involve more proximal regions. It usually follows a viral illness of unknown origin and affects mostly young people. Loss of deep tendon reflexes is also present. Guillain-Barré syndrome is thought to involve antimyelin autoantibodies against motor neurons that evolve after viral illness or influenza vaccine. There is a progressive mixed motor and sensory loss, even though motor neurons are the target of these antibodies, due to the inflammation of spinal nerves in which both motor and sensory fibers travel together.

Myasthenia gravis is a disease of the neuromuscular junction and most commonly presents with ocular symptoms, such as ptosis, diplopia, and dysarthria. It manifests as muscle fatigue without sensory symptoms. Deep tendon reflexes are diminished but not lost in this disease. Myasthenia gravis is an autoimmune disease, which involves acetylcholine (ACh) receptors in the postsynaptic neuromuscular junction.

Poliovirus is a picornavirus, which usually causes an intestinal disease that can progress to viremia and cause the destruction of anterior horn cells of the spinal cord, resulting in paralysis of the innervated muscles. It usually manifests as a purely muscular disorder, and deep tendon reflexes are absent only if the muscles involved in the reflex lose their motor innervation.

Raynaud's phenomenon is a peripheral vascular syndrome manifested by sensitivity to cold, livedo reticularis, and acrocyanosis. It occurs primarily in women in their late teens. The cause is unknown, but the condition is associated with vasospasms.

79–83. The answers are: 79-D, 80-E, 81-B, 82-C, 83-B. *(Respiratory physiology; chronic bronchitis; emphysema)*

Flow–volume curves from forced expiratory maneuvers provide useful information about the dynamic function of airways in health and disease. In the patient depicted in the figure, residual volume (and functional residual capacity) are elevated due to his underlying obstructive disease (bronchitis or emphysema). Loss of elastic recoil (due to underlying disease) and prolongation of expiration (in association with obstruction) usually lead to an increased functional residual capacity and total lung capacity and a decrease in vital capacity. A common pathophysiologic finding is a reduction in the flow rate at all lung volumes during expiration.

Although the clinical manifestations of obstructive disease are quite variable, many patients with bronchitis tend to retain CO_2 at some time during their disease. Patients of this type apparently have a diminished ventilatory drive secondary to peripheral or central chemoreceptors or altered afferent pathways. In spite of an increased work of breathing, these subjects attempt to conserve oxygen expenditure by not adequately increasing ventilation at the cost of an increased partial pressure of CO_2 (P_{CO_2}) (and decreased P_{O_2}). In contrast to those patients that increase their minute volume (and thus maintain a normal P_{CO_2}), subjects such as this patient do not have very large physiologic dead spaces. However, patients with obstructive lung disease do perfuse poorly ventilated regions of lung. These high physiologic shunts generally have only modest effects on arterial P_{CO_2} (although they do contribute to the hypoxemia).

Chronic hypoxemia (often in conjunction with nocturnal desaturation during sleep apnea) leads to erythropoiesis and hypoxic pulmonary vasoconstriction. This desaturation and erythrocytosis produce cyanosis and can lead to right ventricular hypertrophy and right-sided heart failure. In such an event, functional tricuspid regurgitation may be detected by neck vein distention characterized by large v waves (and brisk y descents) as well as the heart sounds described above. Right-sided heart failure leads to an elevation in venous pressure. In spite of an increase in hematocrit, cyanosis and edema secondary to such failure produce the so-called "blue bloater" manifestation.

Although chronic bronchitis and emphysema often co-exist, CO_2 retention and right-sided heart failure are more consistent with a diagnosis of bronchitis. The pathologic hallmark of this disorder is hyperplasia and hypertrophy of mucus-producing glands in the submucosa of large airways. Other destructive changes in proximal and distal airways are manifestations of other pulmonary diseases including emphysema and tuberculosis.

An important familial factor in the development of emphysema is an inherited disorder leading to a deficiency in the production of the protease inhibitor α_1-antitrypsin. Many factors have been associated with an increased incidence of chronic bronchitis, including smoking, air pollution (e.g., sulfur dioxide), occupational exposures (e.g., toluene diisocyanate) and exposure to pathogens (e.g., bacteria, mycoplasma, and viruses).

84–86. The answers are: 84-D, 85-D, 86-B. *(Melanoma diagnosis and therapy)*

The lesion shown in the photograph is that of a superficial, spreading melanoma. This form of melanoma often involves a rapidly expanding superficial lesion that contains shades of brown mixed with bluish-red or black. The border of the lesion is visible or palpably elevated. It is grossly distinguishable from other common pigmented lesions based on color, shape, and rate of growth. Although the back and extremities are common sites for detection of such a lesion, melanomas can arise in other areas of the body.

Melanomas are tumors that are of great concern because of their propensity for metastasis. The liver, brain, and lungs are likely target organs. The process of metastasis is not well understood but involves the elaboration of a number of tissue-degrading enzymes, including collagenase and lysosomal hydrolase, and profibrinolytic compounds, such as plasminogen activator. Interaction with extracellular matrix via laminin and fibronectin molecules is also important. The target organ often elaborates a surface molecule with a high affinity for the disseminating tumor cell.

Adoptive immunotherapy is the current protocol with the most promise after failure to respond to common chemotherapeutic modalities. In this procedure, lymphocytes are removed from the patient, expanded in culture, and treated with interleukin-2 (IL-2) in an attempt to generate lymphokine-activated killer (LAK) cells. These treated cells are returned to the patient and IL-2 is also administered in vivo. The other cytokines (i.e., interleukin-1, interleukin-6, interferon-γ, and tumor necrosis factor) do not generate LAK cells.

87. The answer is B. *(DNA replication)*

Topoisomerase enzymes are important for regulating the equilibrium between supercoiled and relaxed DNA. Okazaki fragments are annealed by the actions of a ligase, and the newly synthesized DNA is "proofread" by a subunit of DNA polymerase III. The RNA primer is required to initiate DNA synthesis and is thought to be synthesized by RNA polymerase.

88–90. The answers are: 88-A, 89-E, 90-A. *(Cystic fibrosis)*

Inheritance via autosomal recessive genetic transmission suggests that each parent must have been a carrier. Since the parents of the patient in question are disease-free, they are heterozygous; thus, their chances of having another child with cystic fibrosis is one in four, according to mendelian genetics.

A deficiency in pancreatic lipases reduces the absorption of fat-soluble vitamins (A, D, and K). Vitamin K is critically important in the synthesis of clotting factors II, VII, IX, and a deficiency in vitamin K leads to bleeding diatheses manifested by a prolonged prothrombin time. Vitamins B_6 and C are water soluble and are less likely to be affected by pancreatic lipase deficiency.

Although clinical improvement from respiratory infections in cystic fibrosis occurs without eradication of bacteria from sputum during antibiotic therapy, it is standard procedure to treat the readily identifiable microorganisms. The gram-positive and particularly difficult to eradicate gram-negative bacteria (e.g., *Pseudomonas aeruginosa*) are often cultured from sputum, and a common regimen includes a β-lactam antibiotic, such as gentamicin, with a gram-negative antibiotic, such as the third-generation cephalosporin, ceftazidime. *P. aeruginosa* is often resistant to nitrofurantoin or nalidixic acid. Pentamidine is used for the treatment of protozoal infections, such as *Pneumocystis carinii*. Rifampin and isoniazid are used in the therapy of tuberculosis.

91. The answer is C. *(Neoplasia of the reproductive tract)*

Twenty-five percent of males in the United States have a tumor in the prostate gland. A prostatic tumor rarely occurs before age 40 years, but the incidence rises rapidly with advancing age. Seventy-five percent of prostatic tumors arise in the posterior lobe, are easily palpable, and, therefore, are detectable.

92–93. The answers are: 92-D, 93-D. *(Pheochromocytoma)*

The paroxysmal symptoms and detection of an abdominal mass within the adrenal gland are consistent with a diagnosis of pheochromocytoma, a relatively rare tumor of the chromaffin cells of the adrenal medulla. The cells of the adrenal cortex are generally not affected, although extra-adrenal chromaffin cells are often involved.

Pharmacotherapy to manage the clinical symptoms includes the use of an α-adrenergic receptor blocker (phenoxybenzamine) either alone or in combination with a β-blocker. β-blockers alone are contraindicated as they may leave the α-adrenoreceptor–mediated effects of the disorder unopposed. Clonidine is a useful test for the disorder; peripheral catecholamine levels will not be depressed after patients with pheochromocytoma take clonidine, whereas normal subjects will show a prompt decline. Methyldopa is likely to be converted in significant amounts to the weak vasoconstrictor alpha methyl norepinephrine, which may exacerbate the symptoms.

94. The answer is B. *(Organophosphate exposure)*

Organophosphates are highly toxic insecticides that occasionally affect agricultural workers. They are also frequently the primary agent in chemical weapons. They are highly lipid-soluble and are absorbed through virtually all body parts, including the skin. They produce a cholinergic crisis secondary to inhibition of acetylcholinesterase, which involves nicotinic and muscarinic receptors, both centrally and systemically. Atropine decreases some of the muscarine effects, including the bronchospasm and increased secretions of the airways. Mechanical ventilation may still be required if respiratory muscles are paralyzed. Pralidoxime, if given early enough, will help regenerate new cholinesterase and ultimately hasten reversal of the overdose.

95. The answer is C. *(Self-tolerance)*

The thymus is an antigenically privileged site, and thymocytes pass through only once; therefore, peripheral tolerance may be a necessary mechanism. There is no evidence that T cells leave and then come back to the thymus. Tolerance seems to be a negative-selection phenomenon, and it is believed that all selection initially takes place in the thymus.

96. The answer is A. *(Protein structure)*

Many polypeptides have a distinctive tertiary structure that provides insight into their function. Zinc fingers and leucine zippers are structural motifs that seem to be crucial in most proteins with DNA-binding functions. Current research indicates that the zinc fingers insert into the major groove of DNA between the bases. EF hands are structural motifs that are important in the calcium-binding properties of molecules like calmodulin, troponin C, and the ryanodine receptor. β-pleated sheets are frequently involved in the transport of hydrophobic molecules: α_1-microglobulin carries porphyrin rings, and apolipoproteins transfer cholesterol esters via β-pleated sheets. Gly-X-Y repeats are important in producing the tight triple helix of collagen. Glycine has only a hydrogen as its side chain and therefore allows the individual helices to be wound tightly without a bulky structure in the center. Immunoglobulin folds are important in the superfamily, which includes immunoglobulins, epidermal and nerve growth factors, and other proteins that have diverse functions.

97. The answer is D. *(Retroviruses)*

The retroviruses are unique in their diploid genetic structure, with two identical RNA molecules per virion. To initiate an effective infection, the virion-associated reverse transcriptase must produce a double-stranded DNA copy of the viral RNA, and that copy must be integrated into the host genome. Infectious virus then is produced from the integrated copy. The various viral antigens are made from messenger RNA (mRNA) produced from the DNA copy, and these antigens include both group-specific and host-specific reactive antigens. The viral RNA has plus polarity.

98. The answer is B. *(Chronic hemolytic anemia and iron overload)*

Patients with a long-standing history of chronic hemolytic anemia (e.g., sickle cell disease or β-thalassemia major) generally have a substantially enlarged spleen, which exacerbates their condition by destroying abnormal but functional erythrocytes. Splenectomy, however, greatly increases the patient's susceptibility to infection by encapsulated organisms because the spleen is a major site of antigen presentation. Congestive heart failure can result from many factors, including iron overload, chronic high-output demand, and mild hypoxia. The heart rate is typically fast and has an enlarged stroke volume in an effort to increase tissue oxygenation. These increased demands are made in the presence of blood, which is poor at delivering oxygen to the overworked myocardium. Increased absorption, as well as regular transfusions, combine to cause fairly severe iron overload. Cardiac myocytes, particularly in the conducting system, suffer damage principally related to iron toxicity. The liver and pancreas are also susceptible to the effects of systemic iron excess. Emphysema is not related to iron toxicity, high-output cardiac failure, or chronic hypoxia.

99. The answer is D. *(Immunoglobulin properties)*

The biological significance of immunoglobulin D (IgD) remains obscure. It has no properties that set it apart from any other immunoglobulin, and it has not yet been implicated in any specific disease states. Immunoglobulin M (IgM) antibodies against immunoglobulin G (IgG) are known as rheumatoid factors and are frequently seen in a variety of autoimmune related diseases. IgG is the main serum antibody, and it remains elevated long after the antigen has disappeared. IgM is the ''first responder'' in the body's production of humoral immunity and is found in the highest titers during the first 10 days following antigen presentation. IgA is especially important in defending against enteric pathogens, and IgE-mediated hypersensitivity results in allergic rhinitis.

100. The answer is D. *(α-Thalassemias)*
None of the common hemoglobinopathies are sex-linked because none of the subunits are encoded on the X chromosome. Two copies of the α-globin subunit gene are located on chromosome 16, and there are two chromosomes from each parent. On each chromosome, the proximity of the two identical α-subunit genes results in a high frequency of recombination, which, in turn, leads to an increased frequency of nonhomologous recombination and deletion. Thus deletions are the most common cause of α-thalassemia. Because restriction fragment length polymorphisms are very sensitive to deletions, they are useful in identifying the genotypes for genetic counseling. The α-thalassemias are most common in Asians and blacks, with the most severe cases occurring in Asians. The severity is governed by the number of normal genes remaining; when one of the genes is missing, it is a completely silent carrier state. Deletion of two genes results in a mild hypochromic anemia, which is clinically silent and is detected only by a routine complete blood count. The more severe forms of the disease (i.e., hemoglobin H disease (Hb H), and hydrops fetalis) result from a loss of three or four of the genes, respectively. Hb H is the abnormal hemoglobin composed of four β subunits instead of two β and two α. Hb H disease causes a hemolytic anemia that is generally well compensated. Hydrops fetalis is incompatible with life, and these infants usually die in utero. The severe forms are more common in Asians because they more often carry the homozygous deletion haplotype (αα/--); therefore, they can pass on a chromosome that has no functional α genes. Black people with the carrier state are more frequently heterozygous in both alleles (α-/α-).

101. The answer is E. *(Multiple endocrine neoplasia)*
Zollinger-Ellison syndrome is a gastrin-secreting, pancreatic islet-cell tumor often associated with multiple endocrine neoplasia (MEN) type I. The primary components of MEN IIa are pheochromocytoma and medullary carcinoma of the thyroid, whereas MEN IIb is characterized by pheochromocytoma and medullary carcinoma as well as the unusual neural tumors of the facial mucosal surfaces. MEN I is characterized by parathyroid tumors, pituitary adenomas, and pancreatic islet-cell tumors. All three types of MEN are hereditary, and the genes have been tentatively assigned to chromosome 10 for type II and chromosome 11 for type I. The patterns of inheritance are variable, as is the expression of disease phenotypes. Some patients have all of the characteristic tumors, whereas others have only one or two of the classically described neoplastic growths. The medullary cells (e.g., adrenal and thyroid), as well as the glia involved in the neuromas, arise embryologically from the neural crest. Thus, it is thought that a neoplastic clone may give rise to all three types of tumors.

102. The answer is B. *(Nephrotic syndrome)*
Nephrotic syndrome is the name given to the set of clinical symptoms that includes proteinuria, generalized edema, hypoalbuminemia, and hyperlipidemia. Several different pathologic lesions of the kidney can be seen when a renal biopsy is performed on a patient with nephrotic syndrome, but the most common is focal segmental glomerulosclerosis. People with systemic diseases (e.g., diabetes and systemic lupus erythematosus) can also have nephrotic syndrome. Nephrotic syndrome specifically excludes hematuria, whether microscopic or gross, which indicates a more serious lesion of the glomerular filtration apparatus and is indicative of nephritis, not nephrosis.

103. The answer is E. *(Effects of chronic alcohol abuse)*
Alcoholism is a major source of morbidity and mortality in the United States. Cerebellar degeneration and ataxia, often seen in association with profound anterograde amnesia, is known as the Wernicke-Korsakoff

syndrome. Demyelination seems to be critical to the cerebellar component of the disease, but the lesion causing the memory loss is still ill-defined. Esophagitis associated with vomiting and chronic reflux is a common complaint of alcoholics, but the more serious Mallory-Weiss tears (usually secondary to fierce retching) involve the rupture of a submucosal vein resulting in acute, voluminous blood loss. Testicular atrophy and amenorrhea are often the result of liver degeneration and the concomitant reduction in steroid metabolism. High estrogen levels result in feedback inhibition of hypothalamic gonadotropin releasing hormone (GnRH) secretion. Chronic alcohol abuse also results in mild hypertension for reasons that are still unclear. Protein malnutrition and the synthesis of fatty acids from ethanol combine to produce the commonly seen elevation in serum triglycerides. Bronchogenic carcinoma is one of the few serious pathologic entities not associated with alcoholism.

104. The answer is D. *(Acute pancreatitis)*
α_1-Antitrypsin deficiency is commonly associated with damage to the liver and lungs, but not the pancreas. Clearly, alcohol ingestion can cause acute pancreatitis, and several bouts of alcohol-induced subacute pancreatitis may allow chronic pancreatic failure to emerge without a clinically symptomatic episode of acute pancreatitis. Elevated serum triglycerides are found more often in people with pancreatitis than in the general population, but the reason for this phenomenon is not understood. The backup of bile into the pancreatic duct may be the reason for pancreatitis associated with biliary tract disease, but the complete sequence of events is poorly understood. Cholestasis is probably part of the reason for the increased incidence of pancreatitis following abdominal surgery, but again, the exact mechanism is not clear. Trauma or surgery, which lead to damaged pancreatic tissue, almost invariably cause some level of pancreatitis because the pancreas is full of digestive enzymes that are extraordinarily destructive if inappropriately released.

105. The answer is C. *(Immunology; immunoglobulins)*
Immunoglobulin E (IgE) has a serum half-life of 2 days, making it the shortest lived immunoglobulin. The low serum levels of this class of immunoglobulin are due to both a high affinity for mast cells and basophils and a low rate of synthesis. It is elevated in certain parasitic infections, such as *Ascaris* infections, and is not an agglutinating or complement-fixing antibody.

106. The answer is E. *(Antimicrobials and pseudomembranous colitis)*
The patient is likely suffering from antibiotic-associated pseudomembranous colitis (note the patient's diarrhea and deterioration following antibiotic therapy). Sigmoidoscopic examination, Gram stain of feces for white blood cells, a *Clostridium difficile* toxin test, and isolating the patient are appropriate procedures to follow for this patient. However, changing the antibiotic from a cephalosporin to clindamycin is inappropriate because *C. difficile* is not sensitive to clindamycin.

107. The answer is D. *(Agnogenic myeloid metaplasia)*
Bone marrow hypocellularity and teardrop-shaped erythrocytes are pathognomonic for agnogenic myeloid metaplasia with myelofibrosis. Leukocyte alkaline phosphatase levels are normal or elevated until the final stages of the disease. The liver does not usually undergo any significant change in size, whereas the spleen is almost always markedly enlarged as it becomes the principal site of extramedullary hematopoiesis.

108. The answer is A. *(Characteristics of warfarin)*
Warfarin affects normal synthesis of clotting factors in the liver, and its coagulant effects can be reversed by vitamin K. It is well-absorbed orally but will cross the placenta and may affect the fetus. It is used on a chronic basis for deep venous thrombosis and long-term care postmyocardial infarction because its onset of action is slow. Another useful anticoagulant is heparin, which is a large water-soluble polymer that must be given parenterally and does not cross the placenta. It is primarily used for acute anticoagulant therapy because its

onset of action is rapid. It can be reversed by the administration of protamine. The main action of heparin is thought to involve catalyzing the activation of antithrombin III in blood, thereby inhibiting thrombin and factor Xa.

109. The answer is D. *(Antioxidants)*
Transketolase is a part of the nonoxidative phase of the hexose monophosphate shunt and has no known role in protecting red blood cells from oxygen insult. A number of enzymes are involved in the protection of red blood cells from oxygen insult by hydrogen peroxide. Glutathione peroxidase catalyzes the reduction of hydrogen peroxide to water. The reduced nicotinamide-adenine dinucleotide phosphate (NADPH) utilized by glutathione reductase to regenerate reduced glutathione is produced in the 6-phosphogluconate dehydrogenase reaction. Catalase results in the decomposition of hydrogen peroxide to water and molecular oxygen.

110. The answer is D. *(Immunology; Arthus reaction)*
The Arthus reaction requires relatively large amounts of antibody and antigen, which then form insoluble complexes and begin to accumulate endogenously. When the aggregates are large enough, the complement cascade is activated. The formation of complement fragments C3a and C5a causes an increase in vascular permeability with resulting edema. Neutrophils and platelets accumulate at the site of the reaction. The activated neutrophils release a host of proteases and collagenases, resulting in rupture of the vessel wall, hemorrhage, and local necrosis. Serum sickness is the most common type III reaction, and the Arthus reaction is the least common.

111. The answer is D. *(Mechanism of action of zidovudine and treatment of AIDS)*
Zidovudine (ZDV) is currently the most important agent available for the palliation of AIDS. ZDV is phosphorylated to a deoxynucleoside derivative, which inhibits viral RNA-dependent DNA polymerase. Its selectivity is a function of its specificity for reverse transcriptase compared to human DNA polymerase. Granulocytopenia and anemia occur in up to 45% of treated patients, and resistance does occur to the drug after prolonged therapy. ZDV delays the development of signs and symptoms of AIDS in patients who are asymptomatic and improves the clinical symptoms of patients with AIDS at most stages in their disease. Thus, the incidence of opportunistic infections decreases, and there are some improvements in neurologic deficits, AIDS-associated thrombocytopenia, psoriasis, and lymphocytic interstitial pneumonia.

112. The answer is B. *(Vascular permeability; inflammation)*
Eosinophil chemotactic factor (ECF) is a set of tetrapeptides that produces a chemotactic gradient to attract eosinophils but has no effect on vascular permeability. Histamine and serotonin increase vascular permeability by causing post-capillary venular contraction. Slow-reacting substance of anaphylaxis (leukotrienes C_4 and D_4) are the only eicosanoids that directly increase vascular permeability. Both serotonin and slow-reacting substance of anaphylaxis increase vascular permeability.

113. The answer is E. *(Chronic obstructive pulmonary disease)*
Risk for chronic obstructive pulmonary disease (COPD) with various degrees of emphysema or chronic bronchitis is strongly associated with cigarette smoking and exposure to irritating substances in the environment (e.g., sulfur dioxide) or workplace (e.g., silica, cotton or grain dust, toluene diisocyanate). Usually, it is associated with older age-groups, especially individuals with preexisting lung disease. A genetically linked deficiency in α_1-antitrypsin is strongly linked to premature obstructive pulmonary disease. Although intravenous drug abuse is associated with pulmonary complications, including acute respiratory failure and opportunistic infections accompanying immunodeficiency-like syndromes in certain individuals, it is not usually considered a risk factor for COPD.

114. The answer is C. *(Human genetics and Duchenne muscular dystrophy)*
In Duchenne muscular dystrophy (DMD) the amount of dystrophin (a 400-kilodalton protein of unknown function but thought to be involved in Ca^{2+} regulation) is reduced from its normal 0.002% of total protein. Derangement of Ca^{2+} homeostasis is thought to be the cause of the excessive shortening of the sarcomeres. The affected muscle groups hypertrophy due to replacement of muscle mass by fibrofatty tissue. DMD is most often transmitted from a female carrier to the affected male (about 1 per 3500 liveborn males) by X-linked recessive inheritance (myotonic dystrophy is associated with mutations on chromosome 19), although approximately one-third of the cases appear to be due to spontaneously arising mutations.

115. The answer is D. *(Virulence factors; group A streptococci)*
The symptoms and clinical microbiology results indicate that the child has scarlet fever caused by a group A streptococcus (*Streptococcus pyogenes*) infection. This organism causes hemolysis by producing extracellular hemolysins such as streptolysin O. Other important virulence factors of this organism include membrane-bound protein (M protein) [which is antiphagocytic and also helps mediate adhesion], lipoteichoic acid (which also mediates adhesion), and a hyaluronic acid capsule. The erythrogenic toxins responsible for scarlet fever rash are not hemolytic.

116. The answer is E. *(Cushing's syndrome)*
Cushing's syndrome may be caused by hypothalamic or pituitary pathology or both, adrenal adenoma (or carcinoma), and exogenous glucocorticoid administration. In pediatric cases, severe growth retardation may occur before closure of the epiphysis during puberty. Hypersecretion of adrenocorticotropic hormone (ACTH) from the pituitary gland, due to either an underlying tumor or overstimulation from corticotropin releasing factor (CRF) of hypothalamic origin, stimulates the adrenal cortex to release excessive amounts of glucocorticoids (and mineralocorticoids). Other sites of excessive ACTH secretion, including tumors of nonendocrine origin, may be important. A useful initial screen to detect the presence of the syndrome is to inject dexamethasone and then to monitor the expected suppression of cortisol (due to pituitary inhibition) in plasma the following day. Patients with various forms of Cushing's syndrome and a responsive adrenal cortex will not undergo the predicted suppression until considerably higher amounts of dexamethasone are administered. Subsequent tests [including urinary secretion and administration of metyrapone (cortisol synthesis inhibitor)] and diagnostic procedures will help to identify the source of the excessive cortisol production.

117. The answer is E. *(Protein synthesis)*
Protein synthesis occurs in both the cytoplasm and the mitochondria of cells and requires large amounts of energy. In addition to requiring adenosine triphosphate (ATP) for the formation of aminoacyl transfer RNA (tRNA), guanosine triphosphate (GTP) is required for initiation, formation, translocation, and termination of the peptide bond. Protein synthesis requires messenger RNA (mRNA), tRNA, and ribosomal RNA (rRNA). Peptide-bond formation involves the transfer of the nascent polypeptide chain from one tRNA to the amino group of another aminoacyl tRNA. This reaction is accomplished by the enzyme complex known as peptidyltransferase, which is an integral part of the 50S ribosomal subunits.

118. The answer is C. *(Osteoclasts; bone metabolism)*
Osteoclasts are stimulated by parathyroid hormone and inhibited by calcitonin. Osteoclasts are multinucleated cells found on the surface of bone, often in Howship's lacuna. They are bone-resorbing cells involved in remodeling bone and in calcium homeostasis, and probably are derived from the macrophage–monocyte system.

119. The answer is C. *(Antibacterial drug use during pregnancy)*
High levels of amoxicillin in the urine can be achieved because penicillins are eliminated mainly unmetabolized via the kidney. There is minimal risk for the fetus using this or other penicillins, although these agents

do cross the placental barrier. Sulfonamides should be avoided due to displacement of bilirubin from serum albumin and resultant deposition of bilirubin in the central nervous system (CNS) [kernicterus] of the fetus and newborn, who do not yet have an intact blood–brain barrier. Minocycline should be avoided since tetracyclines are possibly teratogenic and can cause altered bone growth due to high calcium binding. Gentamicin can damage the eighth nerve in the fetus, leading to hearing impairment.

120. The answer is D. *(Immunologic disorders)*
Graves' disease is a thyroid disorder, but it is not known to be associated with thymomas. Thymomas, 90% of which are benign, are associated with myasthenia gravis, systemic lupus erythematosus, hypogamma-globulinemia, neutrophil agranulocytosis, and polymyositis. The significance of the association with these diseases, in particular myasthenia gravis, remains obscure, although removal of the thymus sometimes leads to regression of this disease.

121. The answer is C. *(Human immunodeficiency virus)*
The human immunodeficiency virus (HIV) has a demonstrated ability to infect any cell with a CD4 receptor, which includes T-helper cells, macrophages, and a subset of brain cells. The virus particle attaches to the cell via the CD4 receptor and gains entry through membrane fusion; it does not require endocytosis. During the replication process, a large amount of viral glycoprotein is produced, which becomes integrated into the host cell membrane. This can either lead to a budding of new virus or fusion with another uninfected CD4$^+$ cell. One infected cell can fuse in this fashion with a large number of uninfected cells, rendering them immunologically inactive.

122. The answer is E. *(Chlamydia trachomatis)*
Chlamydia trachomatis cannot synthesize adenosine triphosphate (ATP) or oxidize the reduced form of nicotinamide–adenosine dinucleotide (NADH) and is an obligate intracellular parasite. *C. trachomatis* organisms are internalized by host cells but evade destruction by preventing lysosomal fusion with the phagosome. *C. trachomatis* infections can be treated with tetracyclines, erythromycin, sulfonamides, sulfamethoxazole–trimethoprim, or rifampin.

123–127. The answers are: 123-E, 124-B, 125-C, 126-A, 127-D. *(Brain function evaluation)*
Short-term memory is dependent on an ability to concentrate. Information for short-term memory is stored in the hippocampus and temporal lobe. Digit repetition measures attention and requires an intact RAS in the pons and midbrain. (Rare deep medial frontal lobe lesions can cause indifference and inattention.) Interpretation of proverbs requires the use of brain areas where the highest cortical function appears to be located. The analytic and conceptual skills are largely based in the prefrontal cortex.

The copying of a design requires many areas of the brain—namely, the visual or occipital cortex, the parietal association areas, and the prefrontal and frontal cortices. Damage to the right parietal lobe results in greater impairment in this task than a similar lesion on the left side. A good performance indicates integrity of many neural structures; therefore, this test is a good screening method. Poor performance requires appraisal of each area involved (e.g., is the problem related to poor motor control of writing? is there a problem with the analysis of the design?).

Although serial 7s subtraction is used by some as a test of concentration (i.e., a test of brain stem RAS integrity), this utilization is an underestimate of the complexity of the task. The ability to calculate is highly dependent on intelligence and education; therefore, the task is calling on brain areas other than the RAS—namely, calculating abilities in the left parietal lobe and recall of mathematical facts in memory storage areas.

128–131. The answers are: 128-F, 129-B, 130-E, 131-G. *(Pulmonary function tests)*
Pulmonary function tests are a critical part of the evaluation in any patient with a breathing disorder. In the diagram, *A* is total lung capacity, *C* is the inspiratory reserve, and *D* is the inspiratory capacity. The residual

volume (*F*), tidal volume (*B*), vital capacity (*E*), and functional residual capacity (*G*) are the most critical because they tend to give information relevant to the patient's pulmonary status.

132–136. The answers are: 132-C, 133-B, 134-A, 135-B, 136-C. (*Family therapies*)
The family therapies can be roughly divided into three schools. The behavioral–psychoeducational approaches are grounded in social learning theory and frequently will instruct patients in the principles of this theory during treatment. The structural–strategic therapies view family problems as misguided and dysfunctional attempts to adapt to current life circumstances. Clarification of current relationship patterns, such as alliances and coalitions, and cognitive reframing are techniques associated with these therapies. The intergenerational–experiential therapies view family problems as rooted in the family's fixation at a particular stage of development; therapy attempts to discover the cause of this fixation by examining transgenerational patterns and elaborating the family's identity.

137–139. The answers are: 137-C, 138-B, 139-B. (*Anatomy of abdominal fascia*)
The abdominal superficial fascia (subcutaneous tissue) has two layers: The superficial fatty layer is called Camper's fascia; the deep membranous layer is called Scarpa's fascia. Both are especially prominent over the abdominal wall. Of these two layers, only Scarpa's fascia can support sutures. Scarpa's fascia continues over the pubis and perineum as Colles' fascia.

140–144. The answers are: 140-D, 141-A, 142-B, 143-B, 144-C. (*Genetics of insulin-dependent diabetes mellitus*)
Approximately 95% of patients with insulin-dependent diabetes mellitus (IDDM) have human leukocyte antigen (HLA) DR4. HLA DR3/DR4 heterozygotes are particularly susceptible to IDDM, and the DR3/DR4 antigens account for more than half the genetic contribution underlying IDDM.

If a proband with IDDM and his sibling share no haplotype, the risk to the sibling of developing IDDM is approximately 2%. The risk is 5% to a sibling who does share one HLA haplotype with a proband affected with IDDM. Approximately half of the normal population has HLA DR3 or HLA DR4; the empiric risk for developing IDDM is approximately 5% to a sibling for whom no HLA typing is available.

If the proband and sibling both share DR3 and DR4, the risk to the sibling of developing IDDM is approximately 20%. Clearly, the HLA haplotype alone does not underlie the genetics of IDDM, and there must be other genes that also contribute to the development of the disease.

145–149. The answers are: 145-E, 146-A, 147-B, 148-E, 149-A. (*Heavy metal poisoning*)
Elemental mercury is volatile at room temperature and is efficiently absorbed through the lungs. Other inorganic and organic forms of mercury are found in industrial processes, foodstuffs, medicines, paints, and cosmetics. These forms usually cause toxicity after gastrointestinal exposure. Metallothionein synthesis is increased after exposure to mercury, and this results in a protective effect against tissue damage. Exposure to the vapor results in airway inflammation and pneumonitis; chronic exposure to the vapor produces toxicity principally in the central nervous system (CNS) [The neuropsychiatric signs commonly observed in felt hat workers, who were exposed to mercury vapor, led to the expression, "mad as a hatter."]. The other forms of mercury can cause corrosive damage to the skin and gastrointestinal tract as well as the CNS manifestations. Gastric lavage and chelation therapy (with N-acetylpenicillamine or dimercaprol) should be considered in the treatment protocol.

The toxic metal arsenic is commonly encountered in a variety of forms (i.e., inorganic, organic, vapor); it produces toxicity in nearly every organ system by tightly binding to sulfhydryl groups as well as by interfering with oxidative phosphorylation. Exposure to arsenic vapor can lead to the rapid onset of severe hemolysis and hematuria. Exposure to the organic and inorganic forms (i.e., through skin or gastrointestinal absorption) can produce acute or chronic symptoms depending on the dose and duration of exposure. Gastric lavage, penicillamine, dimercaprol, and hemodialysis all should be considered for the effective management of arsenic toxicity.

The largest epidemic of lead poisoning in history followed the introduction of lead into paints as a color stabilizer. More than 2 million preschool children are annually affected in the United States. Lead toxicity in all tissues is related to its disruption of sulfhydryl groups in proteins. In adults, chronic exposure leads to abdominal pain, anemia, renal disease, ataxia, and memory loss. Childhood poisoning frequently presents with abdominal pain and anemia, but the CNS effects are most important. Unfortunately, subclinical toxicity is most common; the lead poisoning retards CNS development without causing any symptoms that might bring an affected patient to medical attention. Mental retardation, language deficits, cognitive dysfunction, and abnormal behavior are all common manifestations of long-term exposure to lead during the critical preschool years.

Exposure to cadmium is generally related to occupation or pollution from local refining or mining operations. Toxicity can follow ingestion or inhalation; acute symptoms can quickly follow relatively large doses, whereas chronic symptoms are often associated with cumulative exposure.

Tin is not a common cause of heavy metal toxicity.

150–154. The answers are: 150-D, 151-F, 152-A, 153-B, 154-C. *(Hormonal regulation of the menstrual cycle)*

The outer, stratified squamous epithelia are characteristic of thecal cells (*D*), and the inner, columnar epithelia are characteristic of granulosa cells (*E*). Luteinizing hormone (LH; *B*) exerts its primary effects on thecal cells, whereas follicle-stimulating hormone (FSH; *C*) exerts its primary effects on granulosa cells.

Thecal cells play a key role in estrogen synthesis because granulosa cells cannot produce estradiol from cholesterol: They need the androgen precursors from the thecal cells. During the follicular phase, estradiol participates in both a positive and negative feedback loop with the hypothalamic-pituitary-ovarian axis. Follicular estradiol (*F*) increases the pituitary gland's LH response to hypothalamic gonadotropin-releasing hormone (GnRH) while decreasing its FSH response. The same GnRH (*A*) pulsatile secretions during this period result in progressively larger LH (*B*) secretions until the LH surge occurs, which induces ovulation. FSH also has a surge, which corresponds with the LH surge and ovulation, but the LH surge alone is sufficient to induce ovulation.

FSH (*C*) is responsible for recruiting follicles at the beginning of the menstrual cycle. According to the current model, the follicle with the greatest sensitivity to FSH quickly develops the capacity to increase its estradiol production despite the negative feedback effect of estradiol on pituitary FSH secretion. Thus, as other follicles stop the maturation process due to decreased availability of FSH, one follicle produces increasing amounts of estradiol independent of FSH stimulation.

155–158. The answers are: 155-A, 156-C, 157-D, 158-C. *(Characteristics of lung carcinomas)*

Oncogene amplification and mutation are in the initial phases of study. However, adenocarcinoma has been shown to have a high incidence of K-*ras* oncogene abnormalities, while small cell carcinoma has an association with c-*myc* gene amplifications. Small cell carcinoma differentiates along neuroendocrine cell lines, which is reflected in the presence of membrane-bound, dense-core neurosecretory granules within the cell cytoplasm. The cytoplasm contains peptide hormones, which induce paraneoplastic syndromes. Bronchioloalveolar adenocarcinoma shares histologic similarity to a virus-induced carcinoma in sheep, called jaagsiekte. Bronchioloalveolar adenocarcinoma is characterized by lepidic growth by mucin-secreting cells and by bronchorrhea.

159–163. The answers are: 159-B, 160-E, 161-C, 162-A, 163-B. *(Vitamin biochemistry)*

Coenzyme B_{12} (cobalamin) is the only macromolecule with a metal–carbon bond; cobalt is coordinated with five nitrogens and a methylene group of adenine nucleotide in the active state of the vitamin. Coenzyme B_{12} is important in two kinds of mammalian cellular biosynthetic reactions: intramolecular rearrangements and methylations. The cobalt–carbon bond is sufficiently weak to be a convenient source of free radicals in the rearrangement of methylmalonyl CoA to succinyl CoA, a reaction that is important for shuttling amino acids into the Krebs' cycle. A similar reaction is utilized in its transfer of a methyl group to homocysteine in the formation of methionine; *S*-adenosylmethionine is an important carrier of methyl groups for a variety of methylation reactions, and coenzyme B_{12} is important in the cyclic regeneration of active *S*-adenosyl-methionine.

Vitamin E (α-tocopherol) is essential for protecting unsaturated membrane lipids from oxidation. Unsaturated lipids are susceptible to oxidation by the extracellular environment (e.g., oxygenated blood) as well as by oxygen free radicals, which are generated by a variety of normal cellular metabolic processes. Vitamin E has a remarkable capacity for scavenging oxygen free radicals and may be useful in protecting membrane lipids from oxidative damage. Because oxygen free radicals have been implicated in the progression of Parkinson's disease, clinical trials with high dose vitamin E are being conducted.

Vitamin C (ascorbic acid) was first identified as an essential nutrient when it was discovered that scurvy, a common ailment of European sailors, could be prevented if oranges were kept aboard ships. Vitamin C is essential for maintaining the enzyme proline hydroxylase in its reduced state. In the absence of sufficient vitamin C, proline hydroxylase becomes oxidized and loses its activity. Hydroxylation of proline is critical in helping to maintain the triple-helical structure of collagen. Thus, the symptoms of scurvy (i.e., vitamin C deficiency) are related to the structural weakness of the insufficiently hydroxylated collagen.

Vitamin A (retinol) is an important precursor for the pigment molecule rhodopsin. A deficiency of vitamin A frequently manifests as night blindness. Insufficient production of rhodopsin results in a decreased sensitivity to light, which first affects night vision. Sufficient quantities of vitamin A are especially important during childhood development. High doses of vitamin A analogues have been useful in both the topical [tretinoin (Retin-A)] and oral [isotretinoin (Accutane)] treatment of cystic acne.

Riboflavin (vitamin B_2) is the precursor for the flavin nucleotides, flavin mononucleotide (FMN) and flavin-adenine dinucleotide (FAD). FMN is involved in the mitochondrial electron transport chain, and FAD is critical in forming double bonds between carbon atoms in fatty-acid metabolism.

164–168. The answers are: 164-B, 165-D, 166-E, 167-C, 168-A. *(Blood typing)*
The couple in family 164 can only be the parents of infant B. Infant A, C, D, or E cannot be their child because those children are Rh$^+$, and both the mother and father are Rh$^-$.

The couple in family 165 can only be the parents of infant D. The child of family 165 must have just the N antigen in the MN group. Infant D is the one who has only the N antigen.

The couple in family 166 could be the parents of infant B, C, or E. However, infant B must belong to family 164, and infant C must belong to family 167, since infants A, B, D, and E all have the N blood group antigen, which neither the mother nor the father in family 167 has. Therefore, infant E must belong to family 166. The couple in family 166 cannot be the parents of infant A, who has blood type O, because the child must inherit the gene for either the A or the B antigen from his mother. The couple in family 166 cannot be the parents of infant D, because he must have inherited the gene for either the A or the B blood group antigen from his father, and the father has the O antigen.

The couple in family 168 could be the parents of infant A or B, but infant B must belong to family 164, therefore infant A must be family 168's child. The couple in family 168 cannot be the parents of infant C because he did not inherit the gene for the N blood group antigen, which the father must have transmitted to his son. The couple in family 168 cannot be the parents of infant D or E because both infants have a gene for the B blood group, which neither the mother nor the father in family 168 has.

169–172. The answers are: 169-E, 170-A, 171-C, 172-B. *(Psychological stages of neoplastic disease)*
It is important for the physician to recognize the psychosocial stages that patients with neoplastic disease may experience, because the goals and difficulties of each phase differ. The diagnostic phase requires the

physician's attention to possible patient denial of the disease and to ultimate acceptance of the need for treatment. The actual treatments of neoplastic disease often involve serious side effects (malaise, nausea, vomiting) that may promote noncompliance. The period of remission may involve anxious waiting for signs of the disease, which can lead to hypochondriacal complaints and lack of return to full functioning. Patients in the terminal phase of cancer need to be in a supportive setting with adequate palliation of pain and discomfort.

173–177. The answers are: 173-D, 174-C, 175-A, 176-F, 177-B. *(Protein synthesis, post-translational modification, and targeting)*
Protein synthesis begins in the nucleus, where the gene in question is first transcribed into messenger RNA (mRNA). The nascent transcript generally contains introns, which are pieces of the transcript that do not code for amino acid sequences. The introns are removed in a process known as exon splicing. The correctly spliced mRNA transcript leaves the nucleus and is bound to a free ribosome.

After the correct addition of the first eight to twenty amino acids, a special signal is encountered in most of the proteins that are destined for lysosomes, secretion, or the plasma membrane. This signal peptide causes the ribosome to stop translating the transcript and move to the endoplasmic reticulum (ER). ER with aggregations of ribosomes is frequently called ''rough ER'' because of its dense, speckled appearance. Proteins that are ultimately destined for the cytoplasm (e.g., hexokinase) do not have a special signal, and their translation is finished on free ribosomes void of any ER interaction.

Following synthesis on the rough ER, proteins destined for one of the three special targets frequently have sugar moieties added to asparagine on the nitrogen side chain. This N-linked glycosylation occurs in the lumen of the rough ER; then the protein is sent to the Golgi complex. Although its function is still being studied, it is clear that the Golgi complex is the key site for sorting proteins that are emerging from the rough ER. The N-linked sugars are modified, and additional sugars are frequently added to the oxygen-based side chains of serine or threonine (O-linked glycosylation). Fatty acids and other lipid moieties are often added in the lumen of the Golgi complex, too (i.e., acylation). These various modifications may contribute to the protein's function or structural stability. Sometimes, they serve as signals for targeting mechanisms.

Mannose 6-phosphate was the first targeting signal to be well established. Mannose 6-phosphate moieties are essential for an enzyme to be transferred into the lysosomal lumen. Patients with lysosomal storage diseases frequently have a defect in this targeting mechanism. Usually, the enzyme has a defective signal so that it is synthesized but not concentrated in the site where it serves its degradative function.

Proteins destined for the mitochondria and nucleus are nearly all synthesized in the cytosol on free ribosomes. Therefore, they are generally not glycosylated or acylated. The signal for transporting these proteins to their respective compartments is usually found in the amino acid sequence. A very short nuclear localization sequence causes proteins to be sequestered in the nucleus; one of several signals targets a mitochondrial protein to its appropriate destination (e.g., the inner membrane, matrix, outer membrane, intermembranous space).

178–182. The answers are: 178-B, 179-E, 180-A, 181-D, 182-C. *(Neuropathology)*
Neurofibrillary tangles are not unique to Alzheimer's disease as they are also seen in Down syndrome, normal aging, and pugilistic dementia; however, they uniquely occur in high concentrations in the hippocampus of Alzheimer's patients. Multinucleated giant cells occur in patients with AIDS who have encephalitis. Lewy bodies and eosinophilic cytoplasmic inclusions in the substantia nigra are characteristic of Parkinson's disease. Prions, proteins devoid of nucleic acid that are infectious, are associated with Creutzfeldt-Jakob dementia. Pick's bodies stain silver and are inclusions within neurons.

183–187. The answers are: 183-C, 184-F, 185-A, 186-B, 187-G. *(Structure of messenger RNA)*
The AUG sequence (C) codes for methionine; in eukaryotes, the first AUG following the methylguanylate cap is the site of translation initiation. The 5′ N7-methylguanylate cap is a post-translational modification that involves an unusual high-energy phosphate bond. This cap seems to enhance translation by interacting with the ribosome. It also stabilizes the message against the action of phosphatases and nucleases.

A stem–loop (or hairpin) structure (B) is, so far, the only important secondary structure described for the linear, single-stranded RNA. These stem–loops are created by sequences that are rich in standard Watson-Crick base-pairing ability. They can be found in introns and exons, at the beginning of the message, in the middle, or at the end. Their importance has been demonstrated in prokaryotes (e.g., attenuation, tryptophan operon) as well as in eukaryotes (e.g., the half-life of transferrin).

Exons (D) are the blocks of nucleotide sequence that code for amino acids in the protein. The intervening sequences, or introns (E) do not code for amino acids. Although their role is not fully understood, it is clear that in some cases they can regulate termination of translation as well as the half-life of the message.

The elucidation of the splicing process by which introns are removed and adjacent exons attached marked a major milestone in molecular genetics. Some messages have the capability to splice themselves independent of protein interaction (e.g., autocatalytic activity of RNA). In other messages, the activity of the small nuclear ribonucleoproteins (snRNPs) [F] is essential for exon splicing. The drawing illustrates the lariat intermediate, which is important in both types of splicing.

The 3′ polyadenylate (poly-A) tail (G) is a post-transcriptional modification; adenosine nucleotides are not formally coded in the gene. However, it is clear that genomic sequences indicate the length of the poly-A tail, and many researchers believe that the poly-A tail performs additional functions other than regulation of message half-life.

188–192. The answers are: 188-C, 189-A, 190-B, 191-B, 192-D. *(Neurochemistry)*
Cholinergic neurons of the basal nucleus of Meynert degenerate in Alzheimer's dementia with an associated decrease in choline acetyltransferase. Tyrosine hydroxylase is the rate-limiting step for synthesis of dopamine, norepinephrine, and epinephrine; it forms dopa from tyrosine. The monoamine oxidase (MAO) enzyme for the breakdown of catecholamines and serotonin is located on the mitochondria. Because MAO levels increase with age after 35 years, MAO inhibitors may be particularly useful antidepressant drugs in the elderly. The dorsal raphe nuclei of the pons and medulla constitute an important serotoninergic area of the brain. Tryptophan-5-hydroxylase is the rate-limiting enzyme in the synthesis of serotonin.

193–195. The answers are: 193-B, 194-A, 195-D. *(Inflammatory heart disease)*
Chronic rheumatic heart disease refers to the long-term cardiac complications (especially valvular) of acute rheumatic fever. Typically, the mitral and aortic valve leaflets become thickened and deformed by fibrosis, with commissural fusion. The damaged valves represent a fertile ground for the development of infective endocarditis (subacute type).

Chronic rheumatic heart disease is a complication of acute rheumatic fever, which is a nonsuppurative systemic disorder related to an untreated pharyngitis caused by group A β-hemolytic streptococci. Although the precise mechanism of acute rheumatic fever is unknown, the presence of antistreptococcal antibodies that cross-react with heart antigens in these patients suggests an autoimmune basis for this disorder.

Subacute bacterial endocarditis most commonly is caused by α-hemolytic (viridans) streptococci, organisms that are a normal component of the oral flora. Typically, the organism gains entry to the circulation with minor oral trauma, and a transient bacteremia ensues. The bacteria then colonize a platelet-fibrin thrombus that has formed on a valve previously damaged by chronic rheumatic heart disease, mitral valve prolapse, previous cardiac surgery, or some other cause.

The acute form of bacterial endocarditis, in contrast to the subacute form, typically involves a normal heart valve in the setting of a well-defined bacteremia. In this case, the infectious agent usually is a virulent organism (e.g., *Staphylococcus aureus*) that causes the initial damage to the valves by way of a toxin.

Libman-Sacks endocarditis (also known as nonbacterial verrucous endocarditis) may occur as a complication of systemic lupus erythematosus (SLE). This disorder is characterized by the presence of warty endocardial vegetations along the valve margins and, most distinctively, on the undersurface of the valves.

196–200. The answers are: 196-C, 197-D, 198-A, 199-E, 200-D. *(Hormonal regulation of pregnancy)*
The fetal adrenal cortex lacks a key enzyme required for progesterone synthesis from cholesterol. Thus, maternal and placental progesterone are required for the synthesis of fetal cortisol and aldosterone. Progesterone is also important for stimulating the endometrium to secrete nutrients for the free-floating blastocyst before implantation. Finally, progesterone causes development of the glandular alveoli in the breast.

Estrogen and relaxin act synergistically to relax ligaments and the symphysis pubis. Elevated estrogen levels also suppress follicle-stimulating hormone (FSH) levels throughout pregnancy.

Estrogens and progesterone develop the alveolar and ductal mechanism of the breast; however, they also inhibit the actual production and secretion of milk. Prolactin's ability to stimulate production of milk increases rapidly after parturition, when the steroid inhibitors disappear from the serum.

Human chorionic gonadotropin (hCG) maintains the corpus luteum in much the same way that luteinizing hormone (LH) does during the normal menstrual cycle. The functions of human chorionic somatomammotropin (hCS) have not been well defined, but it appears that hCS gears the maternal metabolism towards supplying a constant level of nutrients to the fetus. Relaxin, which inhibits myometrial contractions and softens the cervix, is produced by the corpus luteum under the influence of hCS.

Test IV

QUESTIONS

DIRECTIONS: Each of the numbered items or incomplete statements in this section is followed by answers or by completions of the statement. Select the ONE lettered answer or completion that is BEST in each case.

Questions 1–5

A child presents to the pediatrician for evaluation of "difficulty walking." Examination reveals a waddling gait, proximal muscle weakness, pseudohypertrophy of the calf muscles, and a Gower maneuver upon standing from a sitting position. A tentative diagnosis of Duchenne muscular dystrophy (DMD) is made, pending the results of serum enzyme studies, electromyography, and muscle biopsy. A family pedigree is illustrated below.

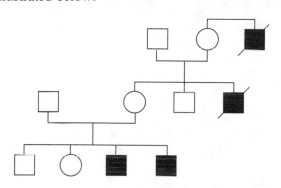

1. According to the pedigree, the mode of inheritance of DMD is

(A) autosomal recessive
(B) autosomal dominant
(C) X-linked
(D) nonpenetrant
(E) none of the above

*mother always carrier for DMD
pass always to only
male child (son)*

2. What is the chance that the mother is a carrier for DMD?

(A) 25%
(B) 50%
(C) 75%
(D) 100%
(E) None of the above

3. What is the chance that the next male child will carry the gene that causes the disease?

(A) None
(B) 50%
(C) 75%
(D) 100%
(E) None of the above

4. The defect in DMD involves a mutation in the gene coding for which of the following proteins?

(A) Actin
(B) Dystrophin
(C) Spectrin
(D) Tropomyosin
(E) None of the above

5. Some DMD can be diagnosed prenatally by which of the following techniques?

(A) Genetic probes
(B) Linkage analysis
(C) Western blot
(D) Southern blot
(E) None of the above

6. The violaceous skin nodule apparent in the photomicrograph below, which was taken from a young individual, is most likely

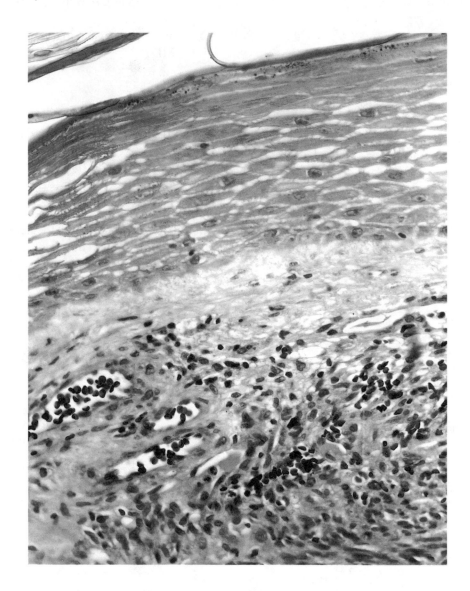

(A) seen on the back of infants' necks

(B) a highly malignant pigmented melanoma

(C) seen in men infected with human immuno-deficiency virus (HIV)

(D) due to radiation therapy that was administered over 10 years ago

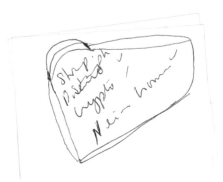

7. Which one of the following statements concerning referred pain is true?

(A) Pain from the transverse colon is usually referred to a midline area below the umbilicus
(B) Somatic pain is usually referred in a diffuse, poorly localized pattern
(C) Diaphragmatic pain is usually referred to the inguinal area
(D) The mechanism of referred pain is well understood

Questions 8–10

An 18-year-old college freshman has been "acting strangely" for several months, according to his roommates. His grades are deteriorating, and he avoids social interactions. He talks about being the devil's accomplice. He is unshaven, and his clothes are messy.

8. The first diagnosis to consider with this patient is

(A) schizophrenia
(B) mania
(C) schizoaffective disorder
(D) major depression
(E) phencyclidine psychosis

9. Further history reveals periods of staring spells and olfactory hallucinations. Based on these symptoms, the physician should order which of the following tests?

(A) Bender Gestalt test
(B) Thematic apperception test
(C) Electroencephalogram
(D) Halstead-Reitan battery
(E) Brain stem evoked potentials

10. A reasonable medication trial for complex partial seizures is

(A) haloperidol
(B) carbamazepine
(C) imipramine
(D) alprazolam
(E) clonidine

11. The term that describes the adherence of neutrophils and monocytes to the vascular endothelium before movement into the extravascular space is

(A) margination
(B) diapedesis
(C) pavementing
(D) migration
(E) clotting

12. A fluorescent probe that binds to glucocorticoid receptors is applied to cells. The probe is freely diffusible throughout the cell and has no effect on the glucocorticoid receptor. If the cell has not been previously stimulated by glucocorticoids, where is the most intense fluorescence?

(A) Cell membrane
(B) Cytosol
(C) Nuclear membrane
(D) Nucleus
(E) Nucleus and cytosol

13. A middle-aged woman presented with a throbbing headache and bilateral tenderness over her forehead. Knobby cords were palpated at the sides and were biopsied. The tissue is pictured in the micrograph below. The correct diagnosis is

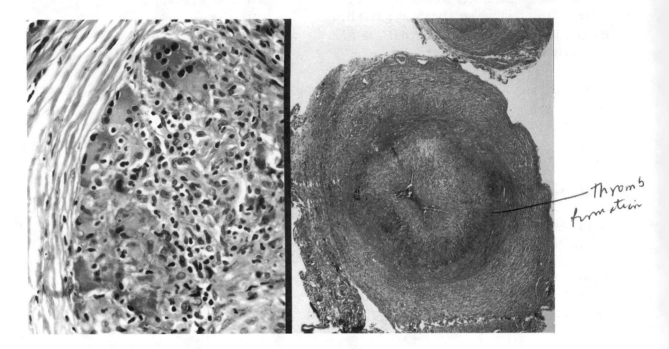

(A) temporal arteritis

(B) foreign body giant cell reaction to an injected substance

(C) Mönckeberg's arteriosclerosis

(D) Takayasu's arteritis

14. Cromolyn sodium is now the first-line agent for the treatment of mild to moderate asthma, especially asthma in children associated with allergenic causes. Although its mechanism of action is unclear, cromolyn sodium's widespread use is due to its

(A) bioavailability after oral administration

(B) direct bronchodilating effect, making it useful in acute emergencies

(C) prophylactic potential secondary to inhibition of the release of inflammatory mediators

(D) immediate effect to reduce bronchospasm

(E) antimuscarinic effects

Questions 15–18

A patient presents with epigastric and right upper quadrant pain. The pain is most intense 2–4 hours after eating and is reduced by the ingestion of antacids. The patient states that he has passed black tarry stools (melena) within the last week.

15. In considering gastric ulcer in the differential diagnosis, the physician should note all of the following risk factors EXCEPT

(A) smoking
(B) elevated secretion of hydrochloric acid (HCl)
(C) caffeine
(D) heredity
(E) gender

16. Fiberoptic endoscopy reveals a yellowish crater surrounded by a rim of erythema that is 3 cm distal to the pylorus. Accordingly, an ulcer has been identified in the patient's

(A) fundus
(B) antrum
(C) duodenum
(D) jejunum
(E) ileum

17. Hypertrophy of which of the following submucosal structures often accompanies denudation of the epithelium in peptic ulcer?

(A) Brunner's glands
(B) Meissner's plexus
(C) Auerbach's plexus
(D) Peyer's patches
(E) Paneth's cells

18. Possible pharmacotherapy for this patient may include

(A) bethanechol
(B) diphenhydramine
(C) indomethacin
(D) ranitidine
(E) dexamethasone

19. The most important prognostic factor for human cancer is

(A) the patient's age
(B) tumor stage
(C) lymphocytic infiltration
(D) vascular invasion
(E) the mitotic index

20. Growth hormone (GH; somatotropic hormone; somatotropin) is synthesized and stored in large amounts in the anterior pituitary gland (adenohypophysis). Which of the following statements accurately describes GH?

(A) It is secreted continuously
(B) Synthesis is stimulated by the action of somatostatin
(C) Receptors have a limited distribution outside the central nervous system (CNS)
(D) It stimulates cartilage and bone growth via somatomedin
(E) It has a proinsulin-like effect in addition to its other actions

21. A 29-year-old intravenous drug abuser presented with bilateral fluffy lung infiltrates. A transbronchial biopsy was performed. A Grocott-Gomori methenamine–silver nitrate stain was performed on the lung tissue (pictured below). The diagnosis is

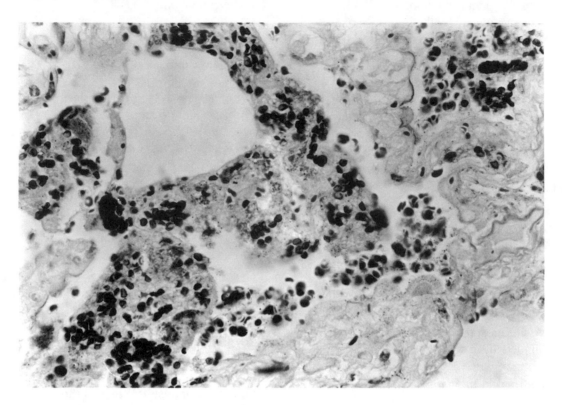

(A) atypical mycobacterial infection

(B) cytomegalovirus (CMV) pneumonitis

(C) nocardial abscess

(D) pneumocystis pneumonia

(E) legionnaires' disease

22. A 24-year-old black woman presented with <u>chest pain</u>; her chest radiograph revealed <u>mediastinal lymph-adenopathy.</u> A lymph node biopsy from the anterior mediastinum was obtained by mediastinoscopy, and the tissue sample is portrayed in the photomicrograph below. The correct diagnosis is

dense collagen

nodular sclerosing Hodgkin disease

multilobated cells

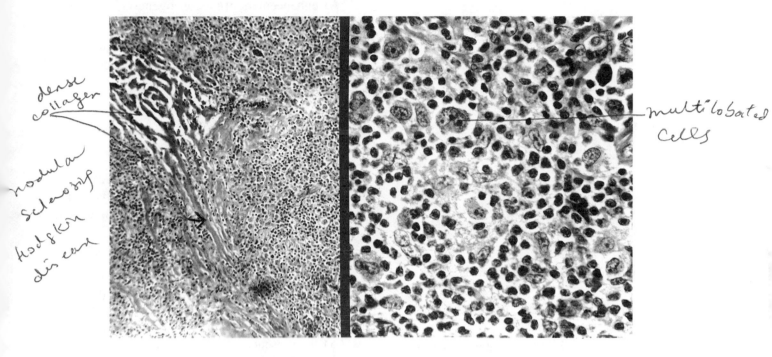

(A) sarcoidosis

(B) thymoma

(C) sclerosing mediastinitis

(D) Hodgkin's disease

23. Which of the following statements regarding the proximal tubular epithelium illustrated below is most likely to be correct?

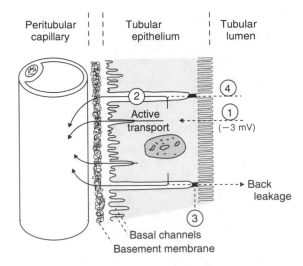

(A) The ion whose movement is depicted in (*1*) is Na$^+$

(B) The process depicted at site (*2*) is aldosterone-sensitive

(C) The cell is impermeable to water because of the tight junctions shown in (*3*)

(D) The process depicted at site (*4*) is affected by antidiuretic hormone (ADH)

(E) The intracellular potential is similar to the tubular lumen potential (−3 mV)

24. Of the following statements regarding thoracic outlet syndrome, which one is true?

(A) It results from an irregularly shaped first thoracic rib

(B) Compression of the left phrenic nerve may occur

(C) Numbness and tingling occur along a median nerve distribution

(D) Compression of the subclavian artery may occur

25. Glucose stimulation of beta cells in the endocrine pancreas subsequently causes

(A) enhancement of gluconeogenesis in the liver

(B) increased glycogenolysis by the liver

(C) stimulation of the release of glucagon

(D) decreased oxidation of amino acids in the liver

Questions 26–27

A 55-year-old patient presents with weakness, weight loss, and bone pain of 3 months' duration. Head x-rays show many well-demarcated osteolytic lesions.

26. All of the following symptoms would help to confirm the diagnosis of this disease EXCEPT

(A) the presence of monoclonal proteins weighing 55,000 daltons in the serum and urine

(B) a history of recurrent bacterial infections

(C) a spike in a particular isotype region in the electrophoretic pattern of serum proteins

(D) the presence of Bence Jones protein in the serum or urine

27. In approximately 55% of patients presenting with multiple myeloma, the major membrane-bound carrier protein, or monoclonal protein, would be

(A) immunoglobulin M (IgM)

(B) IgD

(C) IgE

(D) IgA

(E) IgG

28. Monitoring aminoglycoside serum levels is requisite for the systemic use of the drugs because

(A) they are extensively metabolized by hepatic enzymes
(B) they are rapidly eliminated
(C) they can cause severe hypersensitivity reactions
(D) their therapeutic index is low, and toxicity is easily manifest
(E) they rapidly cross the blood–brain barrier

29. Tamoxifen can control the growth of some forms of female breast cancer by

(A) inhibiting estrogen synthesis
(B) inhibiting androgen-induced DNA transcription
(C) competing for estrogen receptors
(D) inhibiting the secretion of luteinizing hormone (LH)
(E) stimulating nuclear transcription

30. Propranolol (a β-blocker) may be used with nitroglycerin (glyceryl trinitrate; GTN) in concurrent therapy for typical (exertional) angina because propranolol

(A) is a potent vasodilator of coronary arteries
(B) increases conduction in the atria and atrioventricular node
(C) blocks the reflex tachycardia that occurs with the use of GTN
(D) dilates constricted airways
(E) is positively inotropic

31. Phenytoin (Dilantin) is effective in most forms of epilepsy (with the exception of absence seizures) because it

(A) directly binds to chloride channels in the central nervous system (CNS)
(B) enhances the inhibitory actions of γ-aminobutyric acid (GABA) at its receptor in the CNS
(C) affects Na^+ conductance in neurons via voltage-sensitive Na^+-channel inhibition
(D) is usually started concurrently with phenobarbital therapy

32. Which one of the following statements concerning the synthesis of different types of RNA molecules in eukaryotic cells is true?

(A) RNA polymerase I produces mainly messenger RNA (mRNA)
(B) RNA polymerase III produces ribosomal RNA (rRNA)
(C) RNA polymerase II produces transfer RNA (tRNA)
(D) None of the above

33. Which one of the following drugs or chemicals has been associated with the induction of aplastic anemia?

(A) Acetaminophen
(B) Methyldopa
(C) Benzene
(D) Penicillin
(E) Thiouracil

34. A monoclonal antibody (immunoglobulin G; IgG) that neutralizes endotoxin has been produced. This antibody has tremendous therapeutic potential for patients suffering septic shock from endotoxemia, and it might be useful in treating patients who have which one of the following diseases?

(A) Pulmonary anthrax
(B) Whooping cough
(C) Cholera
(D) Leprosy
(E) Bubonic plague

35. Which of the following proteins bind to penicillin?

(A) Alanine racemase
(B) 30S Ribosomes
(C) Peptidoglycan
(D) Porin
(E) Transpeptidase

36. A medical student received a deep laceration in an altercation at a party. He reports having had a DTP (diphtheria-tetanus-pertussis) series in childhood. The most appropriate treatment would be

(A) injection of human tetanus immunoglobulin G (IgG)
(B) injection of equine tetanus IgG
(C) intravenous administration of an aminoglycoside
(D) injection of tetanus toxoid

37. Which of the following statements concerning acetylsalicylic acid (aspirin), the prototype of a group of nonsteroidal anti-inflammatory agents that are also analgesic and antipyretic, is correct?

(A) Aspirin is a potent lipoxygenase inhibitor
(B) The major adverse effect of aspirin is gastrointestinal bleeding
(C) Aspirin can reduce normal body temperature
(D) Aspirin is a competitive inhibitor of platelet cyclooxygenase

38. Which one of the following statements concerning messenger RNA (mRNA) splicing is true?

(A) Alternate splicing, producing two different mRNA molecules from the same gene, is a common occurrence in most mammalian genes
(B) Spliceosomes are collections of small nuclear ribonucleoproteins (snRNPs) located near ribosomes on the rough endoplasmic reticulum
(C) U1 snRNP binds to a nucleotide segment on the 5′ end of the intron to be spliced
(D) Spliceosomes recognize splicing sites by the large 50–80 base-pair sequences on the 5′ and 3′ regions of introns

39. The most common tumor of the appendix, which is pictured below, is

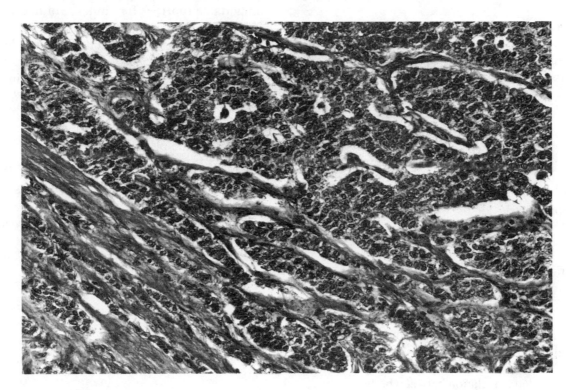

(A) a carcinoid tumor

(B) an adenocarcinoma

(C) a mucocele

(D) an inflammatory pseudotumor

40. Which one of the following conditions would result in a negative nitrogen balance?

(A) Consumption of dietary proteins that are deficient in glycine

(B) Normal intake of dietary protein accompanied by defective cholecystokinin–pancreozymin (CCK–PZ) production

(C) Nitrogen consumption that exceeds nitrogen excretion

(D) A tyrosine supplement in the diet of a child with phenylketonuria (PKU)

(E) A 50% reduction in the hydrochloric acid (HCl) content of gastric juice

41. Translation of a synthetic polyribonucleotide containing the repeating sequence CAA in a cell-free protein synthesizing system produced three homopolypeptides: polyglutamine, polyasparagine, and polythreonine. If the codons for glutamine and asparagine are CAA and AAC, respectively, which of the following triplets is a codon for threonine?

(A) AAC

(B) CAA

(C) CAC

(D) CCA

(E) ACA

Questions 42–43

It is hypothesized that nocturnal body temperatures are linearly related to body weight in 60- to 70-year-old women. Nursing records are reviewed for weights in kilograms and 4 A.M. temperatures in degrees Celsius.

42. These variables are considered to be

(A) continuous
(B) nonparametric
(C) constants
(D) reciprocal
(E) outliers

43. The null hypothesis for the study question described would state that there is

(A) an expected correlation between body weight and temperature
(B) an effect of aging on temperatures in obese elderly women
(C) no relation between temperature and body weight
(D) an inverse relation between body weight and nocturnal temperature
(E) a probability ($P < 0.05$) that body weight is related to nocturnal temperature

44. *Pseudomonas aeruginosa, Staphylococcus aureus,* and *Serratia marcescens* all produce which one of the following substances?

(A) Endotoxins
(B) Enterotoxins
(C) Lipoteichoic acids
(D) Mycolic acids
(E) Pigments

45. Resistance to phagocytosis is among the most important properties for virulence of many bacteria. *Mycobacterium tuberculosis* is very resistant to phagocytic killing and actually grows in macrophages. The successful antiphagocytic strategy employed by *M. tuberculosis* clearly involves which one of the following mechanisms?

(A) Production of protein exotoxins to kill or impair the phagocyte
(B) Prevention of phagosome–lysosome fusion
(C) Elaboration of immunoglobulin A (IgA) protease
(D) Production of the antiphagocytic polysaccharide capsule
(E) Escape from the phagolysosome into the cytoplasm

46. Injection of a pharmacologically effective amount of an antimuscarinic agent, like atropine, may

(A) increase bronchial glandular secretions
(B) increase heart rate
(C) cause paralysis in some skeletal muscles
(D) constrict the pupil
(E) promote sweating

47. G proteins are involved with various cellular signaling pathways and are known to hydrolyze

(A) adenosine triphosphate (ATP)
(B) guanosine triphosphate (GTP)
(C) adenosine diphosphate (ADP)
(D) guanosine diphosphate (GDP)
(E) adenosine monophosphate (AMP)

48. A peripheral lung nodule was resected from a 50-year-old man. The tumor, pictured below, is best classified as

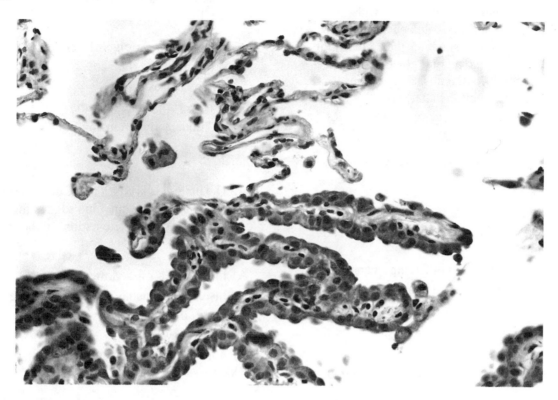

(A) small cell carcinoma

(B) undifferentiated large cell carcinoma

(C) adenoid cystic carcinoma

(D) bronchioloalveolar carcinoma

(E) diffuse large cell lymphoma

49. A lymph node removed from a 32-year-old man shows diffuse large cell lymphoma. Which of the following clinical scenarios most likely characterizes this patient? *non- hodgkin lymphoma*

(A) Disseminated disease at presentation; prolonged survival and eventual death owing to lymphoma or its complications

(B) Rapid development of circulating immature blasts, requiring aggressive cytotoxic therapy

(C) Greater than 90% chance of being alive 10 years after diagnosis

(D) Rapid death if therapy is unsuccessful; approximately 50% chance for long-term survival if therapy achieves complete response

(E) Spontaneous remission in 20% of patients

Questions 50–54

A young adult visits his physician with complaints of polyuria and unexplained weight loss. Fasting plasma glucose is greater than 140 mg/dl (on two occasions), and an oral glucose tolerance test is consistent with a diagnosis of type I insulin-dependent diabetes mellitus (IDDM). *lente insulin*

50. The likely histologic site underlying this patient's disorder is

(A) pancreatic acini
(B) zymogen-containing cells of the pancreatic acinus
(C) alpha cells of the islets of Langerhans
(D) beta cells of the islets of Langerhans
(E) delta cells of the islets of Langerhans

51. An important aspect of treatment in this patient is

(A) a single daily injection of an insulin zinc suspension (Lente insulin)
(B) glipizide
(C) abstinence from dietary carbohydrates
(D) increased intake of saturated fats
(E) avoidance of exercise

52. An endogenous hormone that tends to decrease circulating blood glucose is

(A) glucagon
(B) growth hormone (GH)
(C) somatostatin
(D) epinephrine
(E) thyroid hormone

53. Despite vigorous therapy, all of the following are potential chronic complications of IDDM EXCEPT

(A) intercapillary glomerulosclerosis
(B) proliferative retinopathy
(C) atherosclerosis
(D) peripheral polyneuropathy
(E) pulmonary hypertension

54. The patient is brought to the emergency room in a coma. An important clue suggesting that the coma is the result of ketoacidosis rather than hypoglycemia is

(A) history of a missed meal
(B) history of unusual vigorous exercise
(C) rapid, deep ventilatory pattern
(D) profuse sweating
(E) normal hydration status

55. Halothane has blood:gas and oil:gas partition coefficients of 2.4 and 220, respectively. Methoxyflurane has blood:gas and oil:gas coefficients of 13 and 950, respectively. Which of the following statements regarding these volatile anesthetics is correct?

(A) Both result in faster induction than does nitrous oxide (blood:gas partition coefficient of 0.47)
(B) The minimal alveolar concentration of halothane is less than that of methoxyflurane
(C) Both agents are useful because they do not have any cardiodepressant effects
(D) Recovery from methoxyflurane is faster than that from halothane
(E) An increase in ventilatory rate makes the onset of anesthesia more rapid for either agent

56. Restriction enzymes have which one of the following characteristics? They

(A) can cleave only circular DNA
(B) generate either staggered (sticky) or blunt ends upon cleaving DNA
(C) cleave different DNAs randomly
(D) can cleave different DNAs only once
(E) can cleave both DNA and RNA

57. A chronically ill 43-year-old patient with a relapse of multiple sclerosis has been in the hospital for 4 weeks. He has angered the nurses by being very demanding, including calling them "every 5 minutes" for minor reasons and complaining that they do not respond promptly. To remedy this situation, the physician must

(A) instruct the patient to behave better
(B) order a sedating medication
(C) arrange for the nurses to visit the patient for 3 minutes every hour
(D) warn the patient that he will be transferred to another hospital if he does not straighten out

58. A 74-year-old man presents with hypertension, diabetes mellitus with retinopathy, and chronic obstructive pulmonary disease (COPD). He admits to drinking four bottles of beer a day. He has been living alone for the past year since his wife died. His primary care physician should be especially and immediately concerned about the risk of

(A) renal insufficiency
(B) silent myocardial infarction
(C) suicide
(D) peripheral neuropathy
(E) pneumonia

59. The graph below measures the number of viable bacterial cells in a control culture and cultures of exponentially growing cells to which antibiotics were added at the point indicated by the *arrow*. The antibiotic added to the culture to produce *curve A* was which one of the following?

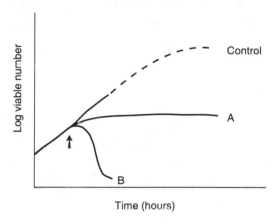

(A) Polymyxin B
(B) Cephalothin
(C) Chloramphenicol
(D) Methicillin
(E) Vancomycin

60. According to the Henderson-Hasselbalch equation:

$$pH = 6.1 + \log [HCO_3^-]/0.03 \times P_{CO_2}$$

The apparent dissociation constant, pK', in blood is 6.1; and the solubility constant for CO_2 in plasma at 38°C is 0.03 mmol/L/mm Hg. If a patient has a plasma $[HCO_3^-]$ of 37 mmol/L and arterial P_{CO_2} of 60 mm Hg, then the patient is most likely to have (recall log 10 = 1; log 20 = 1.3; log 30 = 1.5; normal values of $[HCO_3^-]$ = 25 mmol/L; P_{CO_2} = 40 mm Hg)

(A) respiratory alkalosis
(B) respiratory acidosis
(C) fully compensated respiratory acidosis
(D) metabolic alkalosis
(E) metabolic acidosis

61. The ability of erythrocytes to pump Na^+ from the cytoplasm into the plasma compartment would be compromised most directly by a total deficiency of

(A) stearoyl coenzyme A (CoA) desaturase
(B) diphosphoglycerate kinase
(C) pyruvate carboxylase
(D) glucose 6-phosphatase
(E) malate dehydrogenase

62. A total of 25 hypertensive patients are followed over a 2-week period for the effects of a diuretic drug on K^+ concentrations. The statistical test used to compare the K^+ serum levels before and after medication is most likely to be

(A) discriminant analysis
(B) paired t-test
(C) regression analysis
(D) chi-squared test
(E) Pearson correlation

Questions 63–64

A 22-year-old male college student visits the student health service complaining of extreme fatigue, sore throat, difficulty concentrating, and fever to 39°C over the last week. Physical examination is unremarkable except for mild lymph node enlargement in the axillary, cervical, and inguinal regions and a palpable spleen tip. A blood count shows hemoglobin of 10 g/dl, platelets of 105,000/μl, and white cell count of 22,000/μl with 60% lymphoid cells. The laboratory blood profile also shows an absolute red cell count of 2.3×10^6/μl, mean red cell volume of 125 femtoliters (fl), and mean cell hemoglobin concentration of 43 g/dl.

63. What is the most likely diagnosis for this patient?

(A) Infectious lymphocytosis
(B) *Bordetella pertussis* infection
(C) Cytomegalovirus (CMV) mononucleosis syndrome
(D) Mononucleosis secondary to Epstein-Barr virus (EBV) infection (infectious mononucleosis)
(E) Mononucleosis secondary to *Toxoplasma gondii* infection

64. Which of the following is the most likely cause of this patient's anemia (Hb 10 g/dl)?

(A) Immune-mediated
(B) Compromise of erythroid production secondary to EBV infection of bone marrow precursors
(C) Virus-associated hemophagocytic syndrome
(D) Slow gastrointestinal blood loss since the start of illness owing to thrombocytopenia
(E) Disseminated intravascular coagulation (DIC)

65. The eclipse phase of the virus replication cycle has which one of the following characteristics? It

(A) is defined as that time period after which the first virus particles are assembled
(B) denotes the time between virus entry into the cell and the time virus particles appear extracellularly
(C) is that part of the replication cycle during which virus particles cannot be recovered from the infected cells
(D) is comparable to the metaphase portion of mitosis

66. Light microscopy requires the use of special techniques, such as stains, to visualize cells and cell components. Which of the following cellular components can be visualized after staining for catalase?

(A) Golgi complex
(B) Lysosomes
(C) Rough endoplasmic reticulum
(D) Smooth endoplasmic reticulum
(E) Peroxisomes

67. Dinitrochlorobenzene was applied to a patient's skin over a 1-cm^2 area on the right forearm. Approximately 2 weeks later, a pruritic rash occurred at the site. It can be concluded that

(A) the patient lacks all T-cell–mediated immune function
(B) the patient suffers from DiGeorge syndrome
(C) the reaction would require an additional 2 weeks to develop on subsequent exposure to dinitrochlorobenzene
(D) the reaction observed was most likely caused by CD4$^+$ T cells

Questions 68–70

An ophthalmologic examination of a 60-year-old man complaining of vision problems reveals increased intraocular pressure (25 mm Hg) with optic disk changes and visual field defects. These findings strongly suggest primary open-angle glaucoma for which pharmacotherapy is considered.

68. The underlying cause of the patient's condition is a decreased outflow facility of the aqueous humor. A primary anatomic structure involved with the histopathologic changes that account for this problem is the

(A) conjunctiva
(B) cornea
(C) canal of Schlemm
(D) ciliary process
(E) choroidal vessel

69. Pharmacotherapy for the patient is initially designed to open trabecular meshwork by contracting the ciliary muscle. A useful agent for this purpose is

(A) atropine
(B) succinylcholine
(C) pilocarpine
(D) dexamethasone
(E) tubocurarine

70. After the initial pharmacotherapy fails, the patient is switched to an anticholinesterase agent, echothiophate. Absorption of this agent from the eye may be associated with which of the following adverse systemic effects?

(A) Tachycardia
(B) Urinary retention
(C) Decrease in gastrointestinal motility
(D) Bronchoconstriction
(E) Inappropriate decrease in sweating

71. The peripheral nerve tumor pictured below is best classified as a

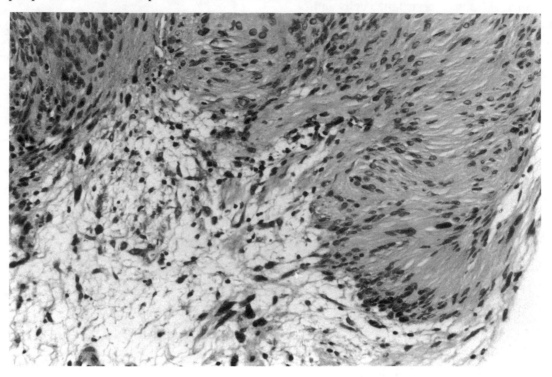

(A) neurofibroma

(B) traumatic neuroma

(C) neurilemoma

(D) triton tumor

72. Triglycerides are neutral fats of animals and food plants; they make up approximately 90% of the dietary intake of fats. An important step in their digestion in the gastrointestinal tract is

(A) significant hydrolysis by gastric lipases

(B) breakdown by biliary enzymes

(C) formation of fatty acids and monoglyceride by pancreatic lipase

(D) active transport of fatty acid products in the intestinal brush border

73. Which of the tracts listed below, whose fibers traverse the spinal cord, brain stem, and higher structures, is thought to cross to the opposite side of the central nervous system (CNS) twice?

(A) The anterior spinocerebellar tract, which conveys unconscious sensory information from joints, tendons, and muscles

(B) The spinal thalamic tract, which conveys conscious sensory information of pain and temperature

(C) The cuneocerebellar tract, which conveys conscious muscle and joint sensory information

(D) The vestibulospinal tract, which conveys efferent fibers

74. A 29-year-old white woman comes to the physician's office stating that she recently discovered a gap in her memory of 2 hours. She tells the physician that her friends informed her that she has been acting inappropriately. Suddenly the patient becomes confused but remains docile. She asks the physician from where the overwhelming smell of rotten food is emanating. The patient most likely suffers from

(A) Klüver-Bucy syndrome of the temporal lobes
(B) temporal lobe epilepsy
(C) jacksonian epileptic seizures
(D) petit mal seizures

75. A 5-year-old child in Bangladesh drinks untreated river water and develops cholera. Which of the following scenarios is most likely to occur?

(A) Recovery following treatment is slow because *Vibrio cholerae* causes chronic intracellular infections
(B) Microscopic examination of stools reveals leukocytes
(C) Disease symptoms arise due to cholera toxin-mediated elevation in cyclic adenosine monophosphate (cAMP) levels in intestinal cells
(D) *V. cholerae* attaches to the dental flora

76. Centrioles are replicated in which phase of the cell cycle?

(A) G_0 phase
(B) G_1 phase
(C) S phase
(D) G_2 phase
(E) M phase

77. Which one of the following statements about energy storage and transfer is true?

(A) Adenosine triphosphate (ATP) can be synthesized from adenosine diphosphate (ADP) by phosphate transfer from 3-phosphoglycerate
(B) Phosphocreatine is an important energy source for muscle tissues
(C) Reactions that have a $K_{eq} > 1$ have a positive $\Delta G°$
(D) When ATP is hydrolyzed to adenosine monophosphate (AMP) and inorganic pyrophosphate (PP_i), the reaction is endergonic and will proceed spontaneously
(E) The energy of hydrolysis for phosphoenolpyruvate is less than that for pyrophosphate

78. The extraction of β-hydroxybutyrate from blood and its oxidation to carbon dioxide and water requires the participation of

(A) β-hydroxybutyrate dehydrogenase and 3-hydroxy-3-methylglutaryl coenzyme A (HMG CoA) lyase
(B) acetoacetate thiokinase and β-hydroxybutyrate dehydrogenase
(C) HMG CoA synthase and thiolase
(D) short-chain fatty acetyl CoA dehydrogenase and thiolase
(E) succinyl CoA: acetoacetate acyltransferase and HMG CoA lyase

Questions 79–81

A 43-year-old man who is being treated with hydrochlorothiazide for control of mild edema presents to the physician complaining of malaise, fatigue, muscular weakness, and muscle cramps. Blood tests reveal elevated creatinine with an even greater elevation in blood urea nitrogen, high blood urate, and altered blood electrolytes.

79. What is the primary anatomic site of action of hydrochlorothiazide?

(A) Proximal tubules
(B) Early distal tubules
(C) Late distal tubules
(D) Thick ascending limb of the loop of Henle
(E) Collecting ducts

80. The patient's complaints most likely reflect the most serious adverse effect of diuretic therapy, which is

(A) hyperglycemia
(B) hyperuricemia
(C) drug hypersensitivity
(D) hyperkalemia
(E) hypokalemia

81. To correct this patient's problem, the physician must consider all of the following therapeutic choices EXCEPT

(A) K^+ supplementation
(B) digitalis
(C) spironolactone
(D) reduced dosage of hydrochlorothiazide
(E) amiloride

82. A 60-year-old woman is brought to the hospital because of fever and confusion. One week ago, she received chemotherapy for lymphoma. In the emergency room, she is noted to have rapid breathing, cool, clammy skin, and a blood pressure of 70/40. Complete blood count shows a white blood cell count of 200/μl. Gram stains of urine and sputum are negative. Which of the following empiric therapies would be most appropriate for this patient?

(A) Gentamicin
(B) Amikacin
(C) Chloramphenicol/gentamicin
(D) Piperacillin/gentamicin

83. An adolescent patient attends weekly individual, psychodynamic psychotherapy sessions. When he begins to feel too close to and dependent on the psychiatrist, he often misses a scheduled appointment. This behavior is an example of

(A) acting out
(B) antisocial personality
(C) repression
(D) suppression
(E) identification with the aggressor

84. Which of the statements concerning the disaccharide pictured below is most accurate? It

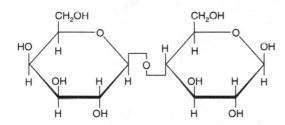

(A) yields a negative result in the Fehling-Benedict reducing sugar test
(B) is cleaved by isomaltose
(C) is a β-galactoside
(D) is digested and absorbed by a lactase-deficient child
(E) is a good source of calories for a 2-week-old child with galactosemia

85. A 42-year-old woman with breast cancer was treated with radiation and currently is receiving chemotherapy. She complained of some left-sided chest pain, which was determined not to be of cardiac origin. On the fourth day, several vesicles appeared on her left thorax, following a rib in distribution; she also had several smaller vesicles at other sites (scalp, leg, forearm). Her physician diagnosed varicella-zoster virus (VZV) infection and <u>started</u> treatment with acyclovir. Which one of the following statements best describes the VZV in this case?

(A) Thymidine kinase–negative VZV mutants are likely to render the treatment ineffective
(B) The initial exposure to VZV in childhood could not have led to viral latency in the dorsal ganglia
(C) The lesions outside the dermatomal distribution are likely explained by depressed cell-mediated immunity

86. A 62-year-old woman died of congestive heart failure due to severe mitral stenosis. At autopsy, sections of the heart revealed the lesions shown in the photomicrograph below. This suggests a previous history of which one of the following conditions?

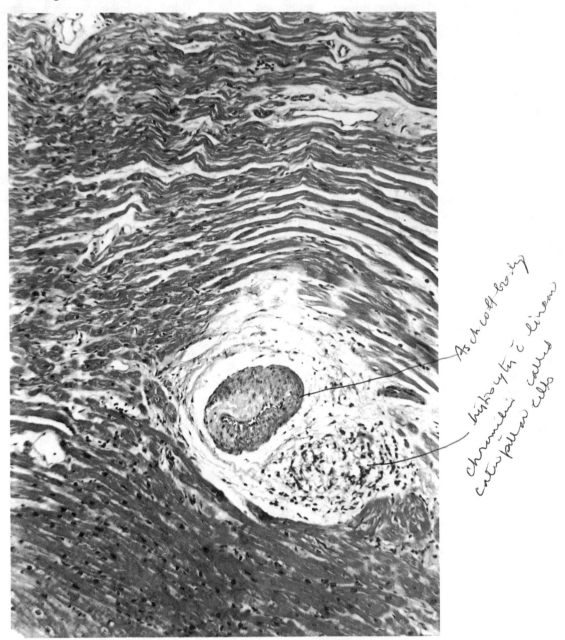

(A) Amyloidosis

(B) Rheumatic fever

(C) Polyarteritis nodosa

(D) Myocardial infarction

87. Which of the following tests is the major projective instrument of personality assessment?

(A) Rorschach inkblot test
(B) Minnesota Multiphasic Personality Inventory
(C) Thematic apperception test
(D) Sentence completion test
(E) Projective drawings

88. Proof of the presence of active disease caused by *Mycobacterium tuberculosis* is provided by which one of the following diagnostic measures?

(A) The tuberculin test
(B) Clinical findings (e.g., weight loss, night sweats, cough, low-grade fever)
(C) Finding acid-fast organisms in sputum
(D) Isolation of *M. tuberculosis*

89. Several workers at a chemical manufacturing facility were referred to a physician for evaluation of connective tissue neoplasms. This physician could expect to find

(A) antigenic cross-reactivity between tumors
(B) distinct antigenic specificity for each tumor
(C) antigenic cross-reactivity between these tumors and those induced by ultraviolet light
(D) distinct antigenic specificity for different cells from the same tumor

90. Hodgkin's lymphoma can be distinguished from other forms of lymphoma by the presence of

(A) Reed-Sternberg cells
(B) the Philadelphia chromosome
(C) Auer rods
(D) decreased quantities of leukocyte alkaline phosphatase

91. An 86-year-old man has diminished vibratory sensation at the knees and toes, although his reflexes are intact, temperature sensation is normal, and he feels well, aside from having headaches. What is the most likely explanation?

(A) Peripheral neuropathy
(B) Normal age-related change
(C) Spinal cord lesion
(D) Small strokes
(E) Brain or brain stem tumor

92. The pressor response to an indirect-acting sympathomimetic agent, such as amphetamine, is

(A) associated with marked tolerance (tachyphylaxis)
(B) decreased in the presence of a monoamine oxidase (MAO) inhibitor
(C) potentiated by an uptake 1 inhibitor, such as imipramine
(D) potentiated by pretreatment with reserpine
(E) related to its direct effects on postsynaptic receptors

93. The introduction of foreign DNA into bacteria is an important tool in molecular biology. Which of the following statements concerning nucleic acid transfer is true?

(A) Transformation is the technique whereby a bacteriophage is used to introduce DNA into a bacteria
(B) Transduction is the technique whereby "competent" bacterial cells are suspended in a solution of calcium chloride and DNA
(C) The most common DNA used in transformation is plasmid DNA
(D) Conjugation is the technique whereby a bacteriophage is used to introduce DNA into a bacteria

Questions (94–100)

A 27-year-old man who has torn his anterior cruciate ligament (ACL) while skiing is sent to the operating room for ACL replacement and reconstruction. The anesthesiologist selects halothane.

94. Important adverse effects of halothane include all of the following EXCEPT

(A) depression of respiratory drive
(B) lowering of ventilatory response to carbon dioxide
(C) malignant hyperthermia in genetically sensitive individuals
(D) lowering of the seizure threshold
(E) depressed myocardial contractility

95. Induction of anesthesia is smooth, and the operation begins. Before any incision is made, the surgical resident informs the surgeon that this surgery is to be performed on the

(A) ankle
(B) knee
(C) hip
(D) elbow
(E) shoulder

96. The ACL stabilizes this joint by attaching the

(A) medial malleolus of the tibia to the talus
(B) lateral malleolus of the fibula to the talus
(C) head of the femur to the innominate (hip) bone
(D) femur to the fibula
(E) femur to the tibia

97. The head of the femur is attached to the innominate bone at the cup-shaped region known as the

(A) ilioischial fossa
(B) iliofemoral fossa
(C) ischial depression
(D) acetabulum
(E) sella turcica

98. The primary site of long bone growth occurs at the

(A) epiphysis
(B) diaphysis
(C) epiphyseal plate
(D) medullary cavity
(E) primary ossification center

99. All of the following bones are carpal bones EXCEPT

(A) capitate
(B) cuboid
(C) navicular
(D) trapezium
(E) trapezoid

100. All of the following statements are true for compact bone EXCEPT that it

(A) is made up of parallel bony columns
(B) contains neurovascular channels
(C) is composed of a network of trabeculae
(D) contains haversian canals
(E) contains osteocytes that communicate via gap junctions

101. Which of the following tests is contraindicated in patients with intracranial neoplasms?

(A) Computed tomography (CT) of the head because of the use of contrast dye

(B) Nuclear magnetic resonance (NMR) because of the length of time a patient must remain supine during testing

(C) Lumbar puncture to examine cerebrospinal proteins and relieve hydrocephalus

(D) X-ray imaging of the skull because the radiation may shrink the tumor and cause hemorrhaging

102. For the past 8 weeks, a scientist has developed rhinorrhea, conjunctival itching, a cough, and wheezing within 5–10 minutes of entering the animal facility where her experimental mice are housed. In the past week, she has begun to have wheezing and shortness of breath at night from 4–8 hours after working in the animal facility. Which of the following describes the late symptom complex? It is

(A) induced by mast cells triggered by rodent antigen with immunoglobulin E (IgE)

(B) a result of complement-mediated cytotoxicity

(C) not blocked by corticosteroids

(D) blocked by antihistamines

103. The figure below is a stylized diagram of the juxtaglomerular apparatus of the kidney. A decrease in the flow of glomerular filtrate into the tubules might cause which one of the following actions?

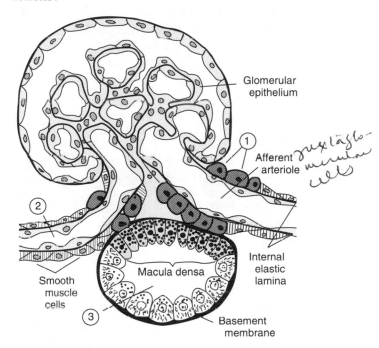

(A) Renin released from *1*

(B) Vasodilation of *2*

(C) An increase in Na$^+$ concentration at *3*

(D) A reflexive vasoconstriction of the afferent arteriole

104. A quantitative Gram stain revealed many fewer cells than expected from the turbidity of a bacterial culture. The decrease in cells was most likely due to

(A) inactivation of the cytochromes

(B) digestion of the bacterial cell wall by autolytic processes

(C) presence of gram-negative organisms in the culture

(D) presence of bacterial spores in the culture

105. According to Fick's law, oxygen consumption is equal to the product of blood flow and arteriovenous oxygen difference. If the lungs absorb 300 ml/min of oxygen, arterial oxygen content is 20 ml/100 ml blood, pulmonary arterial oxygen content is 15 ml/100 ml blood, and heart rate is 60/min, then stroke volume is

(A) 50 ml

(B) 60 ml

(C) 100 ml

(D) 5 L/min

(E) 6 L/min

106. Capsule production is essential for the virulence of many pathogenic bacteria. Which of the following statements best describes bacterial capsules?

(A) The most important function of the *Streptococcus pneumoniae* capsule is adhesion

(B) The capsule of *Haemophilus influenzae* type B stimulates a T-cell–dependent immune response

(C) Opsonizing antibodies are often directed against *S. pneumoniae* capsules

(D) The capsule of group B *Neisseria meningitidis* is protein

(E) The DTP (diphtheria-tetanus-pertussis) vaccine currently licensed contains purified *Bordetella pertussis* capsules

107. True statements about the side chains of amino acids that are found in proteins include which one of the following?

(A) Serine provides strong buffering capacity at pH 7.0

(B) Alanine absorbs ultraviolet light

(C) Glutamic acid and aspartic acid differ significantly in their isoelectric pH (pI)

(D) Proline often produces a bend in the protein chain

(E) Only D-amino acids are incorporated into protein

108. A 56-year-old woman with a history of ovarian cancer treated by chemotherapy several years ago presents to a clinic with complaints of fatigue and the recent development of small hemorrhages on her arms. She has the following lab values: hemoglobin, 9.6 g/dl; white blood cells, 2900/μl; platelets, 56,000/μl. A bone marrow aspirate is hypercellular and contains approximately 10% blasts (normal < 5%) with megaloblastic morphologic changes in the red cell precursors and megakaryocytes with abnormal nuclei. Cytogenetic analysis reveals a clone with a deletion of the long arm of chromosome 7. What diagnosis best fits this woman's condition?

(A) Preleukemia (myelodysplastic syndrome)

(B) Megaloblastic anemia

(C) Acute lymphocytic leukemia

(D) Acute nonlymphocytic (myeloid) leukemia

(E) Chronic myelogenous leukemia

109. Of the drugs listed below, which one is thought to function through a receptor?

(A) Mannitol

(B) Dimercaprol

(C) Cimetidine

(D) Ethylenediaminetetraacetic acid (EDTA)

110. According to the figure below, which one of the following conditions would result in a shift of the oxygen saturation curve from *a* to *b*?

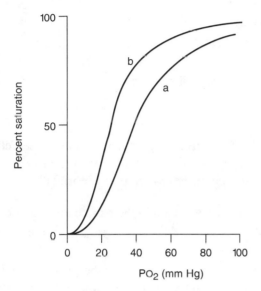

(A) A change in pH from 7.6 to 7.4
(B) A change in P_{CO_2} from 30 to 40 torr
(C) An increase in the concentration of 2,3-diphosphoglycerate (DPG)
(D) The presence of fetal hemoglobin ($\alpha_2\gamma_2$)
(E) The oxidation of the heme iron from Fe^{2+} to Fe^{3+}

111. Which one of the following muscles raises the soft palate during swallowing?

(A) Levator veli palatini
(B) Palatoglossus
(C) Palatopharyngeus
(D) Superior constrictor

112. A 32-year-old man is unemployed and lives in a personal care boarding home. He has a 10-year history of undifferentiated schizophrenia, and has been observed pacing around the house and fidgeting whenever seated. Recently, he received his monthly injection of fluphenazine. The most likely cause of his agitation is

(A) anxiety
(B) restless legs syndrome
(C) akathisia
(D) undiagnosed hyperthyroidism
(E) worsening psychosis

113. Which one of the following statements best describes chondroblasts?

(A) They are endosteal cells capable of secreting proteoglycan
(B) They are perichondrial cells capable of secreting type II collagen
(C) They are periosteal cells capable of secreting type I collagen
(D) They show little mitotic activity
(E) They are filled with rough endoplasmic reticulum but lack a Golgi apparatus

114. A previously healthy 27-year-old woman is seen because of a petechial rash. She denies recent bleeding and has had no recent illnesses. Hemoglobin, hematocrit, and white blood cell counts are normal. Examination of the peripheral blood smear reveals normal red and white blood cells and is remarkable only for a paucity of platelets. The most likely diagnosis in this patient is

(A) aleukemic leukemia
(B) idiopathic thrombocytopenic purpura (ITP)
(C) Glanzmann's thrombasthenia
(D) amegakaryocytic thrombocytopenia
(E) drug-induced thrombocytopenia

Questions 115–120

A 50-year-old man presents to the emergency room with severe epigastric pain, low-grade fever, tachycardia, and mild hypotension. The patient relates a history of moderate to heavy social drinking. The chief resident suspects acute pancreatitis.

115. The single most important laboratory finding to confirm the diagnosis of pancreatitis would be

(A) hyperlipidemia
(B) hyperbilirubinemia
(C) elevated serum amylase
(D) elevated serum phospholipase A
(E) elevated serum alkaline phosphatase

116. Which of the following polypeptide hormones is stimulated by increased acid from the stomach and subsequently stimulates the release of pancreatic juice rich in electrolytes and water?

(A) Gastrin
(B) Secretin
(C) Cholecystokinin
(D) Pancreozymin
(E) Vasoactive intestinal polypeptide (VIP)

117. Which of the following hormones is produced by the duodenal and upper jejunal mucosa and stimulates the release of pancreatic juice rich in digestive enzymes?

(A) Cholecystokinin
(B) Secretin
(C) Glucagon
(D) Pancreatic polypeptide
(E) VIP

118. Neuronal control of pancreatic exocrine function is mediated by

(A) VIP
(B) dopamine
(C) serotonin
(D) substance P
(E) acetylcholine (ACh)

119. Of the following statements about secretin, a polypeptide that has a significant effect on pancreatic secretion, which one is correct?

(A) It is synthesized in the pancreatic acinar cells
(B) It causes the pancreas to secrete large amounts of enzyme
(C) Its release is caused by the presence of fats and amino acids in the upper small intestine
(D) It causes the pancreas to secrete large amounts of bicarbonate ion (HCO_3^-)
(E) It is stored in an active form within S cells of the duodenum

120. The principal reason that the pancreas does not autodigest is that

(A) proteolytic enzymes are secreted as proenzymes
(B) pancreatic acini and ducts secrete a protective mucopolysaccharide, which lines their walls
(C) the pancreas mantains a slightly alkaline pH, rendering the digestive enzymes inactive
(D) pancreatic parenchyma is high in hydroxyproline, which is resistant to proteolysis
(E) proper enzyme substrates are not present

121. A complement fixation test is performed on a patient's serum by first adding influenza type A virus antigen and then adding complement, followed by antibody-coated sheep red blood cells (SRBC), which are then lysed. A possible explanation for this would be

(A) the patient has no immunoglobulin E (IgE) or IgA anti-influenza type A antibodies
(B) the patient's serum contains an antibody that cross-reacts with SRBC
(C) the patient has no complement fixable anti-influenza type A antibodies
(D) the patient's serum contains high levels of IgM, which cause SRBC lysis

122. Volume and pressure (alveolar; pleural) for a normal respiratory cycle are shown in the figure below. Which one of the following statements about respiration is correct?

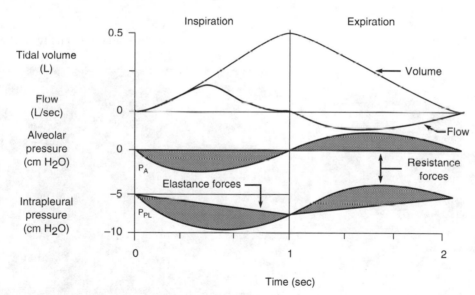

(A) Inspiration is the result of a passive process
(B) Gas flow is greatest at the end of inspiration
(C) Elastic recoil of the lung is identical at the beginning and end of inspiration
(D) During expiration, alveolar pressure becomes greater than atmospheric pressure

123. Which one of the following areas in a eukaryotic cell is a site of RNA processing?

(A) Mitochondria
(B) Golgi complex
(C) Rough endoplasmic reticulum
(D) Nuclear membrane

124. In humans, the major route of nitrogen metabolism from amino acids to urea involves which one of the following sets of enzymes?

(A) Amino acid oxidases and arginase
(B) Glutaminase and amino acid oxidases
(C) Glutamate dehydrogenase and transaminases
(D) Transaminase and glutaminase
(E) Glutamine synthetase and urease

125. A random subject undergoes magnetic resonance imaging (MRI) for an experiment, and a congenital malformation is found: The corpus callosum never developed, leaving the right and left sides of the brain unconnected. Which of the following statements about this man's condition is most likely to be true?

(A) The patient's intelligence and behavior are abnormal
(B) The patient is unable to verbally describe an object placed in his left hand when his eyes are closed
(C) The patient is asymptomatic and shows no neurologic defect on clinical examination
(D) The patient has a positive Romberg sign (i.e., he loses his balance when standing with his eyes closed)

126. The micrograph below is a portion of the liver biopsied from a 42-year-old man. The microscopic features seen are most likely due to

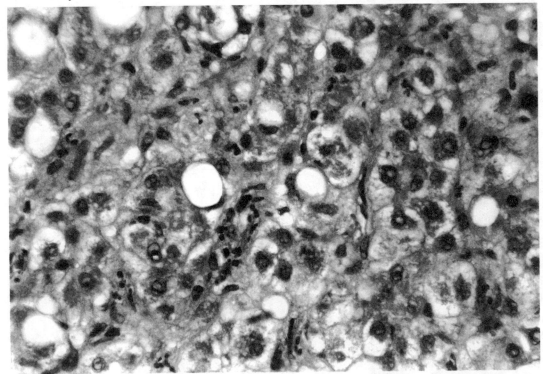

(A) exposure to carbon tetrachloride
(B) acetaminophen toxicity
(C) ethanol use
(D) acute rejection of a liver allograft

DIRECTIONS: Each of the numbered items or incomplete statements in this section is negatively phrased, as indicated by a capitalized word such as NOT, LEAST, or EXCEPT. Select the ONE lettered answer or completion that is BEST in each case.

127. All of the following statements concerning the response of immunoglobulins to viruses in vivo are true EXCEPT that they

(A) displace attached viruses from the host cell
(B) inhibit the action of viral enzymes
(C) induce complement-mediated lysis of infected host cells
(D) retard the infectivity of viruses for host cells

128. Cholesterol biosynthesis occurs in the cytosol of many cells of the body, primarily in the liver, and entails all of the following steps EXCEPT that it

(A) forms lanosterol from squalene and then converts it to cholesterol
(B) requires reduced nicotinamide-adenine dinucleotide phosphate (NADPH) as a source of reducing equivalents
(C) forms 3-hydroxy-3-methylglutaryl coenzyme A (HMG CoA) from acetoacetyl CoA
(D) forms squalene from isoprenoid units
(E) uses HMG CoA reductase for catalysis of HMG CoA to mevinolin

129. Angiotensin-converting enzyme (ACE) hydrolyzes angiotensin I to angiotensin II. Possible explanations why inhibition of this enzyme with specific peptide inhibitors (i.e., captopril) reduces blood pressure in some subjects include all of the following EXCEPT

(A) decreased production of a vasoconstrictor (angiotensin II)
(B) increased synthesis and release of aldosterone
(C) centrally mediated decrease in water uptake
(D) inhibition of synaptic transmission in peripheral sympathetic nervous system

130. All of the following substances readily diffuse through cell membranes EXCEPT

(A) oxygen
(B) carbon dioxide
(C) glucose
(D) water
(E) nitrogen

131. The S_3 heart sound is normally heard only in children or young, thin-chested adults. An accentuated S_3 heart sound can sometimes be heard in either children or adults with all of the following pathologies EXCEPT

(A) mitral regurgitation
(B) patent ductus arteriosus
(C) left ventricular failure
(D) pulmonary stenosis
(E) ventricular septal defects

132. A fecal specimen is cultured from a person with diarrhea, and *Shigella dysenteriae* and *Giardia lamblia* are isolated. All of the following statements about *Shigella* and *Giardia* are true EXCEPT

(A) *Shigella* has a peptidoglycan-containing cell wall but *G. lamblia* does not
(B) *Shigella* and *Giardia* both have DNA and RNA
(C) *Shigella* and *Giardia* both have sterol-containing plasma membranes
(D) *Shigella* has a lipopolysaccharide but *Giardia* does not
(E) *Shigella* has 70S ribosomes but *Giardia* has 80S ribosomes

133. All of the following statements about enzymes are true EXCEPT that

(A) V_{max} is a measure of catalytic efficiency
(B) K_m is a measure of the enzyme's affinity for the substrate
(C) formation of the substrate complex results in rearrangement of specific functional groups of the enzyme
(D) the reaction rate is accelerated by increasing the activation energy
(E) Ionizable amino acid side chains are frequently used as general acids and bases in catalysis

134. Adult respiratory distress syndrome (ARDS) shows all of the following morphologic signs EXCEPT

(A) pulmonary edema
(B) hyaline membrane formation
(C) proliferation of type II pneumonocytes
(D) alveolar wall damage
(E) decreased permeability of the pulmonary capillary endothelium

135. Type II pneumonocytes have all of the following characteristics EXCEPT

(A) they elaborate pulmonary surfactant
(B) they exhibit surface microvilli
(C) they make up most of the alveolar surface area
(D) they contain osmiophilic lamellar bodies
(E) defects in these cells contribute to infant and adult respiratory distress

136. All of the following intracellular substances are second messengers in mammalian cells EXCEPT

(A) inositol 1,4,5-triphosphate (IP_3)
(B) cyclic adenosine monophosphate (cAMP)
(C) Ca^{2+}
(D) diacylglycerol (DAG)
(E) c-*fos*

137. Embolism of a cerebral artery most commonly occurs from all of the following situations EXCEPT

(A) atheromatous plaques of the vertebral artery
(B) atheromatous plaques of the internal carotid artery
(C) endocarditis of the mitral valve
(D) atheromatous plaques of the abdominal aorta

138. Exogenous administration of large amounts of testosterone is likely to produce all of the following effects EXCEPT

(A) masculinization in mature females
(B) feminization in mature males
(C) closure of the epiphysis of long bones
(D) an increase in sperm count

139. All of the following statements about RNA are correct EXCEPT

(A) a messenger RNA (mRNA) molecule is translated once and is then degraded
(B) ribosomal RNA (rRNA) is formed by transcription of a family of repeated nuclear genes
(C) the ribosome, which is a complex of RNA and protein, is the site of protein synthesis
(D) three different RNA polymerase enzymes are required for sustained protein synthesis in human cells
(E) transfer RNA (tRNA) molecules contain an anticodon loop that pairs with the triplet codon of mRNA

140. All of the following statements about hormone receptors are true EXCEPT that they

(A) may elicit their biologic response without being fully saturated with hormone
(B) may be desensitized by phosphorylation
(C) determine the specificity of cellular responses to hormones
(D) are deficient in Addison's disease
(E) are frequently transmembrane proteins

141. All of the following statements concerning the subthalamus are true EXCEPT

(A) it contains the cranial ends of the nerve cells of the red nucleus
(B) it has important connections with the corpus striatum and, thus, is involved with voluntary muscle control
(C) it contains the cranial ends of the nerve cells of the substantia nigra
(D) it has important connections with the cerebellum and, thus, is involved with voluntary muscle control

DIRECTIONS: Each set of matching questions in this section consists of a list of four to twenty-six lettered options (some of which may be in figures) followed by several numbered items. For each numbered item, select the ONE lettered option that is most closely associated with it. To avoid spending too much time on matching sets with large numbers of options, it is generally advisable to begin each set by reading the list of options. Then, for each item in the set, try to generate the correct answer and locate it in the option list, rather than evaluating each option individually. Each lettered option may be selected once, more than once, or not at all.

Questions 142–146

Match each of the following structures with its germ layer of origin.

(A) Ectoderm *N E M P*
(B) Mesoderm
(C) Endoderm *T T T P L P*
(D) Neuroectoderm

142. Melanocytes

143. Adrenal cortex

144. Liver

145. Thyroid gland

146. Gonads

Questions 147–149

Match each description below with the appropriate lettered structure in the scanning electron micrograph of liver parenchymal tissue.

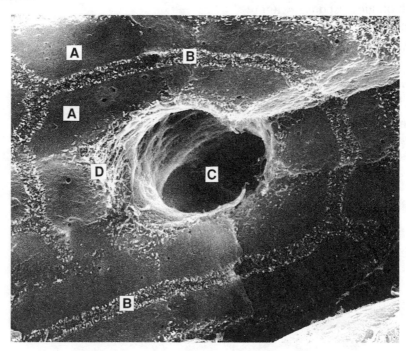

147. Receives blood from the portal vein and hepatic artery and drains blood into the central vein

148. A liver parenchymal cell

149. A bile canaliculus surrounded by tight junctions that form the blood–bile barrier

Questions 150–154

For each lipoprotein type listed below, select the genetic disorder that is most likely to be associated with it.

(A) Combined hyperlipidemia
(B) Hypertriglyceridemia
(C) Type III hyperlipoproteinemia
(D) Hypercholesterolemia
(E) Lipoprotein lipase deficiency

150. Chylomicrons

151. Low-density lipoproteins (LDL)

152. Chylomicron remnants and intermediate-density lipoproteins (IDL)

153. Very low-density lipoproteins (VLDL)

154. VLDL and chylomicrons

Questions 155–159

Match each procedure or operation with the neurotransmitter that it would deplete.

(A) Serotonin and catecholamines in the cerebral cortex
(B) γ-Aminobutyric acid (GABA) and glycine in the spinal cord
(C) Substance P in the dorsal horns
(D) Dopamine in the basal ganglia
(E) Serotonin in the spinal cord

155. Destruction of spinal interneurons (by controlled hypoxia)

156. Section of dorsal roots

157. Section of the medial forebrain bundle

158. Destruction of the substantia nigra

159. Destruction of the medullary raphe

Questions 160–163

Oncogenesis, the production of tumors, occurs because of the loss of cellular signaling, which is frequently caused by a protein that functions as an uncontrolled growth factor receptor. Match the normal physiologic receptor with the oncogene that it most closely resembles functionally and structurally.

(A) *ros*
(B) *erbB*
(C) *trk*
(D) *sis*
(E) *kit*
(F) *jun* — in control of gene transcription

160. Insulin receptor ros

161. Nerve growth factor (NGF) receptor trk

162. Epidermal growth factor (EGF) receptor erbB

163. Platelet-derived growth factor (PDGF) receptor kit

Questions 164–169

Match each disease below with its etiologic agent.

(A) *Treponema pallidum*
(B) *Treponema pertenue*
(C) *Treponema carateum*
(D) *Leptospira interrogans*
(E) *Borrelia recurrentis*

164. Relapsing fever E

165. Bejel A

166. Pinta C

167. Syphilis A

168. Fort Bragg fever D

169. Yaws B

Questions 170–175

The first heart sound (S_1) is composed of sounds from tricuspid and mitral valve closure. The second heart sound (S_2) is the sound of the aortic and pulmonic valves closing. For each cardiovascular abnormality listed below, select the heart sounds with which it is most likely to be associated.

(A) S_1 louder than S_2
(B) S_2 louder than S_1
(C) Aortic valvular ejection sound ✓
(D) Pulmonic valvular ejection sound

170. Mitral valve stenosis

171. Aortic stenosis

172. Acute aortic regurgitation

173. Severe hypertension

174. Anemia

175. Hyperthyroidism

Questions 176–179

Match the forms of joint disease listed below with the characteristic typically associated with it.

(A) Onion-skin thickening of the arterioles
(B) Tophus
(C) Human leukocyte antigen DR4 (HLA-DR4)
(D) Heberden's nodes

176. Rheumatoid arthritis

177. Osteoarthritis

178. Lyme arthritis

179. Gouty arthritis

Questions 180–182

The esophageal and arterial pressure tracings below were made from a normal subject during a voluntary effort to exhale against significant resistance (the Valsalva maneuver), which is a useful test of cardiac function. Match the descriptions that follow with the labeled arterial pressure readings.

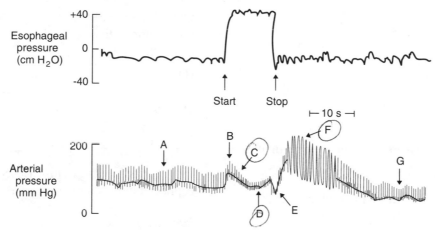

F 180. Loss of this vagally mediated change in arterial pressure is a useful diagnostic aid in assessing autonomic insufficiency

C 181. Changes in arterial blood pressure and pulse pressure are caused by a decrease in venous return

D 182. This area of the arterial blood pressure tracing is consistent with reflex tachycardia

Questions 183–187

Match each disease characteristic with the personality disorder that is most apt to be associated with it.

(A) Obsessive–compulsive
(B) Borderline
(C) Dependent
(D) Narcissistic
(E) Antisocial

E 183. Associated with childhood conduct disorder

A 184. Overly rigid

D 185. Hypersensitive to criticism

B 186. Repetitive self-cutting

A 187. Perfectionistic

Questions 188–192

Based on the clinical information given, select the bone tumor that is most likely to occur in each patient.

(A) Osteosarcoma

(B) Chondrosarcoma

(C) Ewing's sarcoma

(D) Giant cell tumor

(E) Osteoid osteoma

(F) Chondroblastoma

F 188. Epiphyseal lesions in a patient younger than 20 years of age

D 189. Epiphyseal lesions in a patient older than 20 years of age

A 190. Metaphyseal lesions in a patient younger than 20 years of age

E 191. A radiolucent nidus surrounded by sclerotic bone in a patient younger than 20 years of age

C 192. A diaphyseal lesion with concentric onion-skin layering in a patient younger than 20 years of age

Questions 193–200

Match each pathologic feature listed below with the idiopathic inflammatory bowel disease of which it is most characteristic.

(A) Ulcerative colitis

(B) Crohn's disease

(C) Whipple's disease

(D) Hirschsprung's disease

B 193. Segmental lesions

B 194. Fistulae

C 195. Periodic acid-Schiff (PAS)–positive macrophages in the lamina propria

D 196. Megacolon

A 197. Crypt abscesses

B 198. Granulomas

A 199. Superficial ulceration

B 200. Transmural inflammation

ANSWER KEY

1-C	31-C	61-B	91-B	121-C
2-D	32-D	62-B	92-A	122-D
3-A	33-C	63-D	93-C	123-A
4-B	34-E	64-A	94-D	124-C
5-E	35-E	65-C	95-B	125-C
6-C	36-D	66-E	96-E	126 C
7-A	37-B	67-D	97-D	127-A
8-D	38-C	68-C	98-C	128-E
9-C	39-A	69-C	99-B	129-B
10-B	40-B	70-D	100-C	130-C
11-C	41-E	71-C	101-C	131-D
12-B	42-A	72-C	102-A	132-C
13-A	43-C	73-A	103-A	133-D
14-C	44-E	74-B	104-D	134-E
15-B	45-B	75-C	105-C	135-C
16-C	46-B	76-C	106-C	136-E
17-A	47-B	77-B	107-D	137-D
18-D	48-D	78-B	108-A	138-D
19-B	49-D	79-B	109-C	139-A
20-D	50-D	80-E	110-D	140-D
21-D	51-A	81-B	111-A	141-D
22-D	52-C	82-D	112-C	142-D
23-A	53-E	83-A	113-B	143-B
24-D	54-C	84-C	114-B	144-C
25-D	55-E	85-C	115-C	145-C
26-A	56-B	86-B	116-B	146-B
27-E	57-C	87-A	117-A	147-C
28-D	58-C	88-D	118-E	148-A
29-C	59-C	89-B	119-D	149-B
30-C	60-C	90-A	120-A	150-E

151-D	161-C	171-C	181-C	191-E
152-C	162-B	172-B	182-D	192-C
153-B	163-E	173-B	183-E	193-B
154-A	164-E	174-A	184-A	194-B
155-B	165-A	175-A	185-D	195-C
156-C	166-C	176-C	186-B	196-D
157-A	167-A	177-D	187-A	197-A
158-D	168-D	178-A	188-F	198-B
159-E	169-B	179-B	189-D	199-A
160-A	170-A	180-F	190-A	200-B

ANSWERS AND EXPLANATIONS

1–5. The answers are: 1-C, 2-D, 3-A, 4-B, 5-E. *(Duchenne muscular dystrophy)*
Duchenne muscular dystrophy (DMD), or childhood muscular dystrophy, classically occurs only in boys with a pattern of X-linked inheritance. This pattern can be deduced from the pedigree that accompanies the question because all of the affected individuals are males, the mothers and fathers are not affected, and the affected males are on the maternal side of the family.

In X-linked diseases, mothers are always carriers because the mutant gene is on the X chromosome. The male child either receives the X chromosome with the mutant gene and gets the disease or receives a normal X chromosome and does not get the disease. Males cannot be carriers of X-linked disorders. A female carrier has a 50% chance of giving her chromosome that bears the mutant gene to each of her children.

The gene mutation that causes DMD occurs in the dystrophin gene, which is a very large gene located on the short arm of the X chromosome. Most mutations involve deletions of varying lengths. Dystrophin is similar to the cytoskeletal proteins actin and spectrin, both of which are normal in this disease. It is thought that dystrophin plays a role in controlling calcium release, but its true function has not yet been elucidated.

The diagnosis of DMD is confirmed by electromyography, measurement of creatine kinase (CK), which is increased tenfold, and muscle biopsy. CK levels can be measured at birth if DMD is suspected on the basis of family history, but intrauterine diagnosis of all cases of DMD is not yet possible because of the number and types of mutations that occur.

6. The answer is C. *(Histopathology of Kaposi's sarcoma)*
Kaposi's sarcoma was initially described as a cutaneous hemorrhagic nodule usually occurring on the lower extremities of elderly men. Kaposi's sarcoma is now recognized as being associated with human immunodeficiency virus (HIV) infection and afflicting primarily men with the virus. It is recognized histologically by irregular fascicles of spindle cells in the dermis, which are accompanied by extravasated erythrocytes that impart a purple color. Kaposi's sarcoma is believed to be derived from endothelial cells, perhaps lymphatic endothelium. Unlike angiosarcomas, it does not form anastomosing vascular channels.

7. The answer is A. *(Referred pain)*
Referred pain is not well understood. Somatic referred pain is very well localized and intense. Visceral referred pain is the opposite and is thought to be conveyed by autonomic fibers. Diaphragmatic pain is usually referred to the shoulder.

8–10. The answers are: 8-D, 9-C, 10-B. *(Diagnosis and pharmacology of epilepsy)*
Major depression is the first diagnosis to consider because, in the case presented in the question, the subacute time course, self-neglect, social withdrawal, and psychotic symptoms indicate a possible depression. Major depression, even depression associated with psychotic symptoms, is treatable and has a good prognosis. There is no mention of drug abuse to suggest phencyclidine psychosis and no euphoria or increased sociability to suggest mania. The time during which symptoms have occurred has not been long enough to suggest schizophrenia or schizoaffective disorder.

The symptoms listed in the questions suggest complex partial seizures of the temporal lobe. Considering the psychotic symptoms and social withdrawal, epilepsy with schizophreniform interictal disorder might also be considered. The evoked potentials and the projective or cognitive tests would not be helpful.

Carbamazepine is the preferred treatment for complex partial seizures. The antipsychotic drug haloperidol should be added only if the psychotic symptoms do not respond to the antiepileptic agent. Haloperidol and the antidepressant imipramine lower the seizure threshold. The antipanic drug alprazolam is not indicated, although some other types of benzodiazepines are used as antiepileptics.

11. The answer is C. *(Inflammation and cellular margination)*
As the vascular phase of the inflammatory response progresses, neutrophils and monocytes move toward the periphery of the microcirculatory vessels (a process referred to as margination) and adhere to, or pavement, the vascular endothelium in preparation for migration into the extravascular space. To migrate, leukocytes develop pseudopods and move, without accompanying loss of fluid, through gaps between the endothelial cells—a process termed diapedesis. In the latter part of the vascular phase, increased vascular permeability causes loss of plasma with resultant venous stasis and, eventually, clotting in the small capillaries local to the inflamed area.

12. The answer is B. *(Hormone receptors)*
The cytosol would contain the most fluorescence. Glucocorticoid receptors are soluble receptors and are not associated with the plasma membrane. Glucocorticoids diffuse into cells, bind to receptors in the cytosol, and then translocate to the nucleus. Inside the nucleus this hormone-receptor complex regulates transcription via binding to specific sequences of DNA.

13. The answer is A. *(Histopathology of temporal arteritis)*
Temporal (giant cell) arteritis may be one component of the syndrome of polymyalgia rheumatica. Patients present with headache, tenderness over the temporal artery, visual loss (if retinal vessels are affected), and facial pain. Histologically, a granulomatous reaction is seen within the vessel wall associated with a mixed neutrophilic and lymphocytic infiltrate. Giant cells appear to phagocytize portions of elastica, and the vessel may be thrombosed in its late stage (*right*). Clinical response to steroids is excellent. Mönckeberg's arteriosclerosis shows medial calcification of arteries and is not an arteritis, whereas Takayasu's arteritis ("pulseless disease") involves the aortic arch and its major branches.

14. The answer is C. *(Asthma and pharmacology of cromolyn sodium)*
Cromolyn sodium inhibits degranulation of mast cells and, in other poorly understood ways, interferes with the inflammatory process now assumed to be critical to moderate asthma caused by a variety of allergens and other conditions. Cromolyn is not absorbed from the gut and must be administered topically to the lung where it acts prophylactically to inhibit bronchospasm caused by inhaled allergens, exercise, or altered environmental conditions. It does not directly relax bronchial smooth muscle in vivo or in vitro and, thus, is of little use in acute emergencies of bronchial hyperreactivity. However, prophylactically, it will reduce the bronchial response to a number of spasmogens.

15–18. The answers are: 15-B, 16-C, 17-A, 18-D. *(Gastric ulcer disease)*
A number of physiologic, genetic, and other factors increase the risk of gastric (and duodenal) peptic ulcers. Smoking and caffeine are known to adversely affect the morbidity, mortality, and healing rates of peptic ulcers. In general, first-degree relatives of peptic ulcer patients as well as males have a threefold to fourfold increased risk of developing this disorder. Paradoxically, in gastric ulcer disease, acid secretion is not elevated. It is possible that excess secreted hydrogen ion is reabsorbed across the injured gastric mucosa. In general, a defect in gastric mucosal defense is the more important local physiologic factor promoting ulceration at this site.

In the patient described in the question, direct visualization identified a duodenal ulcer, a very common cause of right upper quadrant pain and melena. Denudation of the mucosal epithelium is the hallmark of histologic changes in peptic ulcer disease and, in duodenal ulcer, is often accompanied by hypertrophy of submucosal Brunner's glands (mucus-secreting glands).

The agents of choice for duodenal ulcer include histamine (H_2) antagonists, including ranitidine or cimetidine. Other useful agents, alone or in combination with H_2 antagonists, include anticholinergic drugs, "proton pump" inhibitors (benzimidazoles), antacids, and cytoprotective analogues of prostaglandins E_1, E_2, and prostacyclin.

19. The answer is B. *(Tumor pathology)*
In most human cancers, the stage of the disease, not the age of the patient, is the most important prognostic factor. Stage refers to the extent, or degree of spread, of the disease in the patient (i.e., localized, regional, or distant). Tumor grade (i.e., differentiation), mitotic count, and extent of invasion correlate with the stage of the tumor, in that high-grade (i.e., less differentiated) tumors and highly invasive tumors tend to be high-stage lesions.

20. The answer is D. *(Growth hormone)*
Growth hormone stimulates cartilage and bone growth via somatomedin, an intermediary peptide. It is secreted periodically, like many other pituitary hormones, and is affected in a negative fashion by somatostatin, a hypothalamic peptide. Unlike other anterior pituitary hormones, cellular targets for growth hormone are relatively ubiquitous. Somatomedin, synthesized in the liver and possibly other sites (e.g., muscle), is an important mediator of the growth effects of the hormone on cartilage and bone. Indeed, growth hormone has no direct effects on these cells by itself. Growth hormone has a large array of effects on amino acid, fat, and carbohydrate activities and, in general, displays anti–insulin-like actions.

21. The answer is D. *(Diagnosis of pneumocystis pneumonia)*
Pneumocystis pneumonia is caused by *Pneumocystis carinii*, a microorganism of uncertain classification that belongs to either the protozoa or fungi. It forms four to seven microcysts within a frothy honeycomb-like alveolar exudate in the air spaces. These cysts contain numerous sporozoites, which are released from the cysts at maturation. Pneumocystis pneumonia is commonly seen in individuals infected with human immunodeficiency virus (HIV), a condition that would be suspected in an individual with a history of intravenous drug abuse.

22. The answer is D. *(Histopathology of Hodgkin's disease)*
The photomicrograph of the woman's biopsy shows classic features of nodular-sclerosing Hodgkin's disease. The node is divided into irregular nodules by broad bands of dense collagen (*left*). In the panel on the *right*, the nodal infiltrate is composed of lymphocytes, plasma cells, eosinophils, and multilobated cells with prominent red nucleoli, called Reed-Sternberg cells. Although Reed-Sternberg cells are not pathognomonic of this disease, they are diagnostic when seen in this appropriate inflammatory milieu. The nodular sclerosis type of Hodgkin's disease usually presents with a large mediastinal mass and involvement of adjacent lymph node groups (e.g., supraclavicular nodes).

23. The answer is A. *(Na$^+$ transport and renal epithelial physiology)*
Na$^+$ is transported from the tubular lumen to the peritubular capillary by an electrochemical gradient that is largely generated by the action of the Na$^+$, K$^+$-ATPase activity at the basolateral surface. The cell is freely permeable to water and chloride, thereby reabsorbing a virtually isosmotic fraction of tubular luminal fluid. The attraction of Na$^+$ creates a very large intracellular negative potential (approximately -70 mV). There is no significant hormone dependence of ion transport in these cells on either aldosterone or antidiuretic hormone (ADH).

24. The answer is D. *(Thoracic outlet syndrome)*
Thoracic outlet syndrome describes compression of the lower trunk of the brachial plexus and the subclavian artery by an anomalous thirteenth (cervical) rib. Sensory changes occur over the distribution of the ulnar nerve; the phrenic nerves are not involved.

25. The answer is D. *(Gluconeogenesis and glycolysis)*
Stimulation of beta cells by glucose results in the release of insulin. Insulin has numerous effects on virtually every tissue, and its overall effect is the conservation of body fuel supplies. It does this by promoting the

uptake and storage of glucose, amino acids, and fats. In the liver, it decreases gluconeogenesis and glycogenolysis and promotes glycolysis. In addition, it promotes lipogenesis in the liver and fat cells and is antilipolytic. It is also an important anabolic protein hormone while simultaneously inhibiting the breakdown of amino acids. It inhibits the release of glucagon from neighboring alpha cells.

26–27. The answers are: 26-A, 27-E. *(Multiple myeloma; immunoglobulin abnormalities)*
Well-demarcated or "punched out" osteolytic lesions are almost pathognomonic for multiple myeloma. In 99% of the patients with multiple myeloma, electrophoretic analysis of the serum proteins shows an increase in one of the immunoglobulin classes or light chains, approximately 23,000 daltons (Bence Jones protein), in the urine. The presence of 55,000-dalton monoclonal proteins is indicative of heavy-chain disease, a different type of monoclonal gammopathy that is not associated with osteolytic lesions. Although not specific for this disease, patients with multiple myeloma do suffer from a suppression of synthesis of normal antibodies and are, thus, susceptible to recurrent bacterial and viral infections.

In approximately 55% of people diagnosed with multiple myeloma, the membrane-bound protein (M protein) is immunoglobulin G (IgG), and in 25%, the M protein is IgA and rarely IgM, IgD, or IgE. In the remaining 20%, Bence Jones proteinuria without the serum M protein is seen.

28. The answer is D. *(Pharmacology of aminoglycosides)*
Aminoglycosides can cause severe nephrotoxicity and ototoxicity. Their therapeutic index is low; peak and trough levels are commonly monitored to allow for dose adjustments or a change in timing of administration. Aminoglycosides are eliminated rapidly with a serum half-life of 1–5 hours. However, rapid clearance is not the major determinant for therapeutic monitoring. Aminoglycosides are not extensively metabolized. Because they are polar molecules, they are lipid insoluble and do not cross the blood–brain barrier. The incidence of hypersensitivity reactions is extremely low.

29. The answer is C. *(Neoplasia and hormone action)*
Tamoxifen has become the drug of choice for the initial endocrine management of breast cancer as well as a useful adjuvant therapy for the palliative management of advanced breast cancer. It is relatively nontoxic, and patients with breast tumors containing estrogen receptors are most likely to respond to the drug. The drug binds to the estrogen receptor in the nucleus but does not stimulate transcription. The tamoxifen–estrogen receptor complex does not readily dissociate, thereby affecting estrogen receptor recycling. In premenopausal women, competition with estrogen receptors in the anterior pituitary and hypothalamus disrupts normal feedback inhibition of gonadotropin-releasing hormone, thereby enhancing gonadotropin release.

30. The answer is C. *(Angina therapy)*
Nitroglycerin (glyceryl trinitrate; GTN) is most effective by decreasing preload in angina. At high concentrations, some benefit in angina is obtained from GTN by reducing afterload. However, this latter effect is often accompanied by reflex tachycardia that may disrupt the improvement in myocardial oxygen consumption and supply achieved by GTN. Propranolol is useful in blocking this reflex effect because it is negatively inotropic and negatively chronotropic. Propranolol may be accompanied by coronary artery vasospasm after removing β-receptor–mediated dilation and leaving unopposed a coronary artery α-receptor–mediated vasoconstriction.

31. The answer is C. *(Antiepileptics)*
Phenytoin decreases resting Na^+ flux as well as the flow of Na^+ currents during chemical depolarization or action potential. In the central nervous system (CNS), this results in depression of the generation and transmission of repetitive action potentials in epileptic foci. It is usually the drug of choice for all seizures except absence seizures and, in general, is started alone to assess its efficacy. Phenytoin is associated with

potential teratogenic effects (fetal hydantoin syndrome). Other agents like diazepam or phenobarbital affect chloride channels by interacting with γ-aminobutyric acid (GABA) at its receptor site.

32. The answer is D. *(RNA synthesis)*
RNA polymerase I produces ribosomal RNA (rRNA). RNA polymerase II produces mostly messenger RNA (mRNA). RNA polymerase III makes transfer RNA (tRNA) and other small RNAs. The reason that mammalian cells use three different types of RNA polymerases is not known.

33. The answer is C. *(Toxicology and aplastic anemia)*
Benzene is associated with the induction of aplastic anemia by damaging myeloid stem cells. Thiouracil is associated with agranulocytosis, primarily because of its ability to decrease production or increase destruction of neutrophils. Penicillin acts as a hapten, which produces erythrocyte destruction via warm antibody autoimmune hemolysis. In contrast, methyldopa stimulates the production of antibodies against intrinsic red blood cell antigens. Ingestion of an excessive quantity of acetaminophen is followed by the production of toxic metabolites, which first decrease hepatic glutathione levels and then cause a centrilobular necrosis due to biomolecular adduct formation.

34. The answer is E. *(Monoclonal antibodies and gram-negative bacteria)*
A monoclonal antibody, such as immunoglobulin G (IgG), would be useful only against organisms producing lipopolysaccharide, namely gram-negative bacteria. The organism would have to produce a disease state through bacteremia since IgG would only be present in the circulatory system. Organisms such as *Bordetella pertussis*, the causative agent of whooping cough, and *Vibrio cholerae*, the agent of cholera, are gram-negative but do not invade the bloodstream. Pulmonary anthrax is caused by *Bacillus anthracis*, which is a gram-positive organism. Leprosy is caused by *Mycobacterium leprae*, which is acid-fast, not gram-negative. Bubonic plague, however, is caused by *Yersinia pestis*, a gram-negative organism that multiplies in the bloodstream, spreading through to the lymphatics. *Y. pestis* has many virulence factors, including lipopolysaccharide.

35. The answer is E. *(Mechanism of action of penicillin)*
The principles of antibiotic action are perhaps best exemplified by penicillin. Antibiotics act by specifically binding to macromolecules only found in the parasite. Transpeptidase is the only penicillin-binding protein listed; it is inactivated when binding occurs.

36. The answer is D. *(Passive immunity; vaccination)*
The most appropriate treatment for the medical student described in the question would be an injection of tetanus toxoid, which would trigger an anamnestic response because of the DTP (diphtheria-tetanus-pertussis) administration in childhood. If there is no history of DTP immunization, passive immunity can be induced by the administration of heterologous (e.g., equine) or homologous (i.e., human) antibodies. Type I and type III reactions can result from heterologous administration. Aminoglycosides are given for infections caused by gram-negative bacteria. The tetanus toxoid is produced by *Clostridium tetani*, a gram-positive rod.

37. The answer is B. *(Adverse effects of aspirin)*
The major adverse effect of aspirin is gastrointestinal bleeding. Inhibition of local cytoprotective arachidonic acid metabolites (prostaglandin E_2 and prostacyclin) in the gastric mucosa contributes to this adverse effect and can be offset by simultaneously using exogenous synthetic prostanoids. In addition, aspirin has a direct irritating effect on the mucosa. Nonsteroidal anti-inflammatory agents in general have little effect on lipoxygenase activity but do affect cyclooxygenase. In particular, aspirin is an irreversible inhibitor of this enzyme in platelets (and other cell types) by acetylating the α-amino group of the terminal serine. This irreversible inhibition has significant implications in that platelet function will not be restored to normal until a new

enzyme has been synthesized. Aspirin has little effect on normal body temperature but reduces abnormally elevated body temperatures secondary to alterations in central thermoregulation.

38. The answer is C. *(RNA splicing)*
The splicing reaction takes place in the nucleus of the cell before capping and polyadenylation as part of the post-transcriptional modification of eukaryotic RNA. U1 small nuclear ribonucleoprotein (snRNP) recognizes a 9 base-pair region of the introns involved and is thought to precipitate the organized formation of the large particle termed the spliceosome on the RNA. The splicing reaction then cuts the intron at the 5′ end and forms a "lariat" structure by covalently binding the cut 5′ end of the intron to a sequence on the 3′ end. The intron is then cut again at the 3′ end and thus is cut out of the RNA.

39. The answer is A. *(Carcinoid of the appendix)*
The most common tumor of the appendix is a carcinoid tumor. The neoplastic cells show neuroendocrine differentiation. The cells grow in nests and are associated with a delicate, branching vascular network. The nuclei of the cells have a "salt and pepper" chromatin distribution. Typically, the cytoplasm of the cells contains granules, which are visible by special stains. Silver salts turn the granules black; thus, they are argyrophilic. The behavior of these tumors is related to their depth of invasion into the muscular wall and serosal adipose tissue.

40. The answer is B. *(Nitrogen metabolism)*
Negative nitrogen balance would result from defective cholecystokinin–pancreozymin (CCK–PZ) production when the consumption of dietary protein is normal. Negative nitrogen balance occurs when the excretion of nitrogen exceeds the intake of nitrogen. A number of conditions can cause a negative nitrogen balance, including a deficiency in any one of the essential amino acids or a defect in the intestinal phase of protein digestion and absorption. CCK–PZ is essential for stimulating the secretion of inactive pancreatic zymogens, which become active proteases in the small intestine. The intestinal phase of digestion is essential to maintaining nitrogen balance; the gastric phase appears to have little, if any, impact. For example, gastric resection can be performed without affecting nitrogen balance. In phenylketonuria (PKU), tyrosine becomes an essential amino acid and must be supplied in the diet.

41. The answer is E. *(Protein synthesis)*
The synthetic polynucleotide sequence of CAACAACAACAA... could be read by the in vitro protein synthesizing system starting at the first C, the first A, or the second A. In the first case, the first triplet codon would be CAA, which codes for glutamine. In the second case, the first triplet codon would be AAC, which codes for asparagine; and in the last case, the first triplet codon would be ACA, which codes for threonine.

42–43. The answers are: 42-A, 43-C. *(Biostatistics)*
The variables described in the question are continuous in that their values are along a continuum as are age and IQ, as opposed to being categorical. Categorical variables, such as sex, race, and marital status, require the use of nonparametric statistical tests, such as the chi-squared test.

A null hypothesis is the hypothesis that an observed difference is due to chance alone and not to a systematic cause. In the study question, the null hypothesis is that there is no relationship between temperature and body weight. The study is designed to disprove the null hypothesis. The null hypothesis does not involve a P value, although a cutoff is generally chosen to show the likelihood that an association between variables is not due to chance alone (i.e., $P = 0.05$ means that there is a 5% probability that the two events or measurements are similar due to chance alone).

44. The answer is E. *(Bacterial pigment production)*
Pseudomonas aeruginosa, Staphylococcus aureus, and *Serratia marcescens* are all pigment producers. Pigment production by bacteria is associated with both gram-positive and gram-negative organisms. *P.*

aeruginosa and *S. marcescens* produce endotoxins, and only *S. aureus* produces enterotoxin and lipoteichoic acids. None of the organisms listed produce mycolic acids.

45. The answer is B. *(Mycobacteria)*
Mycobacterium tuberculosis produces factors such as sulfatides, which inhibit the fusion of phagosomes with lysosomes. In addition to inhibiting phagosome–lysosome fusion, *M. tuberculosis* escapes engulfment by lysosomes. The organisms are also resistant to phagocytic killing because of their tough cell surface.

46. The answer is B. *(Autonomic pharmacology and effects of antimuscarinic agents)*
Atropine may abolish the parasympathetic input that normally maintains a relatively slow heart rate. Indeed, atropine is often used intraoperatively (and in emergencies) to increase heart rate. Atropine inhibits secretions from salivary, lacrimal, bronchial, and sweat glands. It causes mydriasis and cycloplegia. It has no effect on skeletal muscle in which neuromuscular transmission involves acetylcholine (ACh) and nicotinic, not muscarinic, receptors.

47. The answer is B. *(G proteins and signal transduction)*
Guanosine triphosphate (GTP)–binding proteins (G proteins) are involved with the process of signal transduction and are the target of toxins, such as pertussis and cholera toxins. G proteins are activated when bound to GTP and deactivate via the hydrolysis of GTP to form guanosine diphosphate (GDP).

48. The answer is D. *(Bronchioloalveolar carcinoma)*
Bronchioloalveolar carcinomas are well-differentiated adenocarcinomas, which grow in a nondestructive fashion over the matrix of the alveolar septa, replacing normal pneumonocytes. This pattern has been called lepidic growth. Bronchioloalveolar carcinomas also have a propensity for aerogenous and lymphatic spread, and widespread intrapulmonary metastases may occur.

49. The answer is D. *(Therapeutic effects in neoplasia)*
Paradoxically, patients with histologically "unfavorable" high-grade lymphomas show long-term survival if a complete clinical remission can be attained. However, it is rare to attain cure in histologically low-grade "favorable" non-Hodgkin's lymphomas: Patients die gradually from bone marrow compromise or lymphoma over many years. Long-term survival after 5 years for diffuse large cell lymphomas is roughly 50%. Those who do not attain complete remission usually die within several years. Spontaneous remissions are rarely seen in aggressive lymphomas.

50–54. The answers are: 50-D, 51-A, 52-C, 53-E, 54-C. *(Diabetes mellitus)*
The beta cells of the islets of Langerhans are the major site of insulin production in the pancreas. In insulin-dependent diabetes mellitus (IDDM), these cells are affected by genetic, autoimmune, viral, or other environmental factors so that they produce inadequate or no insulin.

Patients with type I IDDM are often started on daily injections of an intermediate-acting insulin preparation. Oral hypoglycemic agents such as glipizide are contraindicated in this group. Although abstinence from carbohydrates was initially thought appropriate, dietary manipulations now generally involve maintaining a complex carbohydrate diet with an emphasis on minimizing the intake of fats, especially saturated fats. Exercise normalizes peripheral tissue sensitivity to exogenous insulin.

Alpha cells of the endocrine pancreas secrete glucagon, which increases blood glucose by increasing glycogenolysis and gluconeogenesis in the liver. Growth hormone (GH) opposes the action of insulin by interfering with the body's ability to use glucose. Somatostatin suppresses glucagon secretion and, therefore, tends to decrease blood glucose.

Despite control of blood glucose levels with exogenous insulin, diet, and exercise in patients with IDDM, chronic changes in the microcirculation (especially in the kidney and eye) and macrocirculation (e.g., atherosclerosis) frequently occur. In addition, peripheral polyneuropathy is the most common diabetic neuropathy noted and appears to be associated with accumulation of sorbitol within Schwann cells. Currently, there is no association of IDDM and pulmonary hypertension.

Diabetic ketoacidosis is a common problem, and coma may ensue in 10% of the individuals. Rapid deep breathing (Kussmaul's respiration) is an important sign of such ketoacidosis and is the result of compensatory mechanisms in response to metabolic acidosis. In patients with hypoglycemic coma (from exuberant effects of insulin), a history of a skipped meal or vigorous exercise is helpful. In addition, their coma is often accompanied by profuse sweating rather than dehydration (which may be the case in ketoacidosis). Obviously, discerning between the two causes is critical to establish appropriate emergency therapy, and blood glucose levels will confirm clinical impressions.

55. The answer is E. *(Characteristics of volatile anesthetics)*
Halothane and methoxyflurane are typical inhalational drugs, which tend to depress both the cardiovascular and respiratory systems. Methoxyflurane is more potent (i.e., it has a lower minimal alveolar concentration) than halothane, as predicted from its higher oil:gas partition coefficient. Both result in considerably slower induction than nitrous oxide because their respective blood:gas partition coefficients are greater than that of nitrous oxide. Similarly, recovery from methoxyflurane is slower than that from halothane because its oil:gas partition coefficient is greater than that of halothane. An increase in ventilatory rate will make the onset of anesthesia more rapid for all inhalational anesthetics.

56. The answer is B. *(DNA and restriction enzymes)*
Restriction enzymes recognize specific base sequences in double-helical DNA and cleave both strands of the duplex at specific sites. Most of the cleavage sites contain a twofold rotational symmetry (the recognized sequence is palindromic). The cuts resulting from these enzymes may be either staggered or blunt. Restriction enzymes can cleave DNA molecules into a number of specific fragments. These enzymes are specific for DNA; they do not cleave RNA.

57. The answer is C. *(Physician–patient interactions)*
Regular, structured visits by the nurses can help to reassure a dependent and frightened patient and keep the nurses from feeling resentful. The patient's disease and disability have made him feel angry and out of control, and he is acting out his feelings by bothering the nurses. Punitive actions and indirect warfare with the patient will not remedy the situation.

58. The answer is C. *(Suicide risk)*
Elderly men have the highest suicide rate of any group, especially with the additional risk factors of widowerhood, alcohol abuse, chronic medical problems, and living alone. Although renal insufficiency, silent myocardial infarction, peripheral neuropathy, and pneumonia are valid concerns, suicide has the highest lethal potential and need for active monitoring.

59. The answer is C. *(Antibiotic action)*
Chloramphenicol is bacteriostatic and, therefore, was responsible for the leveling off of *curve A*. All of the agents listed, except chloramphenicol, are bactericidal. Cephalothin, methicillin, and vancomycin all interfere with cell wall synthesis, leading to bursting and to cell death. Polymyxin affects cell membrane function, causing irreversible loss of small molecules from the cell. Chloramphenicol inhibits protein synthesis and is bacteriostatic. Therefore, the cell number in the culture with chloramphenicol does not decrease, and the organisms are viable. Removal of chloramphenicol will result in growth.

60. The answer is C. *(Acid–base balance)*
According to the Henderson-Hasselbalch equation, the patient's pH is approximately 7.4 (normal), and his P_{CO_2} and $[HCO_3^-]$ are elevated. The elevation in P_{CO_2} (respiratory acidosis) has been compensated (i.e., normal pH)

by a rise in $[HCO_3^-]$. This latter phenomenon is brought about by the kidneys excreting more acid and reabsorbing more HCO_3^-. Full compensation as in this example is most likely to be associated with chronic perturbations in acid–base balance. Such changes may be common in chronic obstructive pulmonary disease (COPD).

61. The answer is B. *(Na^+ transport; adenosine triphosphate production)* ✓
The ability of erythrocytes to pump Na^+ from the cytoplasm depends on a source of adenosine triphosphate (ATP). All of the erythrocyte's ATP is generated by glycolysis. The compound 1,3-diphosphoglycerate is a high-energy glycolytic intermediate that is converted to 3-phosphoglycerate with the concomitant phosphorylation of adenosine diphosphate (ADP) to ATP. This reaction is catalyzed by phosphoglycerate kinase. Pyruvate carboxylase and glucose 6-phosphatase are gluconeogenic enzymes and are not present in the erythrocyte. Malate dehydrogenase is a mitochondrial enzyme and is not present in the erythrocyte. Stearoyl coenzyme A (CoA) desaturase is an enzyme in β-oxidation and is not present in the erythrocyte.

62. The answer is B. *(Biostatistics)*
A paired t-test allows a comparison of mean K^+ values before and after treatment by comparing each patient's initial serum level with his or her repeat value.

63–64. The answers are: 63-D, 64-A. *(Differential diagnosis of infectious mononucleosis)*
This patient presents with the classic picture of infectious mononucleosis caused by Epstein-Barr virus (EBV) infection. Extreme fatigue, difficulty concentrating, and fever are generalized systemic symptoms. Pharyngitis reflects the local immunologic response by T cells reactive against viral antigens on infected tonsillar B cells. Splenomegaly is also a consequence of immunologic response to EBV. Morphologic examination of lymphocytosis in the peripheral blood should reveal atypical lymphocytes, which are activated T cells with increased cytoplasm and less mature nuclear chromatin. Lymphocytes of infectious lymphocytosis and pertussis are morphologically normal, albeit increased in number; also pertussis is a disease of young children. Serum from this patient should yield a positive test for heterophile antibodies. The combination of pharyngitis and lymphadenopathy is characteristic of EBV-associated mononucleosis. Cytomegalovirus (CMV) mononucleosis lacks both of these features. Toxoplasmosis, a rare cause of mononucleosis, may have lymphadenopathy but not pharyngitis.

    A not uncommon feature of infectious mononucleosis with EBV-mediated expansion of B cells is the development of antibodies to red cells, usually directed against the Ii antigen system. Most such antibodies are cold agglutinins; that is, they react with erythrocytes at temperatures less than 37°C. Cold agglutinins are usually of the immunoglobulin M (IgM) class, and a Coombs' test may or may not be positive. The virus-associated hemophagocytic syndrome has been seen in patients with EBV infections, although usually in immunocompromised patients. Direct infection of erythroid precursors is not a feature of EBV infection. Disseminated intravascular coagulation is a rare occurrence in infectious mononucleosis, and thrombocytopenia may cause petechiae but not hemorrhagic blood loss.

65. The answer is C. *(Replication cycle of viruses)*
During the eclipse phase, it is impossible to recover the virus particles from infected cells. The eclipse phase of the virus replication cycle is the final stage of adsorption (during which the virus invades the cell, multiplies, kills, and lyses the cell) and the process of penetration and uncoating (during which the virus particles become engulfed by the cytoplasm of the host cell where virus particles are broken down and released).

66. The answer is E. *(Cell function; organelles)*
Catalase is an enzyme that catalyzes the synthesis and degradation of hydrogen peroxide. Peroxisomes, also called microsomes, contain large amounts of catalase and, therefore, can be visualized after staining for catalase. Peroxisomes function in the metabolism of hydrogen peroxide, cholesterol, and lipids.

67. The answer is D. *(Delayed-type hypersensitivity reactions)*
The reaction observed was most likely caused by CD4$^+$ T cells. It is a delayed reaction, demonstrating that the T cells are working fine; therefore, the patient could neither lack all T-cell–mediated immune function nor suffer from DiGeorge syndrome. Sensitization has already occurred; therefore, the secondary exposure would show symptoms faster than the primary reaction.

68–70. The answers are: 68-C, 69-C, 70-D. *(Open-angle glaucoma)*
Primary open-angle glaucoma is a genetically determined disorder that is the most common form of glaucoma in the general population. In the patient described in the question, a decreased outflow facility resulted in an imbalance between aqueous humor inflow and outflow. Outflow of aqueous humor is accomplished primarily by filtration through the trabecular network to the canal of Schlemm and, to a lesser extent, via absorption into iris blood vessels (uveoscleral outflow).

Cholinomimetics contract the ciliary muscle, thereby reducing resistance of aqueous humor outflow through the trabecular mesh and canal of Schlemm. Accordingly, topical administration of pilocarpine is the agent of choice for this patient. Atropine is a muscarinic antagonist and may exacerbate this problem. Succinylcholine is a depolarizing muscle relaxant and may exacerbate this condition by acutely contracting the accessory striated muscles of the eye before its paralyzing effects. Dexamethasone is a glucocorticoid that may exacerbate primary open-angle glaucoma by further reducing aqueous outflow via the trabecular meshwork. Tubocurarine is a nondepolarizing muscle relaxant that has relatively little effect on muscarinic receptors of the ciliary muscle.

Cholinesterase inhibitors, such as echothiophate, are useful for glaucoma therapy but are well absorbed from the eye, and adverse systemic effects secondary to an increase in cholinergic activity are possible. Bronchoconstriction, especially in patients with hyperreactive airways, is a serious concern. In addition, these agents may promote micturition, increased gastrointestinal motility, decreased heart rate, and increased sweating—all physiologic responses typical of cholinomimetic effects secondary to inhibition of acetylcholinesterase.

71. The answer is C. *(Histopathology of peripheral nerve tumors)*
Schwannomas, such as neurilemomas, are solitary encapsulated tumors that form eccentric masses derived from peripheral nerves. The histologic appearance in the photomicrograph reveals Antoni A areas (*at right*), which are cellular regions with spindle cells that have elongated tapered nuclei. These nuclei may palisade to form a picket fence–like array called a Verocay body. The looser, edematous zones with hyalinized blood vessels are called Antoni B areas. In contrast, neurofibromas form unencapsulated, onion-like, bulbous expansions of the nerve and are composed of loose interlacing bands of spindle cells with wavy nuclei.

72. The answer is C. *(Gastrointestinal transport of fats)*
The formation of fatty acids and monoglyceride by pancreatic lipase is an important step in the digestive fate of triglycerides. Although there are gastric lipases, they have a relatively insignificant effect on ingested neutral fats. This is in contrast to a critical role for pancreatic lipase in the pancreatic juice. Neutral fats are emulsified by bile salts, and further agitation within the intestine makes their surface available for significant hydrolysis by the water-soluble pancreatic lipase. The products, fatty acids and 2-monoglyceride, would quickly convert back to fat if they were not made into micelles by bile salts. These bile salts ferry the micelles to the intestinal brush border where the hydrophobic fatty acid (and monoglyceride) rapidly diffuse passively through the lipid membrane.

73. The answer is A. *(Neurophysiology)*
The anterior spinocerebellar tract is thought to cross the spinal cord and ascend to the cerebellum where it crosses the spinal cord again. The spinal thalamic tract crosses the cord only once. The cuneocerebellar tract

contains fibers that run from the nucleus gracilis and cuneatus to the ipsilateral cerebellar hemisphere. The vestibulospinal tract also remains ipsilateral.

74. The answer is B. *(Epilepsy)*
The patient most likely has temporal lobe epilepsy, in which seizures are sometimes preceded by acoustic or olfactory hallucinations. Patients are also confused or anxious and sometimes perform complex and bizarre behaviors with no recall of events after the attack. Klüver-Bucy syndrome results from bilateral destruction of the temporal lobes and manifests as loss of fear and anger as well as docility, increased appetite, and hypersexuality. Jacksonian seizures are the classic tonic–clonic convulsions due to focal activity in the primary motor cortex. Petit mal (or absence) seizures usually occur in children and involve brief myoclonic jerks, sudden loss in body tone with rapid recovery, or brief losses of consciousness during which the patient stares into space.

75. The answer is C. *(Enteric infection by enterotoxigenic bacteria)*
The symptoms of cholera result from the attachment of *Vibrio cholerae* to the intestinal mucosa and production of cholera toxin. The infection is acute, and the bacteria remain extracellular. The action of cholera toxin involves elevation of intestinal cyclic adenosine monophosphate (cAMP) levels, which results in massive fluid loss (diarrhea).

76. The answer is C. *(Cell cycle; organelles)*
Centrioles are made of nine tubular triplets, and they function in mitotic spindle formation and in the production of cilia and flagella. Centrioles are self-duplicated in the S (synthesis) phase of the cell cycle.

77. The answer is B. *(Energy storage and transfer)*
A high-energy bond is defined as a bond that, when hydrolyzed, will release a sufficient amount of energy to drive the synthesis of adenosine triphosphate (ATP) from adenosine diphosphate (ADP) and inorganic phosphate (P_i). This requires approximately 7.3 kcal/mol. There are two intermediates in glycolysis that are high-energy compounds: phosphoenolpyruvate and 1,3-bisphosphoglycerate. In the tricarboxylic acid (TCA) cycle, the conversion of succinyl coenzyme A (CoA) to succinate releases enough energy to synthesize guanosine triphosphate (GTP) from guanosine diphosphate (GDP) and P_i. In muscle tissue, phosphocreatine is a storage form of high energy. The hydrolysis of phosphate from phosphocreatine is coupled with the synthesis of ATP. A reaction that is exergonic is accompanied by a $\Delta G°$ that is < 0. The relationship between $\Delta G°$ and K_{eq} is $\Delta G° = -RT \ln K_{eq}$. For a reaction to proceed spontaneously, the K_{eq} must be > 1 and the $\Delta G°$ must be < 0.

78. The answer is B. *(Oxidative enzymes)*
The extraction of β-hydroxybutyrate from blood, and its oxidation to carbon dioxide and water, requires the participation of acetoacetate thiokinase and β-hydroxybutyrate dehydrogenase. All tissues except the liver use β-hydroxybutyrate as a metabolic fuel. The enzymes required for catabolism of the ketone bodies are localized in the mitochondria. These enzymes are β-hydroxybutyrate dehydrogenase, succinyl coenzyme A (CoA), acetoacetate acyltransferase, and acetoacetate thiokinase. 3-Hydroxy-3-methylglutaryl CoA (HMG CoA) lyase catalyzes a step in fatty acid oxidation that takes place in the kidneys or liver. HMG CoA lyase breaks down (*S*)-3-hydroxy-3-methylglutaryl CoA into acetyl CoA and acetoacetate.

79–81. The answers are: 79-B, 80-E, 81-B. *(Thiazide diuretic therapy)*
The thiazide diuretics, such as hydrochlorothiazide, primarily act in the early distal tubules by binding to a membrane protein that is a Na^+ and Cl^- cotransporter. Thus, both Na^+ and more importantly Cl^- reabsorption in the early distal tubules are blocked. The thiazide diuretics also have a small effect in the late proximal tubules.

Although most diuretics can cause all of the untoward effects listed in the question, the patient's neuromuscular dysfunction is most likely the result of hypokalemia, the most important and most serious side effect listed. Hypokalemia is produced because the diuretics cause a large amount of Na^+ to collect in the distal tubules, which leads to Na^+ reabsorption (sodium avidity) and a concomitant depletion of K^+. This Na^+–K^+ exchange site is a primary mechanism for renal control of K^+ homeostasis.

Because this patient is suffering from classic diuretic-induced K^+ loss, he should be supplemented with K^+. The physician may also prescribe a K^+-sparing diuretic, such as amiloride or spironolactone, to be used in combination with a reduced dosage of the thiazide diuretic to maintain K^+ balance. The altered blood K^+ would lead to an increased sensitivity to digitalis-related cardiovascular toxicity; therefore, digitalis should not be used to treat this patient's edema.

82. The answer is D. *(Empiric antibacterial therapy in an immunocompromised host)*
The most likely diagnosis is septic shock secondary to bacteremia. Chemotherapy for cancer is a common cause of neutropenia, with subsequent fever and infection. The risk is high when the white blood cell count is less than $500/\mu l$. In addition, cold, clammy skin is indicative of peripheral vascular shutdown. Lactic acid buildup will lead to metabolic acidosis and compensatory rapid breathing. Patients with neutropenic fever must be treated with double broad-spectrum antibacterial agents for gram-negative rods, including *Pseudomonas*. The combination of piperacillin, a broad-spectrum β-lactam, and gentamicin, an aminoglycoside that has broad gram-negative activity, is a good choice. In addition, penicillin–aminoglycoside combinations may be synergistic because of the different mechanisms of action of these agents; penicillins are cell wall synthesis inhibitors, and aminoglycosides inhibit protein synthesis. Single aminoglycoside therapy with gentamicin or amikacin would not effectively prevent infection by resistant organisms. Both chloramphenicol and gentamicin are protein synthesis inhibitors and would not be expected to work synergistically.

83. The answer is A. *(Psychotherapy management)*
The patient motorically and nonverbally expresses (acts out) his conflictual feelings and anxiety about the closeness he feels toward his physician by avoiding a scheduled appointment. There is some degree of repression of these feelings, but the motor behavior indicates that the patient is acting out. Suppression is a conscious decision to postpone something, but missing these appointments was not done consciously.

84. The answer is C. *(Disaccharide structure and function)*
The structure shown is that of the milk disaccharide lactose. Lactose is composed of 1 mol of galactose and 1 mol of glucose, which are joined by a β-galactosidic linkage. Lactose is the substrate for the intestinal enzyme lactase, which hydrolyzes the disaccharide. Therefore, lactose would not be digested or absorbed by a lactase-deficient child. Because galactosemia arises from an impaired ability to metabolize galactose, lactose would not be a good source of calories for a child with galactosemia. Additional galactose would augment the problem. Because the only requirement for a reducing sugar is an unsubstituted carbonyl group, the disaccharide would give a positive result in the Fehling-Benedict reducing sugar test. The anomeric carbon of the glucose residue is in equilibrium with the open chain structure, thereby providing an unsubstituted carbonyl group.

85. The answer is C. *(Varicella-zoster virus)*
The lesions outside the dermatomal distribution are explained by depressed cell-mediated immunity. When varicella-zoster virus (VZV) goes outside a dermatomal distribution, it is because the affected person is immunosuppressed either from old age (≥ 65 years) or medication (in this case, chemotherapy). Thymidine kinase–negative mutants rarely occur, except in human immunodeficiency virus (HIV) patients on prolonged prophylaxis with acyclovir. Initial exposure to the infection always leads to viral latency of the dorsal ganglia.

86. The answer is B. *(Histopathology of rheumatic fever)*
The photomicrograph of the heart shows an Aschoff body (*lower right*), which is pathognomonic of a history of rheumatic fever, and the mitral stenosis is also probably a consequence. Aschoff bodies constitute foci of fibrinoid necrosis surrounded by histiocytes, giant cells, and specialized histiocytes with linear chromatin called "caterpillar cells," which are seen with acute rheumatic fever and are eventually replaced by scar tissue. Tissue affected by rheumatic heart disease usually shows pericardial adhesions, valvular deformities, and fusion and shortening of the chordae tendineae.

87. The answer is A. *(Personality assessment)*
The major projective instrument of personality assessment is the Rorschach test. The thematic apperception test, sentence completion test, and projective drawings all are projective tests, but they are less well studied and yield more limited information. The Minnesota Multiphasic Personality Inventory, which is the most frequently used personality test, is an objective instrument, not a projective test.

88. The answer is D. *(Tuberculosis culture; diagnostic tests)*
Isolation of *Mycobacterium tuberculosis* is diagnostic of active tuberculosis. The tuberculin test can be positive in the absence of active disease. The clinical findings are not specifically pathognomonic for tuberculosis, nor is demonstration of acid-fast organisms.

89. The answer is B. *(Tumor immunology)*
Antigens of physically induced tumors, such as those induced by chemical carcinogens, ultraviolet light, or x-rays, exhibit little or no antigenic cross-reactivity. Because random mutations are the most likely explanation for these types of tumors, each tumor displays distinct antigenic specificity. The cells of a given tumor arise from a single cell and are, therefore, antigenically similar.

90. The answer is A. *(Hematopoietic–lymphoreticular system)*
Reed-Sternberg cells are diagnostic for Hodgkin's lymphoma. The Philadelphia chromosome and decreased quantities of leukocyte alkaline phosphatase are commonly observed in chronic myelogenous leukemia. Auer rods are most often seen in increased numbers in acute myelogenous or myelomonocytic leukemia.

91. The answer is B. *(Neurologic diagnosis)*
The selectivity of the deficit makes a supraforaminal lesion and a peripheral neuropathy impossible. Whether position sense is impaired has not been delineated. If it is impaired, the posterior column of the spinal cord becomes a possibility, but an isolated vibratory deficit can occur as a normal aging change. When diminished vibratory sensation is encountered, position sense must be tested carefully to make the branch point.

92. The answer is A. *(Autonomic pharmacology)*
Indirect-acting sympathomimetic agents, like amphetamine, are transported by the uptake 1 mechanism into nerve terminals where they displace norepinephrine to account for the pressor response. Because these agents lack hydroxyl groups on the catechol ring, they are without significant direct effects on synaptic receptors. Thus, their action is affected by the presence of other agents that modify adrenergic transmission. Reserpine depletes norepinephrine stores, and monoamine oxidase (MAO) inhibitors may potentiate norepinephrine levels. Therefore, the pressor response to amphetamine would be potentiated by an MAO inhibitor and decreased by reserpine. Imipramine interferes with uptake of amphetamine and reduces its effect in this and other ways. A hallmark of indirect-acting sympathomimetics is tolerance or tachyphylaxis. This is presumably secondary to depletion of endogenous norepinephrine pools after repetitive application of amphetamine.

93. The answer is C. *(Nucleic acid transfer)*
Transduction is the technique whereby a virus, known as a bacteriophage, is used to introduce DNA into bacteria. Transformation uses high concentrations of calcium chloride to help DNA cross the bacterial plasma membrane. Conjugation refers to direct transfer of DNA between bacteria. Circular, or plasmid, DNA is the form of DNA most commonly used to transfer genes into bacteria via transformation.

94–100. The answers are: 94-D, 95-B, 96-E, 97-D, 98-C, 99-B, 100-C. *(Anatomy of skeletal muscles and properties of halothane)*
Unlike intravenous anesthetics (e.g., methohexital), inhalational anesthetics such as halothane do not possess notable excitatory effects on the central nervous system (CNS), and, therefore, do not lower seizure threshold. All anesthetics tend to depress cardiac function and respiratory drive. Halothane and other anesthetics may induce malignant hyperthermia in certain genetically susceptible individuals.

The anterior cruciate ligament (ACL) is important to the proper functioning of the knee joint. The ACL attaches the femur to the tibia. Damage to this ligament is usually sports-related and caused by rapid deceleration or torque. The ligament is essential to the stability of the knee joint, and surgery is necessary to prevent further injury.

Latin for "little vinegar saucer," the acetabulum is the rounded cavity on the external surface of the innominate bone that receives the head of the femur.

The epiphyseal plate lies between the epiphysis and diaphysis of long bones and is the area of highest mitotic activity. During bone growth, the epiphyseal plates migrate distally, finally becoming epiphyseal lines when growth is completed.

The cuboid is a tarsal bone. The navicular is both a carpal and a tarsal bone. All of the other bones listed (i.e., capitate, trapezium, trapezoid) are carpal bones.

A haversian system, or osteon, is composed of osteocytes, lacunae, canaliculi, and concentric lamellae. It is the fundamental unit of compact bone. Compact bone is made up of lamellae, which are parallel bony columns that surround a central (haversian) canal; these canals are neurovascular channels and interconnect via Volkmann's canals. Osteocytes occupy lacunae and communicate with each other via gap junctions that are formed between tiny cytoplasmic projections found in canaliculi. Trabeculae are characteristic features of cancellous (spongy) bone.

101. The answer is C. *(Diagnostic tests)*
Lumbar puncture is absolutely contraindicated in patients with intracranial neoplasms because it may cause a rapid extrusion of brain tissue of the cerebral hemisphere through the tentorial notch or of the medulla and cerebellum through the foramen magnum. These tumors usually cause cerebrospinal fluid (CSF) pressure buildup, and lumbar puncture causes rapid depressurization of the fluid. Computed tomography (CT) with contrast medium, nuclear magnetic resonance (NMR), and x-ray are all useful tools in imaging brain tumors and do not cause the complications previously mentioned.

102. The answer is A. *(Immunoglobulin E–mediated hypersensitivity)*
The scientist has developed an allergy after repeated exposure to the rodents. The late symptom complex was induced by mast cells triggered by previous interaction of rodent antigen with immunoglobulin E (IgE). This is a typical late phase set of reactions, which are mast cell–mediated; no complement is involved. Corticosteroids will block the late reaction. The involvement of histamine is early, not late.

103. The answer is A. *(Renal physiology)*
If glomerular filtration decreases, excessive reabsorption of Na^+ (and Cl^-) will occur in the ascending limb of the loop of Henle. The decrease in ion concentration within the distal tubules causes the release of renin from the juxtaglomerular cells (*1*), with subsequent formation of angiotensin II and vasoconstriction of the

efferent arteriole (2) to help return filtration to normal values. In addition, there will be afferent arteriolar vasodilation to support glomerular filtration.

104. The answer is D. *(Gram stain; bacterial growth)*
Bacterial spores probably caused the decrease in the number of cells expected from the turbidity of the culture. Spores contribute to turbidity, but they do not stain in Gram's procedure.

105. The answer is C. *(Hemodynamics)*
Under the circumstances described in the question, the stroke volume is 100 ml. Cardiac output is the ratio of oxygen consumption to the arteriovenous difference. In this case, it is:

$$\frac{300 \text{ ml/min}}{20 \text{ ml/100 ml} - 15 \text{ ml/100 ml}} = 6000 \text{ ml/min}$$

Stroke volume is the ratio of cardiac output to heart rate:

$$\frac{6000 \text{ ml/min}}{60 \text{ min}} = 100 \text{ ml}$$

106. The answer is C. *(Antiphagocytic virulence factors)*
Opsonizing antibodies promote phagocytosis and are often directed against the capsules of pathogens, including *Streptococcus pneumoniae*. The most important function of the *S. pneumoniae* capsule is to inhibit phagocytosis (until opsonizing antibodies are produced). The capsules of both *Haemophilus influenzae* type B and *Neisseria meningitidis* are polysaccharides that elicit a poor T-cell–dependent immune response. The existing DTP (diphtheria-tetanus-pertussis) vaccine contains killed whole *Bordetella pertussis* cells, not purified capsules.

107. The answer is D. *(Structure and function of proteins)*
The chemical properties of proteins are determined by the nature of the constituent amino acid side chains. There are no ionizing groups, physiologically speaking, on the side chain of serine to provide buffering capacity. Only those amino acids with aromatic side chains absorb significantly in the ultraviolet range. Both glutamic acid and aspartic acid have a pI of approximately 4.5, and only L-amino acids are incorporated into protein. The side chain of proline contains a cyclic ring that cannot bond hydrogen and, therefore, disrupts the α-helical structure.

108. The answer is A. *(Diagnosis of myelodysplastic syndrome)*
Clinically persistent and unexplained cytopenias associated with morphologically abnormal differentiation in bone marrow precursors define preleukemia, often referred to as the myelodysplastic syndrome. Many of these individuals will have bone marrow blast percentages of less than 5%, and patients suffer from complications of bone marrow failure such as bleeding, infection, and anemia. Others will show an increase in bone marrow blasts between 5% and 30% and have a higher propensity to develop frank acute myeloid leukemia, particularly at the higher levels. Bone marrow blasts greater than 30% define acute leukemia. Cytogenetic changes, if present in myelodysplastic syndrome, are similar to those observed with acute myeloid leukemia, such as an extra chromosome 8, loss of chromosome 5 or 7, or loss of the long arm of chromosome 5 or 7. Despite megaloblastoid morphologic changes, these patients do not resolve with treatment for megaloblastic anemia. It is rare for chronic myelogenous leukemia to present with a low white cell and platelet count and bone marrow dyspoiesis.

109. The answer is C. *(Receptors; histamine (H$_2$) receptor antagonists; toxicology therapy)*
Cimetidine, like most drugs, interacts with a specific receptor, the histamine (H$_2$) receptor. Mannitol is the osmotic diuretic used most frequently in the prevention and treatment of acute renal failure occurring in

conditions such as cardiovascular surgery, trauma, and hemolytic transfusion reactions. Ethylenediamine-tetraacetic acid (EDTA) and dimercaprol chelate heavy metals but do not need to interact directly with any receptor for their pharmacologic actions.

110. The answer is D. *(Hemoglobin–oxygen interaction)*
The affinity of hemoglobin A_1 ($\alpha_2\beta_2$) for oxygen is decreased by an increase in H^+ concentration (a decrease in pH), by an increase in the P_{CO_2}, or by an increase in the concentration of 2,3-diphosphoglycerate (DPG). All of these conditions result in a shift of the oxygen saturation curve to the right. Fetal hemoglobin ($\alpha_2\gamma_2$) has a higher affinity for oxygen than does adult hemoglobin ($\alpha_2\beta_2$) and consequently becomes saturated at a lower P_{O_2}.

111. The answer is A. *(Musculature of the oral cavity)*
During deglutition, the levator veli palatini muscle raises the soft palate to seal the nasopharynx. Contraction of the palatoglossus elevates the base of the tongue and, with help from the palatopharyngeus muscle, closes the oropharyngeal isthmus behind the food bolus. The superior constrictor muscle helps raise the posterior portion of the pharynx over the bolus.

112. The answer is C. *(Side effects of neuroleptics)*
Akathisia, an extrapyramidal side effect of neuroleptics, causes restlessness and an urge to keep moving. The agitation in the man presented in the question seems more motoric than psychic, making worsening psychosis less likely. Although hyperthyroidism causes hyperactivity, this patient has no other symptoms of thyroid disease. Restless legs syndrome is a sleep-related disorder, generally associated with nocturnal myoclonus. It is described as a creepy, crawly feeling in the legs at rest (especially when supine) that is relieved by walking.

113. The answer is B. *(Extracellular matrix production and chondroblasts)*
Chondroblasts are cartilage cells located deep in the perichondrium, the dense connective capsule that surrounds cartilage. As chondroblasts secrete an extracellular matrix rich in type II collagen and cartilage proteoglycan, they become surrounded by their own extracellular matrix and differentiate into chondrocytes. Both chondroblasts and chondrocytes are capable of cell division by mitosis. The endosteum is a layer of osteoblasts in bone. The periosteum is the outer connective tissue covering of bone.

114. The answer is B. *(Pathophysiology of idiopathic thrombocytopenic purpura)*
Idiopathic thrombocytopenic purpura (ITP) is most common in young women, and the usual presentation is of isolated thrombocytopenia without associated illness. Amegakaryocytic thrombocytopenia can occur, but it is much less common, especially in this age-group. Drug-induced thrombocytopenia is also possible but is unlikely in a healthy woman who has no reason to take medications. Patients with thrombasthenia are not thrombocytopenic, and aleukemic leukemia is unlikely to occur without other cytopenias.

115–120. The answers are: 115-C, 116-B, 117-A, 118-E, 119-D, 120-A. *(Exocrine pancreatic function)*
Elevated serum amylase is the single most important diagnostic finding for confirmation of acute pancreatitis. A serum amylase level threefold higher than normal virtually confirms the diagnosis.
Secretin is composed of 27 amino acids, is secreted by the mucosal cells of the duodenum, and promotes the secretion of pancreatic juice rich in electrolytes and water. Cholecystokinin is released by mucosal cells in the upper small intestine in response to peptones and fats. It is absorbed into the bloodstream and stimulates the pancreas to secrete large quantities of digestive enzymes.
Although neuronal control of pancreatic exocrine function is secondary to hormonal control, parasympathetic stimulation of pancreatic secretory activity occurs via vagal fibers, which release acetylcholine (ACh).
Secretin and cholecystokinin are secreted by the mucosa of the small intestine into the bloodstream. They

exert their effects after entering the pancreatic circulation. Secretin is stored in an inactive form in the S cells of the duodenum and is released and activated in response to acid. It causes the pancreas to secrete copious amounts of bicarbonate ion (HCO_3^-); but unlike cholecystokinin, which is secreted in response to food, secretin does not significantly affect pancreatic enzyme secretion. The proteolytic enzymes are synthesized as proenzymes, inactive precursors that must be processed before they are active. Many proenzymes, including chymotrypsinogen, procarboxypeptidase, and prophospholipase, are activated by trypsin. Trypsinogen is activated by enterokinase.

121. The answer is C. *(Immunology; complement fixation)*
The complement fixation test is composed of sheep red blood cells (SRBC), antibodies to SRBC, and complement. The concentration of complement is limiting, and any loss of complement is reflected by a decrease in the extent of SRBC lysis. This loss of complement could occur during preincubation of the complement with an antigen–antibody complex not related to the SRBC, which would cause fixation and activation of the cascade. All or most of the complement would be consumed so that the introduction of SRBC does not result in lysis. In this case, because lysis did occur, the patient's serum possesses no complement-fixable [immunoglobulin G (IgG)] anti-influenza type A antibodies. A cross-reactive antibody has no bearing on the complement fixation test.

122. The answer is D. *(Pulmonary mechanics)*
Inspiration is an active process brought about by contraction of the diaphragm. This contraction results in increased chest volume, thereby lowering pleural and alveolar pressure and creating a gradient for the movement of air. At the end of inspiration, flow is zero and alveolar pressure equals atmospheric pressure. The difference between alveolar and pleural pressure is the recoil pressure of the lung, which is always greatest at higher lung volumes and, thus, is greater at the end of inspiration. During expiration, inspiratory muscles relax, and the elastic forces of the lungs compress alveolar gas, which raises alveolar pressure to values greater than atmospheric pressure and creates a pressure gradient to expel gas from the lung.

123. The answer is A. *(RNA processing)*
RNA processing occurs in two locations within cells. The most common site is the cell nucleoplasm, where the majority of RNA transcribed in the nucleus is spliced, capped, and polyadenylated. The other site is the mitochondria, each of which contains a ring of DNA that codes for two ribosomal RNA (rRNA) molecules, proteins, and all the transfer RNA (tRNA) required to synthesize the encoded proteins.

124. The answer is C. *(Urea metabolism; amino acid enzymes)*
The pathway by which the α-amino groups of the amino acids are incorporated into urea involves a number of transaminases that transfer the amino group from the amino acids to α-ketoglutarate, with the concomitant formation of glutamate. The glutamate is converted back to α-ketoglutarate and ammonium by the mitochondrial enzyme glutamate dehydrogenase. The ammonium produced in the reaction is the substrate for carbamoyl phosphate synthesis. This reaction constitutes the first step in urea biosynthesis.

125. The answer is C. *(Neurophysiology)*
Patients born without a corpus callosum show no neurologic defects. Only lesions introduced after the brain has developed would produce symptoms. The Romberg sign is indicative of cerebellar disease and has no bearing in this case.

126. The answer is C. *(Histopathology of alcohol-induced acute liver damage)*
The liver biopsy shows the typical features of alcohol-induced acute liver injury, which include steatorrhea, acute inflammation, and Mallory bodies. Mallory bodies are intracellular filamentous material believed to be

related to prekeratin, which is normally produced by the liver. This injury to the liver is a direct effect of alcohol.

127. The answer is A. *(Viral immunity)*
Antibodies cannot displace attached viruses from the host cell. The role of antibodies in preventing diseases caused by viruses is demonstrated by the effectiveness of the polio vaccine. For the poliovirus, and other viruses as well, antibodies bind to proteins on the surface of the viruses, which inhibits the virus from entering host cells. This attachment of immunoglobulins [most notably immunoglobulin G (IgG)] to the virus particle also leads to phagocytosis by attachment of the Fc portion of the antibody to macrophages. Attachment of the antibody to an infected host cell presenting viral antigens leads to complement-mediated lysis. Antibodies have been found that inhibit critical viral enzyme functions, such as neuraminidase of the influenza virus.

128. The answer is E. *(Cholesterol biosynthesis)*
The synthesis of cholesterol uses acetyl coenzyme A (CoA) as the sole source of carbon atoms and reduced nicotinamide-adenine dinucleotide phosphate (NADPH) as a source of reducing equivalents. The NADPH is supplied primarily through two reactions, which are catalyzed by a glucose 6-phosphate dehydrogenase and 6-phosphogluconate dehydrogenase. The formation of 3-hydroxy-3-methylglutaryl CoA (HMG CoA) results from the condensation of acetoacetyl CoA and acetyl CoA. The step that is committed to cholesterol synthesis is the conversion of HMG CoA to mevalonic acid. This step is catalyzed by HMG CoA reductase. HMG CoA is used to synthesize activated isoprenoid units, which are subsequently condensed to form squalene. Squalene is converted to lanosterol and then to cholesterol by a series of reactions that involve the addition of oxygen, cyclization to give the sterol ring structure, and elimination of three carbon atoms as carbon dioxide. Mevinolin is an inhibitor of HMG CoA reductase.

129. The answer is B. *(Blood pressure regulation)*
Angiotensin-converting enzyme (ACE) hydrolyzes the decapeptide angiotensin I to the vasoconstrictor octapeptide, angiotensin II. Inhibition of this enzyme by a number of competitive antagonists is a new and useful way to lower blood pressure in some individuals. In addition to reducing circulating levels of the endogenous angiotensin II peptide, inhibition of ACE may have central effects, including a decrease in the dipsogenic effect of angiotensin II. Furthermore, angiotensin II appears to facilitate neurotransmission in the central and peripheral sympathetic nervous systems. Although angiotensin II is a potent stimulator of aldosterone secretion in the zona glomerulosa of the adrenal cortex, and inhibition of this effect might be expected to reduce blood pressure (by enhancing Na^+ excretion by the kidneys), there usually is little change in aldosterone levels because other endogenous secretagogues, including steroids, K^+, and minimal levels of angiotensin II, can maintain aldosterone secretion. Nonetheless, there is little indication to believe that the aldosterone level would actually increase, and if it did, this would result in NA^+ reabsorption, water retention, and an increase in arterial blood pressure.

130. The answer is C. *(Cell structure; membranes)*
The cell membrane is composed of a variety of proteins scattered within a phospholipid bilayer. The phospholipid molecules contain a hydrophilic head and a hydrophobic tail and, therefore, are amphipathic. The cell membrane readily allows the diffusion of molecules such as oxygen, carbon dioxide, nitrogen, and water; however, glucose does not diffuse through the cell readily, and entry into the cell is enhanced by carrier proteins (facilitated diffusion and active transport).

131. The answer is D. *(Cardiac mechanics and sounds)*
Pulmonary stenosis and pulmonary hypertension are associated with a prominent S_4 heart sound. Left-to-right shunts involving the left ventricle (e.g., ventricular septal defects and patent ductus arteriosus) are associated with a prominent S_3 heart sound, as are mitral regurgitation and left ventricular failure.

132. The answer is C. *(Prokaryotic and eukaryotic differences)*
Because shigellae are gram-negative prokaryotic bacteria, they have peptidoglycan-containing cell walls, lipopolysaccharide, 70S ribosomes, RNA, and DNA, but they do not have sterols in their plasma membranes. *Giardia* species are eukaryotic protozoa with 80S ribosomes, RNA, DNA, and sterol-containing plasma membranes.

133. The answer is D. *(Enzyme catalysis)* ✓
The activation energy is the amount of energy required to pass into the transition state; the rate of the reaction depends on the number of molecules in the transition state. Increasing the activation energy lowers the reaction rate. Each enzyme has two kinetic parameters: V_{max} is an index of catalytic efficiency, and K_m is a measure of the affinity of the enzyme for the substrate. The binding of substrate to enzyme induces a conformational change in which the functional group that participates in catalysis is appropriately juxtaposed with the substrate bonds that are to be altered in the reaction. General acid–base catalysis is a catalytic mode frequently used by enzymes.

134. The answer is E. *(Respiratory failure)* ✓
Adult respiratory distress syndrome (ARDS) is a model of acute alveolar injury with pulmonary edema and respiratory failure. A number of conditions can lead to ARDS, particularly if high concentrations of oxygen are used as supportive respiratory therapy. Focal atelectasis and alveolar collapse occur with the development of pulmonary edema; hyaline membranes appear, type II pneumonocytes proliferate, and there is variable damage to the alveolar walls. The mechanisms of ARDS are not completely understood. The permeability of the endothelium of the pulmonary capillary and the epithelium of the alveolar wall is increased in ARDS, → pulm. and it is responsible, in part, for the characteristics of the syndrome. edema

135. The answer is C. *(Anatomy of the respiratory system)*
Type II pneumonocytes cover less than 5% of the alveolar surface, but they form a reserve for replacement of damaged type I pneumonocytes. These multilamellar bodies are the source of the phospholipid-containing pulmonary surfactant. Defects in these cells contribute to infant and adult respiratory distress.

136. The answer is E. *(Cellular signal transduction)*
The nuclear oncogene product *c-fos* assists in the regulation of gene expression. Although its expression is affected by second messengers, it is not thought of as a second messenger. Inositol 1,4,5-triphosphate (IP_3) and diacylglycerol (DAG) are important second messengers generated by phospholipase C from phosphatidylinositol biphosphate. IP_3 causes the release of intracellular stores of Ca^{2+}, which is also an important second messenger, and DAG activates a Ca^{2+}-dependent protein kinase, protein kinase C. Cyclic adenosine monophosphate (cAMP) is synthesized by adenylate cyclase from adenosine triphosphate (ATP) and can act as a second messenger to activate enzymes such as cAMP-dependent protein kinase.

137. The answer is D. *(Embolism)*
Thrombi from the left side of the heart to the parent vessels of the cerebral arteries all may embolize to occlude a cerebral artery; however, the abdominal aorta is beyond these vessels that lead to the brain and, thus, is unlikely to cause an embolism in the brain. Severe fracture of any long bone may result in a fat embolus to ✓ the cerebral arteries.

138. The answer is D. *(Effects of exogenous testosterone)*
Although testosterone is required for normal spermatogenesis, it is involved in an important feedback inhibition pathway. Accordingly, introduction of high concentrations of testosterone can inhibit gonadatropin-releasing hormone production in the hypothalamus and interfere with important steps in spermatogenesis induced by luteinizing hormone. In addition, testosterone can be metabolized to estrogens in men as well

as women, and this estrogen formation can add to the inhibition of normal spermatogenesis. This effect is usually reversible in most mature men but can persist in a subset of anabolic steroid abusers. Testosterone is very likely to produce its well-known masculinization effects in mature women and can produce feminization in men. Although testosterone has a significant myotrophic effect on muscle mass in children, it is never used in this age-group because it causes closure of the epiphysis of long bones.

139. The answer is A. *(RNA function)*
The synthesis of RNA in eukaryotes requires three different RNA polymerases: one each for the synthesis of messenger RNA (mRNA), ribosomal RNA (rRNA), and transfer RNA (tRNA). All of these RNAs are required for protein synthesis. The ribosome is a complex made up of approximately 75 proteins and several types of rRNA and is the site where mRNA and tRNAs come together to participate in protein synthesis. The triplet base codons for amino acids are contained in mRNA; tRNA contains a complementary anticodon, which promotes interaction between mRNA and tRNA during protein synthesis.

140. The answer is D. *(Hormone receptors; Addison's disease)*
Addison's disease is caused by an overall atrophy of the adrenal cortex and is not related to an abnormality in hormone receptors. Many peptide hormone receptors are transmembrane proteins that may elicit their full biologic response when only a small fraction of the receptors are occupied by hormone. The specificity of the response of a particular cell or tissue is defined, at least in part, by the types of receptors localized on or in the cell. Some hormone receptors are desensitized by phosphorylation. Following phosphorylation, dissociation of the hormone from the receptor may occur without a corresponding decrease in the biologic response.

141. The answer is D. *(Neuroanatomy)*
The subthalamus is located (not surprisingly) below the thalamus. It is an exceedingly complex area of the brain connected to many areas to integrate motor control, but it is not connected with the cerebellum.

142–146. The answers are: 142-D, 143-B, 144-C, 145-C, 146-B. *(Embryology)*
Ectoderm gives rise to the nervous system, sensory epithelia, epidermis, mammary glands, and the pituitary gland. Melanocytes in the dermis arise from neuroectoderm. Mesoderm gives rise to cartilage, bone, connective tissue, muscles, the cardiovascular system, kidneys, gonads, spleen, and the adrenal cortex. Endoderm gives rise to gastrointestinal and respiratory mucosa, and the parenchyma of the tonsils, thyroid gland, parathyroid glands, thymus, liver, and pancreas.

147–149. The answers are: 147-C, 148-A, 149-B. *(Hepatic histology)*
This is a scanning electron micrograph of the liver. Liver parenchymal cells (*A*) secrete bile into the bile canaliculi (*B*) and blood proteins, such as serum albumin and transferrin, into the liver sinusoids (*C*). Liver sinusoids are modified fenestrated and discontinuous capillaries that receive blood from the portal vein and hepatic artery in the portal canals and carry it to the central veins.

150–154. The answers are: 150-E, 151-D, 152-C, 153-B, 154-A. *(Lipoproteins and genetic disorders)*
Lipoprotein lipase is an enzyme normally located within the capillary endothelium; it is involved in converting chylomicrons to chylomicron remnants. A deficiency in lipoprotein lipase leads to elevated circulating levels of chylomicrons. Chylomicron levels may also be elevated in systemic lupus erythematosus (SLE). Familial hypercholesterolemia, caused by mutation within a single gene, is one of the most common human mendelian disorders. Low-density lipoprotein (LDL) levels are elevated in the serum because this disorder markedly decreases the number of high-affinity LDL receptors within the liver. LDL levels may also be elevated in nephrotic syndrome and hyperthyroidism.

Familial (type III) hyperlipoproteinemia has been traced to a single amino acid substitution within the receptor for apoprotein E. Because the apoprotein E receptor is required for the normal metabolism of both chylomicron remnants and intermediate-density lipoproteins (IDL), both of these molecules accumulate in the blood.

The biochemical defect underlying familial hypertriglyceridemia is unknown. In this disorder, serum levels of both very low-density lipoprotein (VLDL) and triglycerides are elevated. VLDL and triglyceride levels may also be elevated in diabetes mellitus and chronic alcoholism.

The defect underlying familial hyperlipidemia is unknown, although research suggests a deficiency in apoprotein CII. In this disorder, serum levels of VLDL and chylomicrons are elevated; alcoholism, diabetes mellitus, and oral contraceptives are also capable of elevating VLDL and chylomicron levels.

155–159. The answers are: 155-B, 156-C, 157-A, 158-D, 159-E. *(Neuroanatomy)*

Many neuroanatomic pathways now can be specified by their neurotransmitters. Thus, selective depletion of the neurotransmitters can be caused by sectioning the pathways or by destroying the perikarya that produce the neurotransmitter.

Destruction of interneurons of the spinal cord would deplete γ-aminobutyric acid (GABA) and glycine, inhibitory transmitters produced by interneurons. Dorsal root section would reduce substance P concentration in the dorsal horns. This neurotransmitter presumably transmits pain impulses from the small fibers in the lateral division of the dorsal roots. Destruction of the substantia nigra would deplete dopamine, the major neurotransmitter within the basal ganglia. Section of the medial forebrain bundle would destroy many of the axons that connect the catecholaminergic and serotoninergic nuclei of the brain stem with the cerebral cortex. Destruction of the medullary raphe would destroy the serotoninergic neurons of the medulla that project to the spinal cord.

Not only can the neurotransmitters be depleted by actual anatomic destruction of axonal pathways or the destruction of neuronal perikarya, but various drugs and chemicals can also selectively block neurotransmitters either by inhibiting their formation, inhibiting their release, or competing with binding sites on the postsynaptic membrane. By combining anatomic lesions with chemical blockade and direct chemical analysis, various lines of evidence can be developed to establish the transmitters involved in the various layers and regions of the cortex and the different nuclei of the central nervous system (CNS).

160–163. The answers are: 160-A, 161-C, 162-B, 163-E. *(Oncogenes; oncogenesis; signal transduction; growth factor receptors)*

Alteration of virtually any cellular signaling system has the potential for causing oncogenesis. The *ros* oncogene product is an activated insulin receptor. The homolog of one of the two subunits of the nerve growth factor (NGF) receptor is *trk*. The oncogene *erbB* has activated tyrosine kinase, which is also activated when epidermal growth factor (EGF) binds to the EGF receptor. The oncogenic homolog of the platelet-derived growth factor (PDGF) receptor is *kit,* whereas *sis* binds to the PDGF receptor. The nuclear oncogene *jun* is involved in the control of gene transcription.

164–169. The answers are: 164-E, 165-A, 166-C, 167-A, 168-D, 169-B. *(Etiology of spirochetal diseases)*

Borrelia recurrentis is the etiologic agent of relapsing fever in humans. The disease occurs worldwide and is characterized by a febrile bacteremia. The disease name is derived from the fact that there can be 3–10 recurrences, apparently from the original infection. The disease is transmitted to humans from infected animals by ticks and from human to human by lice.

Bejel is nonvenereal, endemic syphilis caused by a variant of *Treponema pallidum*. The disease usually is seen in children in the Middle East and Africa. Transmission appears to be through the shared use of drinking and eating utensils; bejel is not transmitted sexually. The disease develops in primary, secondary, and tertiary stages.

Pinta is a tropical disease caused by *Treponema carateum*. It occurs primarily in Central and South America, where it appears to be spread by person-to-person contact. Unlike other treponemal diseases, the lesions of pinta remain localized in the skin.

The etiologic agent of syphilis is *T. pallidum*. Humans are the only natural host of the spirochete, and venereal transmission is the most common means of acquiring the infection. Congenital syphilis occurs when the fetus is infected transplacentally and survives to delivery. Accidental laboratory infections occasionally occur.

Fort Bragg fever is a localized name of pretibial fever caused by *Leptospira interrogans* serogroup *autumnalis*. The disease is characterized by a rash on the shins. Humans probably acquire the infection by contact with the urine of infected animals.

Treponema pertenue is the etiologic agent of yaws. The disease occurs primarily in children in tropical regions, where it appears to be transmitted by direct contact or by vectors such as flies. This potentially disfiguring disease has primary, secondary, and tertiary stages.

170–175. The answers are: 170-A, 171-C, 172-B, 173-B, 174-A, 175-A. *(Abnormal heart sounds)*
The first heart sound, S_1, is composed of the sounds of tricuspid and mitral valve closure. Mitral valve closure is normally almost silent, and S_1 is normally quieter than the second heart sound, S_2, which is the sound of the aortic and pulmonic valves closing. S_1 is better heard at the apex of the heart, and S_2 is better heard at the base of the heart. With mitral valve stenosis, the left ventricle is underfilled at the end of diastole, and its systolic contraction has force sufficient to cause the mitral valve leaflets to close audibly. During ventricular systole, the presence of aortic stenosis produces a high flow rate through the stenotic valve, which is appreciated as a pansystolic murmur. The sound is heard well at both the base and apex of the heart and is relatively unchanged by respiratory movements. In acute aortic regurgitation, the left ventricle is overfilled, and the ejection fraction is reduced. During ventricular systole, the pressure buildup is more sluggish than normal due to the leaking aortic valve. The mitral valve closure becomes even quieter than normal; thus, S_1 is quieter than normal. In systemic hypertension, the higher than normal pressure within the aortic bulb at the end of systole causes the very forceful closure of the aortic valve, which produces an S_2 that is louder than usual. In cases of severe anemia or hyperthyroidism, the heart rate is increased along with cardiac output. The increase in heart rate causes the heart to spend a greater portion of its time in systole and less time in diastole. The reduction in diastolic time means that the left ventricle may be relatively underfilled at the beginning of systole. As stated above, the contraction of an underfilled ventricle allows the mitral valve to close with force sufficient to cause S_1 to be louder than S_2.

176–179. The answers are: 176-C, 177-D, 178-A, 179-B. *(Degenerative joint disease)*
Rheumatoid arthritis is a common chronic inflammatory disease affecting the joints. Initially, the small joints of the hands and feet are involved. The disease is strongly associated with genetic factors—over 75% of Caucasians affected have human leukocyte antigen DR4 (HLA-DR4).

Osteoarthritis is characterized by progressive deterioration of the articular cartilage of weight-bearing joints. Erosion of cartilage eventually leads to thickening of the underlying bone and to knobby protruding of the bone. These protrusions are called Heberden's nodes. They may break off the bone surface and form intra-articular bodies called "joint mice."

Lyme disease (Lyme arthritis) is caused by *Borrelia burgdorferi*, which is transmitted by ticks, whose reservoirs are field mice and deer. The disease has a spectrum of symptoms similar to those of rheumatoid arthritis, principally affecting the knees. Symptoms may last for a long period of time (months) and may lead to a chronic insidious polyarthritis.

Gout is manifested by hyperuricemia, arthritis (gouty arthritis), and the deposit of tophi (urate crystals) in and around the joints. The tophi are surrounded by histiocytes, giant cells, and fibroblasts, causing inflammation.

180–182. The answers are: 180-F, 181-C, 182-D. *(Valsalva maneuver)*
The subject described in the question exhaled against a small leak, requiring the use of thoracic and abdominal muscles to maintain voluntarily an elevated esophageal (and intrathoracic) pressure of 40 cm H_2O. Transmission of applied pressure causes a rise in blood pressure (*B*) followed quickly by a decrease in arterial pressure and pulse pressure (*C*) as venous return is cut off. A reflex change during the maneuver prevents further decline in blood pressure with accompanying reflex tachycardia (*D*). When the strain ends, the blood pressure falls, and venous return is restored (*E*). In a normal subject, an overshoot in pressure followed by a vagally mediated bradycardia ensues (*F*).

183–187. The answers are: 183-E, 184-A, 185-D, 186-B, 187-A. *(Personality disorders)*
Antisocial behavior in an adult has roots in similar behavior as a child or teenager; such children are termed conduct-disordered. Obsessive–compulsive individuals are rigid, perfectionistic, overly organized, and have difficulty relaxing or having fun. Narcissistic individuals are self-centered with a grandiose sense of self, yet they have underlying poor self-esteem and become enraged when they perceive criticism, even if slight. Individuals with borderline personalities frequently cut themselves, even superficially, and often have multiple scars.

188–192. The answers are: 188-F, 189-D, 190-A, 191-E, 192-C. *(Tumors of the musculoskeletal system)*
A chondroblastoma is a benign tumor composed of small immature chondrocytes, each with a single nucleus, dispersed among benign-appearing, multinucleated giant cells and chondroid matrix. This tumor most often occurs within the epiphyseal region of long, tubular bones of individuals between the ages of 10 and 20 years. Males are affected twice as often as females.

A giant cell tumor is a benign, but locally invasive, lesion characterized by many multinucleated giant cells distributed in a stroma of neoplastic, smaller, mononucleated cells. Over 50% of these "brown" tumors develop in the distal femur or proximal tibia or fibula. The majority of individuals with this tumor are between 20 and 40 years of age. Females are affected slightly more often than males. The tumor frequently recurs many years after surgical removal.

An osteosarcoma is a malignant tumor that most often arises in the medullary cavity of the metaphyseal end of the long bones of the extremities. It is a tumor of mesenchymal cells in which there is deposition of osteoid or new bone. This tumor is most often seen in adolescent or young adult males. Deletions of the long arm of chromosome 13, which are associated with retinoblastoma, are hypothesized to be associated with osteosarcoma development. Radiographs of osteosarcomas often show Codman's triangle—an angle formed between the elevated periosteum and the plane of the outer surface of the cortical bone.

Osteoid osteoma is a small, extremely painful benign tumor without the potential for malignant transformation. Radiographically, it appears as small, radiolucent foci surrounded by dense sclerotic bone. Most lesions are intracortical and arise near the ends of the femur or tibia. The lesion appears most often in individuals between 5 and 25 years of age, and it occurs twice as often in males as in females.

Ewing's sarcoma is a malignant neoplasm, most often seen in the pelvis and long tubular bones. It is characterized radiographically by "onion-skin" layering of the cortex and widening of the diaphyseal region. Ewing's sarcoma usually arises before the age of 20 years, and it appears twice as often in males as in females. This tumor is associated with translocation of portions of the long arms of chromosomes 11 and 22.

The majority of chondrosarcomas affect the pelvis and ribs; they most often occur between the middle and the end of the life span.

193–200. The answers are: 193-B, 194-B, 195-C, 196-D, 197-A, 198-B, 199-A, 200-B. *(Intestinal diseases)*

Ulcerative colitis usually involves the large intestine, where it commonly causes a diffuse inflammatory reaction that stops abruptly at the terminal ileum. The rectum is invariably involved. The inflammatory reaction involves the mucosa and superficial submucosa and results in crypt abscesses and pseudopolyps. Ulcerative colitis is associated with an increased risk of colonic adenocarcinoma.

Crohn's disease affects the large and small bowel in a segmental fashon, resulting in "skip" lesions. The inflammatory process is transmural, leading to fistulae between adjacent segments of intestine. The characteristic histologic finding is the non-necrotizing granuloma, which may be seen in the inflammatory reaction within the bowel wall or in pericolonic lymph nodes.

Extra
Practice
Questions

QUESTIONS

DIRECTIONS: Each of the numbered items or incomplete statements in this section is followed by answers or by completions of the statement. Select the ONE lettered answer or completion that is BEST in each case.

1. Fetal hemoglobin (Hb F) is able to bind oxygen well because

(A) Fetal red blood cells have high levels of 2,3-bisphosphoglycerate (2,3-BPG)
(B) Fetal red blood cells have low levels of 2,3-BPG
(C) Hb F binds 2,3-BPG tightly
(D) Hb F does not bind 2,3-BPG well
(E) The oxygen partial pressure (Po_2) levels of the placenta are high

2. Select the statement that best describes the relationship of nerve roots to somites.

(A) Somites retain their original nerve root when they migrate
(B) Somites receive their innervation from the level to which they migrate
(C) Nerve roots migrate rostrally or caudally with their somites
(D) Nerve roots exchange somites when the somites migrate
(E) None of the above

3. An investigator has isolated a bacterium that, in the absence of glucose, constitutively produces the proteins coded for by the *lac* operon. Which of the following statements explains this observation?

(A) The promoter has a mutation that prevents RNA polymerase from binding
(B) There is a missense mutation in the gene for β-galactosidase
(C) The gene for the catabolite activator protein is mutated and inactive
(D) There is a mutation in the attenuator sequence
(E) The gene for the repressor protein is mutated and inactive

4. To withdraw cerebrospinal fluid (CSF) [i.e., perform a spinal tap], a needle tip must pass successively through the

(A) pia mater, dura mater, epidural space, and arachnoid membrane
(B) arachnoid membrane, epidural space, dura mater, and subdural space
(C) subdural space, dura mater, epidural space, and arachnoid membrane
(D) arachnoid membrane, subdural space, dura mater, and epidural space
(E) epidural space, dura mater, subdural space, and arachnoid membrane

5. Fluid that collects during acute inflammation and has a protein content exceeding 3 g/dl and a specific gravity exceeding 1.015 is referred to as

(A) edema
(B) an effusion
(C) a transudate
(D) serum
(E) an exudate

6. Which of the following statements concerning hair follicles is correct?

(A) They form by mesenchymal proliferation
(B) They form by epithelial invagination and are induced by underlying mesenchymal condensations
(C) They are rarely associated with sebaceous glands
(D) They form lanugo hairs after birth
(E) They contribute to the vernix caseosa

Questions 7–10

A 29-year-old black man presents to a clinic for a routine examination. His family history is significant for cardiovascular disease, including a father who died of a myocardial infarction at 49 years of age and a grandfather who is presently 70 years old and has severe congestive heart failure. Physical examination is unremarkable except that the patient is 20 pounds heavier than ideal body weight, and his blood pressure is 160/100. Repeat blood pressure evaluation confirms this reading.

7. First line therapy for this patient should be

(A) initiation of captopril therapy
(B) initiation of propranolol therapy
(C) initiation of verapamil therapy
(D) dietary restriction
(E) initiation of hydralazine therapy

8. The recommended therapy made little difference. Which therapy should be tried next?

(A) Reserpine
(B) Dietary restriction
(C) Methyldopa
(D) Thiazide diuretic
(E) Diltiazem

9. Two months later, the patient's blood pressure is 156/98. The physician discontinues previous therapy and initiates therapy with a selective β blocker, such as

(A) atenolol
(B) propranolol
(C) nadolol
(D) timolol
(E) labetalol

10. One month later, the patient's blood pressure is 140/86. However, the patient reports persistent dizziness. The physician stops the current therapy and initiates therapy that was initially well tolerated but ultimately caused bronchospasm and cough. An agent capable of producing these effects is

(A) methyldopa
(B) captopril
(C) diltiazem
(D) reserpine
(E) propranolol

11. Assuming support of breathing and blood pressure, if required by the site of the lesion, which surgical lesion would abolish consciousness?

(A) Transection of the rostral part of the cervical cord
(B) Transection of the pontine basis
(C) Hemispherectomy
(D) Transection of the midbrain tegmentum
(E) Removal of the cerebellum

12. A biopsy should be sent to the pathology laboratory in which of the following modes?

(A) Fixed in formalin
(B) Fixed in alcohol
(C) Fresh in saline
(D) Frozen
(E) Fixed in a generic fixative

13. The following graph shows the tubular loss of glucose (excretion rate) plotted against the rate at which glucose is filtered at the glomerulus (filtered load). Which lettered point on the curve corresponds to the Tm for glucose?

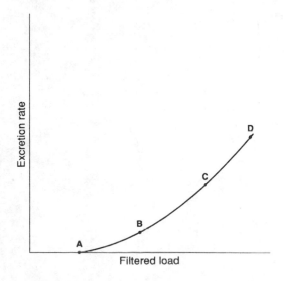

14. Reciprocal innervation is most accurately described as

(A) inhibition of flexor muscles during an extension
(B) activation of contralateral extensors during a flexion
(C) reduction of Ia fiber activity during a contraction
(D) simultaneous stimulation of alpha and gamma motoneurons
(E) inhibition of alpha motoneurons during a contraction

15. The region of the brain that is most involved in problem solving is the

(A) parietal lobe
(B) frontal lobe
(C) temporal lobe
(D) cerebellum
(E) occipital lobe

Questions 16–21

A hyperventilating patient is suffering from untreated diabetes. Over the past several days, he has experienced thirst, frequent urination, weight loss, and fatigue. Analysis of his blood reveals below normal pH, bicarbonate level, and partial pressure of carbon dioxide (P_{CO_2}) and above normal glucose level.

16. The acid–base abnormalities of this patient can best be described as

(A) respiratory acidosis with metabolic alkalosis
(B) respiratory alkalosis with metabolic acidosis
(C) metabolic acidosis with respiratory alkalosis
(D) metabolic alkalosis with respiratory acidosis
(E) metabolic acidosis with respiratory acidosis

17. What is the primary cause of the below normal pH in this patient?

(A) Hyperventilation
(B) Water loss because of frequent urination
(C) Lactic acidosis
(D) Renal failure
(E) Ketoacidosis

18. Which of the following metabolic pathways is most active in the liver of this patient?

(A) Gluconeogenesis
(B) Glycolysis
(C) Glycogenesis
(D) Fatty acid synthesis
(E) Lipolysis

19. Which of the following processes is most likely occurring in the skeletal muscle of this patient?

(A) Glycolysis
(B) Proteolysis
(C) Gluconeogenesis
(D) Urea cycle
(E) Ketone body synthesis

20. Most of the glucose 6-phosphate (G6P) formed in the liver of this patient will be converted to

(A) ribose 5-phosphate
(B) glucose 1-phosphate
(C) glucose
(D) pyruvate
(E) fructose 6-phosphate

21. This patient is initially treated with insulin and hydration therapy, but no decrease in blood glucose levels occurs. How can this be explained?

(A) The β-cells of the pancreatic islets have been totally destroyed
(B) The diabetes is type I
(C) The diabetes is type II
(D) The low blood pH is interfering with the insulin treatment and must be returned to normal before treatment is effective

22. A renal allograft recipient presents with fever and adenopathy 3 months after engraftment. Serum studies show markedly elevated anti–Epstein-Barr virus (EBV) titers. A biopsy of the allograft is most likely to show

(A) fibrinoid necrosis of the small vessels
(B) vascular sclerosis
(C) interstitial fibrosis
(D) a dense lymphoplasmacytic interstitial infiltrate with cytologic atypia
(E) isometric vacuolar change in the tubular epithelial cells

Questions 23–24

The left ventricular and aortic pressure tracings below were recorded during cardiac catheterization of a 62-year-old patient who complains of chest pain and dizziness on exertion.

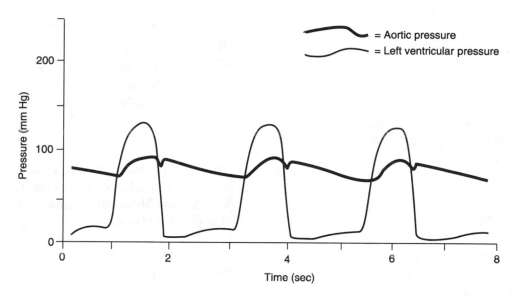

23. The left ventricular and aortic pressure tracings indicate that this patient has

(A) pulmonary stenosis
(B) aortic stenosis
(C) mitral stenosis
(D) aortic insufficiency
(E) mitral insufficiency

24. The most likely physical sign of this patient's condition is

(A) a systolic murmur
(B) a diastolic murmur
(C) a presystolic murmur
(D) a mid-diastolic murmur

25. A renal allograft recipient develops bloody diarrhea. A colonic biopsy shows focal necrosis and hemorrhage. Individual endothelial cells are large with prominent nuclear inclusions. The expected copathogen is

(A) Epstein-Barr virus (EBV)
(B) *Candida*
(C) *Pneumocystis*
(D) toxoplasmosis
(E) *Giardia*

26. The primary screening method in the detection of AIDS carriers is

(A) virus isolation
(B) Western blot followed by immunoassay
(C) immunoassay followed by Western blot
(D) immunoassay for viral antigen
(E) DNA hybridization for viral RNA

27. The coronary arteries in a failed heart allograft are likely to show

(A) fibrinoid necrosis indicating vascular rejection

(B) granulomatous arteritis indicating vascular rejection

(C) no change, because the coronary arteries are not a target for rejection

(D) transmural hemorrhage indicating vascular rejection

(E) a subintimal and focally transmural infiltrate of macrophages and lymphocytes indicating vascular rejection

Questions 28–30

A physician who has recommended urography for her competent, 68-year-old male patient is trying to decide whether or not to disclose the remote risk (1 in 10,000) of a fatal reaction.

28. If the physician favors nondisclosure, reasoning that it would not be in the patient's best interests to worry him with such remote risks, the physician is guided by the principle(s) of

(A) beneficence but not nonmaleficence

(B) nonmaleficence but not beneficence

(C) both beneficence and nonmaleficence

(D) justice

(E) gratitude

29. If the physician believes that her decision should be determined by what other physicians would do in similar circumstances, she is guided by

(A) both beneficence and nonmaleficence

(B) strong paternalism

(C) weak paternalism

(D) respect for autonomy

(E) the professional practice standard

30. If the physician bases her decision on her assessment of whether or not the patient would want to learn about such remote risks, the physician is guided by

(A) respect for autonomy

(B) beneficence

(C) nonmaleficence

(D) both beneficence and nonmaleficence

(E) the professional practice standard

31. A renal allograft recipient fails to produce urine in the first 48 hours after engraftment. Imaging studies reveal that the allograft is normal size. The graft is well matched. A biopsy is performed and shows needle-shaped crystals within vascular lumens. What is the most likely diagnosis?

(A) Hyperacute rejection

(B) "Harvest injury"

(C) Preexisting atheroembolic disease

(D) Acute cellular rejection

(E) Acute vascular rejection

Questions 32–33

A 52-year-old man presents with the complaint of blood in his stools. He reports that he has experienced some changes in his bowel habits over the last 18 months and recently has become aware of the sensation that his evacuations are not complete. Proctoscopic examination reveals a large ulcerating mass in the descending colon. Biopsy results confirm the diagnosis of carcinoma of the colon, and the malignant mass is surgically removed. The patient is placed on appropriate chemotherapy and discharged 2 weeks later to be followed up in the oncology clinic. Monthly blood specimens taken during the next year reveal the following carcinoembryonic antigen (CEA) levels:

	CEA (ng/ml)
Preoperative sample	50
Postoperative sample (day 1)	65
Month 1	15
Month 2	5
Months 3–9	<2.5
Month 10	10
Month 11	25
Month 12	40

32. The patient's serum CEA levels were assayed periodically because of the usefulness of CEA in

(A) localization of certain tumors in vivo
(B) diagnosing carcinoma of the colon
(C) diagnosing carcinoma of the pancreas
(D) diagnosing carcinoma of the prostate
(E) follow-up for the recurrence of certain malignancies

33. The CEA levels obtained during months 10 to 12 for this patient indicate that

(A) metastases have developed
(B) the initial diagnosis of colon cancer was incorrect
(C) surgical removal of the tumor was complete
(D) a revised diagnosis of carcinoma of the pancreas is warranted
(E) the patient is having an anamnestic response to the tumor

Questions 34–38

In a study designed to test the effect of a new knee brace on running speed, eight college athletes who wore the brace turned in the following times (in minutes) in a 1000-meter speed trial: 4, 2, 5, 2, 4, 5, 5, and 9.

34. The mean finishing time for this group of subjects is

(A) 8.0 minutes
(B) 5.0 minutes
(C) 4.0 minutes
(D) 4.5 minutes
(E) none of the above

35. The median finishing time is

(A) 3.0 minutes
(B) 4.0 minutes
(C) 4.5 minutes
(D) 5.0 minutes
(E) none of the above

36. The modal finishing time is

(A) 2.0 minutes
(B) 4.0 minutes
(C) 5.0 minutes
(D) 9.0 minutes
(E) none of the above

37. The range of times is

(A) 7.0 minutes
(B) 4.0 minutes
(C) 5.0 minutes
(D) 9.0 minutes
(E) none of the above

38. The standard deviation for these data is

(A) 34/7
(B) $\sqrt{34/8}$
(C) $\sqrt{191.5/7}$
(D) $\sqrt{34/7}$
(E) none of the above

39. Which condition is most likely to respond to corticosteroid therapy?

(A) Acute vascular rejection
(B) Cyclosporine nephrotoxicity
(C) Acute cellular rejection
(D) "Harvest injury"
(E) Recurrent glomerulosclerosis

Questions 40–42

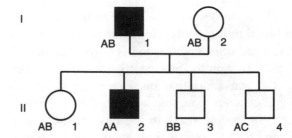

The figure above shows the DNA typing for a family that has Huntington's disease (HD). I-1 has HD, as does his son II-2. Family members II-1, II-3, and II-4 want to know what their risk is of having inherited the abnormal gene. The family members have had DNA analysis with a marker approximately 2 million base pairs from the mutation causing HD.

40. The risk for HD in II-1 is

(A) significantly increased
(B) significantly decreased
(C) mildly increased
(D) not changed because the markers are uninformative
(E) nonexistent

41. The risk for HD in II-3 is

(A) significantly increased
(B) significantly decreased
(C) mildly increased
(D) not changed
(E) nonexistent

42. The risk for HD in II-4 is

(A) significantly increased
(B) significantly decreased
(C) mildly increased
(D) not changed
(E) nonexistent

Questions 43–44

A hematologist is asked to see a 52-year-old man who has been hospitalized for 6 weeks because of various complications beginning with a bowel obstruction. The patient has had several operative procedures, one of which required transfusion of 3 units of packed red cells. He has been unable to eat and has been receiving broad-spectrum antibiotics almost continuously. Recently performed tests show a prolonged PT and PTT, which were corrected when the patient's plasma was mixed with an equal volume of normal plasma. Quantitative fibrinogen, thrombin time, and platelet count all are normal.

43. The most likely cause of the coagulation abnormality is

(A) an acquired inhibitor
(B) dilution of coagulation factors secondary to transfusions
(C) vitamin K deficiency
(D) folate deficiency
(E) von Willebrand's disease

44. If the patient is not actually bleeding, which of the following therapeutic measures would be best?

(A) Watch and wait
(B) Give fresh frozen plasma (FFP)
(C) Give parenteral vitamin K
(D) Give cryoprecipitate
(E) Discontinue the antibiotics

45. For immunohistochemical (IHC) analysis, employing either immunofluorescence or immunoperoxidase (IP) techniques, which characteristic is true?

(A) IHC can be used to define the origin of many tumor types
(B) Immunofluorescence methods provide a permanent slide
(C) The peroxidase method is less sensitive
(D) IP methods are preferred to identify immune complexes
(E) Polyclonal antibodies cannot be used

46. The anamnestic response is defined as

(A) a gradual rise in antibody titers
(B) true immunologic paralysis
(C) the prompt production of antibodies after a second exposure to antigen
(D) species-specific antibodies
(E) the lag in antibody production after initial antigen exposure

Questions 47–48

Lung compliance in a 32-year-old female patient is studied. Data collected under control and experimental conditions are listed in the following table.

	Respiratory Rate (breaths/min)	Tidal Volume (ml)	Change in Interpleural Pressure during Inspiration (cm H_2O)
Control	15	600	4
Experimental	25	600	10

47. This patient's lung compliance during control and experimental conditions was

(A) unchanged
(B) 40 ml/breath and 24 ml/breath, respectively
(C) 150 ml/cm H_2O and 60 ml/cm H_2O, respectively
(D) 150 cm H_2O/ml and 60 cm H_2O/ml, respectively

48. This patient can be characterized as having frequency-dependent compliance, which indicates

(A) abnormal surfactant function
(B) obstructive lung disease
(C) restrictive lung disease
(D) pulmonary vascular disease

Questions 49–51 refer to the following reaction.

$$R\text{-}CH_2OH + O_2 \rightarrow R\text{-}CHO + H_2O_2$$

49. This reaction exhibits a $\Delta G^{\circ\prime} = 2.8\,kcal/mol$. At equilibrium, what is the ratio of products to reactants?

(A) 100:1
(B) 10:1
(C) 1:1
(D) 0.1:1
(E) 0.01:1

50. Which one of the following types of enzymes catalyzes this type of reaction?

(A) Dehydrogenase
(B) Oxidase
(C) Oxygenase
(D) Peroxidase
(E) Aldolase

51. An enzyme that catalyzes this reaction requires a cofactor to participate in the electron transfer step of the overall reaction. Which of the following cofactors is most likely bound to the enzyme for this purpose?

(A) Pyridoxal phosphate
(B) Biotin
(C) Flavin adenine dinucleotide (FAD)
(D) Thiamine pyrophosphate
(E) Coenzyme A (CoA)

52. A patient presenting with sweating, narrow pupils, a slow heart rate, and low blood pressure is most likely to have been poisoned with

(A) *Amanita muscaria*
(B) methyl alcohol
(C) chloroform
(D) heroin
(E) cocaine

Questions 53–55

The county budget has $10 million remaining to be allocated. One council member urges that it be spent on handicapped children in a county center who have been living in wretched conditions with an overworked, marginally trained staff. She urges that these unfortunate citizens have been neglected in the past and deserve whatever help the state can give them. A second council member argues that $10 million is too much to invest in such a small number of citizens, and that it would be far more productively used to purchase a year's worth of school supplies for all of the county's children enrolled in public schools.

53. The question of how to use the county funds most fundamentally concerns the principle of

(A) autonomy
(B) paternalism
(C) justice
(D) beneficence
(E) none of the above

54. The ethical theory expressed in the viewpoint of the second council member is

(A) libertarianism
(B) a rights theory
(C) a virtue theory
(D) utilitarianism
(E) strict egalitarianism

55. The ethical theory assumed by the first council member could be considered to be any of the following EXCEPT

(A) libertarianism
(B) a rights theory
(C) a virtue theory
(D) socialism
(E) strict egalitarianism

Questions 56–63

A pediatrician wanted to determine the relationship between chronic otitis media in young children and parental history of such infections. From the records of a large pediatric practice, he identified 50 children between 1 and 3 years of age who had experienced at least three middle ear infections during the preceding year. Fifty children in the same age group, treated by the same practice for other illnesses, were also identified. The pediatrician interviewed the parents of subjects in both groups to determine their history of chronic otitis media as young children. Of the children with recurrent ear infections, 30 had a family history of chronic otitis media, compared with 20 of the children treated for other illnesses.

56. This study is an example of a

(A) cross-sectional study
(B) prospective cohort study
(C) case–control study
(D) experimental study
(E) randomized controlled clinical trial

57. Which of the following would be *least* likely to threaten the internal validity of this study?

(A) Selection bias
(B) Confounding variables that compete with family history as explanations for chronic otitis media
(C) Improper control for possible age differences
(D) Recall bias

58. The odds ratio (OR) of chronic otitis media in children between the ages of 1 and 3, given a parental history of such infections, is

(A) 2.25
(B) 1.20
(C) 1.50
(D) 0.60
(E) not able to be directly calculated from the data

59. The relative risk (RR) of chronic otitis media in children between the ages of 1 and 3 with a parental history of such infections is

(A) 2.25
(B) 1.20
(C) 1.50
(D) 0.60
(E) not able to be directly calculated from the data

60. The absolute risk of chronic otitis media in children between 1 and 3 years of age who have a parental history of this disorder is

(A) 2.25
(B) 1.20
(C) 1.50
(D) 0.60
(E) not able to be directly calculated from the data

61. What is the most appropriate statistical test for determining whether a significant association exists between chronic otitis media in children between the ages of one and three and a parental history of otitis media?

(A) Paired *t* test
(B) Chi-square test
(C) Correlation analysis
(D) Analysis of variance
(E) Independent sample (pooled) *t* test

62. The pediatrician conducting this study reports the existence of a statistically significant association between chronic otitis media in children between the ages of one and three and a parental history of such infections ($P < .05$). Which of the following represents the most appropriate interpretation of this finding?

(A) A strong and clinically important association exists between the study variables in the populations from which the samples were drawn
(B) An unbiased comparison was made between the study groups
(C) There is a causal link between chronic otitis media in young children and a family history of this disorder
(D) There is a less than 5% chance that the observed association occurred by random chance

63. All of the following statements about the p value reported by this investigator in question 62 are true EXCEPT

(A) the p value represents the probability that the statistical test will detect a significant association between the study variables when, in fact, such an association does not exist in the populations from which the study samples were drawn
(B) The p value is the probability that samples showing the observed degree of association were drawn by random chance from populations in which the study variables were not associated
(C) the p value defines the probability of rejecting a true null hypothesis (type I error)
(D) the p value measures the strength of the association between the two study variables; the smaller the p value, the stronger the association

DIRECTIONS: Each of the numbered items or incomplete statements in this section is negatively phrased, as indicated by a capitalized word such as NOT, LEAST, or EXCEPT. Select the ONE lettered answer or completion that is BEST in each case.

64. Chronic renal allograft rejection involves all of the following EXCEPT

(A) vascular sclerosis
(B) interstitial fibrosis
(C) tubular atrophy
(D) glomerulosclerosis
(E) tubulitis

65. The development of normal male external genitalia requires all of the following EXCEPT

(A) at least an X and a Y chromosome
(B) testosterone
(C) testes
(D) labioscrotal swellings
(E) paramesonephric duct derivatives

66. All of the following are characteristic of disease EXCEPT

(A) a pathophysiologic alteration in functioning
(B) mood swings
(C) objective biologic changes
(D) changes in the quality of life
(E) signs upon physical examination

67. Ultrasound can be used for all of the following purposes EXCEPT

(A) to detect Down syndrome
(B) to detect neural tube defects
(C) to measure skull size
(D) to guide amniocentesis by visualizing the fetus and placenta
(E) to locate the placenta

68. Acute rejection in lung allografts includes all of the following pathologic features EXCEPT

(A) fibrosing obliteration of respiratory bronchioles
(B) perivascular lymphocytic infiltrate
(C) interstitial and alveolar lymphocytic and neutrophilic inflammation
(D) lymphocytic bronchitis
(E) hemorrhagic necrosis and hyaline membrane formation

69. Drugs known to be teratogenic to the fetus include all of the following EXCEPT

(A) aminopterin
(B) alcohol
(C) birth control pills
(D) phenytoin
(E) heroin

70. All of the following landmarks form an extensive part of the boundary of the parietal lobe EXCEPT

(A) the sylvian fissure
(B) the central sulcus
(C) a line from the superior preoccipital notch to the inferior preoccipital notch
(D) the calcarine sulcus
(E) the limbic lobe

71. Morphologic examination of a heart diseased by pericarditis may reveal all of the following EXCEPT

(A) fibrinous exudate
(B) calcification
(C) fibrosis
(D) malignant cells
(E) hemochromatosis

72. All of the following statements concerning the role of prostaglandin in labor are true EXCEPT

(A) prostaglandin induces uterine smooth muscle contraction
(B) prostaglandin synthetase increases maternal blood prostaglandin levels
(C) a decrease in arachidonic acid causes prostaglandin to increase in maternal blood
(D) lysosomal enzymes cleave arachidonic acid from phospholipids
(E) phosphatidyl ethanolamine cleavage produces a prostaglandin precursor

73. Malnutrition can result in all of the following conditions EXCEPT

(A) numerous infections
(B) emaciation
(C) fatty liver
(D) gastric carcinoma
(E) anorexia

74. Electron microscopy (EM) is useful for all of the following diagnostic purposes EXCEPT

(A) identifying viruses in tissues
(B) classifying a lymphoma as a B-cell or T-cell type
(C) making a diagnosis of Whipple's disease
(D) classifying a bullous skin disease as pemphigus
(E) identifying immune complexes in renal glomerulonephritis

75. Turner syndrome shows all of the following characteristics EXCEPT

(A) absence of menses
(B) numerous ovarian follicles
(C) webbed neck
(D) sterility
(E) 45, X karyotype

76. Black carbon particles, cleared from the blood by the reticuloendothelial system of a laboratory animal, can be seen in cells in all of the following organ components EXCEPT

(A) lymph node sinuses
(B) glomeruli
(C) intestinal epithelium
(D) liver sinuses
(E) splenic cords

77. Renal agenesis can be associated with all of the following causes or clinical features EXCEPT

(A) abnormal allantoic regression
(B) failure of inductive interaction between the ureteric bud and the metanephric blastema
(C) an absence of symptoms
(D) oligohydramnios
(E) death soon after birth

DIRECTIONS: Each set of matching questions in this section consists of a list of four to twenty-six lettered options (some of which may be in figures) followed by several numbered items. For each numbered item, select the ONE lettered option that is most closely associated with it. To avoid spending too much time on matching sets with large numbers of options, it is generally advisable to begin each set by reading the list of options. Then, for each item in the set, try to generate the correct answer and locate it in the option list, rather than evaluating each option individually. Each lettered option may be selected once, more than once, or not at all.

Questions 78–82

Match each of the following descriptions with the most appropriate lettered region of the nephron pictured below.

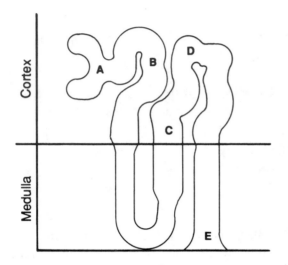

78. Tubular fluid always is hyposmotic at this site

79. The TF/P ratio for glucose is 1.0 at this site

80. The urea concentration is highest at this site

81. The U_{osm} can reach 1200–1400 mOsm/L at this site

82. The macula densa is closest to this site

Questions 83–87

Match the characteristic with the appropriate protozoan.

(A) *Pneumocystis carinii*
(B) *Entamoeba histolytica*
(C) *Naegleria fowleri*
(D) *Toxoplasma gondii*
(E) *Trichomonas vaginalis*

83. Oocysts in cat feces are transmitted to humans by the fecal–oral route

84. Etiologic agent of fulminant meningoencephalitis causing death in 3–5 days

85. Etiologic agent of a sexually transmitted disease

86. Etiologic agent of dysentery and hepatic abscess

87. Etiologic agent of pneumonia in immunocompromised people

Questions 88–92

For each characteristic of a complement component listed below, select the component that is most closely associated with it.

(A) C2
(B) C4
(C) C3bBb
(D) C3e
(E) C3b
(F) C5a
(G) C9
(H) C5b6789

88. Neutralizes virus activities

89. Stabilized by properdin

90. Associated with symptoms seen in hereditary angioedema

91. Provokes release of neutrophils from bone marrow

92. Promotes opsonization

Questions 93–97

Match each description following with the most appropriate organelle.

(A) Primary lysosome
(B) Phagolysosome
(C) Heterolysosome
(D) Autolysosome
(E) Residual body

93. A secondary lysosome containing effete components of the cell that produced it

94. A telolysosome that remains in a cell

95. GERL product before it engages in any other metabolic event

96. The product of a primary lysosome fusing with ingested bacteria

97. The product of a primary lysosome fusing with a substance from the extracellular environment

Questions 98–101

For each of the hematologic disorders presented below, select the diagnostic test by which it can be identified.

(A) Coombs' test
(B) Ham test
(C) Osmotic fragility test
(D) Heinz bodies test
(E) Donath-Landsteiner antibody test

98. Paroxysmal nocturnal hemoglobinuria (PNH)

99. Autoimmune hemolytic anemia with warm-type antibody

100. Glucose-6-phosphate dehydrogenase (G6PD) deficiency, Mediterranean type

101. Hereditary spherocytosis (HS)

Questions 102–106

Match each condition described below with the term of inheritance that best defines it.

(A) Allelic heterogeneity
(B) Variable expressivity
(C) Nonpenetrance
(D) Consanguinity
(E) Locus heterogeneity

102. A man shows no detectable signs of Marfan syndrome (an autosomal dominant disorder of connective tissue), although his father and two daughters are affected

103. Retinitis pigmentosa (a type of retinal degeneration) occurs in an autosomal dominant, an autosomal recessive, and an X-linked form

104. Tay-Sachs disease is seen in high frequency in the Chicoutimi area of Quebec, where most individuals are descended from a few early French settlers

105. Duchenne muscular dystrophy (DMD) is the consequence of either a deletion involving the dystrophin gene or a point mutation of the same gene

106. In a family with myotonic dystrophy, the father has frontal balding, severe weakness, and cardiac arrhythmia; his sister has early-onset cataracts; and his child has electromyographic abnormalities

Questions 107–111

Match the source of the afferent fibers listed below with the part of the cerebellar cortex to which each fiber most strongly projects.

(A) Cerebellar hemisphere
(B) Anterior lobe of the vermis
(C) Tonsil
(D) Flocculonodular lobe
(E) All parts of the cerebellum equally

107. Spinocerebellar tracts

108. Trigeminocerebellar tract

109. Principal inferior olivary nuclei, lateral part

110. Vestibular nerve and nuclei

111. Nucleus locus ceruleus

Questions 112–115

In the diagram below, each letter represents a different metabolite that is derived from glucose 6-phosphate (G6P). Match each compound listed with the correct letter.

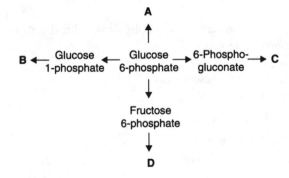

112. Glycogen

113. Pyruvate

114. Ribose 5-phosphate

115. Glucose

Questions 116–119

Match each of the descriptions below with the embryonic structure that it best describes.

(A) Liver diverticulum
(B) Midgut
(C) Dorsal pancreatic rudiment
(D) Cloaca
(E) Vitelline duct

116. This hindgut derivative receives the excurrent ducts of the reproductive and urinary systems

117. This structure forms at the junction between the foregut and the hindgut and differentiates into glucagon-secreting islet tissue

118. This structure forms the ileum and ascending colon

119. This structure forms endocrine and exocrine tissue as it grows into the septum transversum

Questions 120–125

Match the stages of neutrophil maturation with the appropriately lettered cell in the figure below.

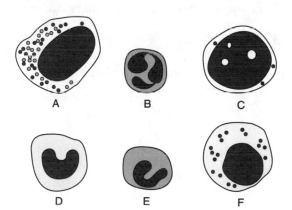

120. Myeloblast

121. Band neutrophil

122. Myelocyte

123. Mature neutrophil

124. Promyelocyte

125. Metamyelocyte

Questions 126–130

Match each lesion listed below with the resultant visual field defect.

(A) Contralateral superior homonymous quadrantanopia
(B) Inferior altitudinal hemianopia (blindness in the inferior half of the visual field of both eyes)
(C) Partial contralateral inferior homonymous quadrantanopia
(D) Complete contralateral homonymous hemianopia without macular sparing
(E) Complete blindness

126. Bilateral destruction of the occipital lobes

127. Unilateral destruction of the inferior part of one parietal lobe

128. Destruction of the anterior to the middle third of the temporal lobe

129. Complete destruction of the calcarine cortex of one occipital lobe

130. Bilateral destruction of the superior bank of the calcarine fissure

Questions 131–135

For each pathologic response, select the disease with which it is most likely to be associated.

(A) Silicosis
(B) Asbestosis
(C) Tuberculosis
(D) Chronic berylliosis
(E) Coal worker's pneumoconiosis (CWP)

131. Caseating granulomas

132. Centrilobular emphysema

133. Noncaseating granulomas

134. Pleural calcifications

135. Polarizable flecks in nodules

Questions 136–144

Match the pathophysiological mechanism of sickle cell disease (Hb SS) with the appropriate clinical manifestation.

(A) Vaso-occlusion in the microcirculation and tissue infarction
(B) Hemolysis and shortened red cell survival
(C) Suppression of bone marrow erythropoiesis due to parvovirus infection
(D) Unstable structure of hemoglobin causing precipitation
(E) Impairment of antibody response and complement activation

136. Sickle cell crisis (painful infarctive crisis)

137. Aplastic crisis

138. Acute chest syndrome

139. Gallstones

140. Growth and development retardation in affected children

141. Infections caused by encapsulated organisms

142. Painless hematuria and papillary necrosis

143. Aseptic necrosis of the hip

144. Retinal detachment and blindness

Questions 145–149

Match each distal lung component described below with the appropriate lettered structure in the micrograph below.

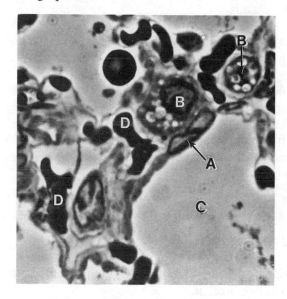

145. A cell that carries carbon dioxide and oxygen

146. A cell that secretes surfactant

147. A squamous type I cell

148. An area that frequently contains macrophages

149. A cell that contains phospholipid-rich multilamellar bodies

Questions 150–152

Match each cause of an acid–base disturbance with the characteristic set of body fluid changes.

	Plasma pH	Plasma [HCO$_3^-$] (mEq/L)	Urine pH
(A)	7.27	37	acid
(B)	7.31	16	acid
(C)	7.40	15	alkaline
(D)	7.40	24	acid
(E)	7.55	22	alkaline

150. Hyperventilation

151. Chronic respiratory tract obstruction

152. Diabetic ketoacidosis

Questions 153–156

The diagram below illustrates the anatomic arrangement for the presynaptic inhibition of an excitatory neuron. Match each of the following descriptions with the appropriate lettered area of the diagram.

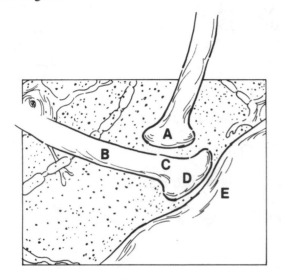

153. A decrease in the entry of Ca^{2+}

154. The release of GABA by exocytosis

155. A decrease in the size of the excitatory postsynaptic potential

156. An increase in the Cl^- conductance

Questions 157–161

Match each functional description with the kind of gametogenic cell it best describes.

(A) Primordial germ cell
(B) Primary oocyte
(C) Primary spermatocyte
(D) Secondary oocyte
(E) Secondary spermatocyte

157. A tetraploid cell produced by the millions after puberty

158. A cell that has a diploid amount of DNA and undergoes an equal cytoplasmic division to form spermatids

159. A cell that has a diploid amount of DNA and undergoes unequal cytoplasmic divisions

160. A cell that is derived from the yolk sac and forms spermatogonia

161. A cell that has a tetraploid amount of DNA and can be arrested in meiosis I for 40 years or more

Questions 162–166

Match the following functions with the associated factor or protein.

(A) Sigma (σ) factor
(B) dnaA protein
(C) Catabolite activator protein (CAP)
(D) Rho (ρ) factor
(E) Transcription factor IID (TFIID)

162. Prokaryotic positive transcription regulatory factor

163. Required for proper initiation of replication in *Escherichia coli*

164. Required for termination of transcription in prokaryotes at particular termination sequences

165. Required for initiation of transcription from TATA box–containing promoters

166. Required for proper initiation of transcription in prokaryotes

Questions 167–171

In this figure, the letters in each box correspond to organs or tissues in the postabsorptive state. Match the listed organs and tissues to the correct letter in each box in the figure.

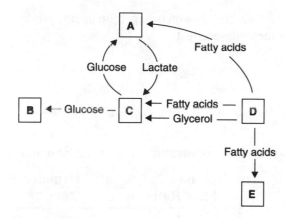

167. Liver

168. Brain

169. Skeletal muscle

170. Heart muscle

171. Adipose tissue

Questions 172–176

Match each phrase describing a feature of inflammatory heart disease with the disease it characterizes.

(A) Acute rheumatic fever
(B) Chronic rheumatic heart disease
(C) Acute endocarditis
(D) Subacute endocarditis
(E) Libman-Sacks endocarditis

172. Fusion of the commissures

173. Infection by group A β-hemolytic streptococci

174. Infection by α-hemolytic (viridans) streptococci

175. Infection by *Staphylococcus aureus*

176. Warty vegetations on the undersurface of the mitral valve

Questions 177–182

Match each description below with the most appropriate adenohypophysial cell type.

(A) Corticotrope
(B) Gonadotrope
(C) Somatotrope
(D) Thyrotrope
(E) Lactotrope

177. A basophil that secretes a hormone that regulates spermatogenesis and ovulation

178. The acidophil that secretes prolactin

179. A basophil that secretes a hormone that regulates basal metabolic rate

180. A basophil that secretes a hormone that regulates the ionic composition of blood and urine

181. An acidophil; the volume of its secretion product is altered in pituitary dwarfs

182. The basophil with the smallest granules

Questions 183–185

Match each statement about drug action with the drug that is most likely to be associated with it.

(A) Cyclophosphamide
(B) 5-Fluorouracil
(C) Cytarabine
(D) Vincristine
(E) Mitomycin

183. In addition to being a natural product, this drug is an alkylating agent because it is reduced intracellularly and alkylates DNA.

184. This drug inhibits DNA polymerase and can be incorporated into DNA and RNA.

185. This drug is a phase-specific agent, producing metaphase arrest.

Questions 186–190

The following information was obtained from a healthy 24-year-old man who was studied in a renal laboratory:

Inulin Concentration (mg/ml)	Glucose Concentration	Urine Flow Rate	Hematocrit Ratio
Urine = 150	Urine = 1 mg/ml	1.2 ml/min	0.40
Renal arterial plasma = 1.50	Plasma = 90 mg/dl		
Renal venous plasma = 1.20			

Using the above data, match each of the following measurements of renal function with the appropriate lettered value.

(A) 0.20
(B) 108 mg/min
(C) 120 ml/min
(D) 600 ml/min
(E) 1000 ml/min

186. Glomerular filtration rate

187. Renal blood flow

188. Filtration fraction

189. Renal plasma flow

190. Filtered load of glucose

Questions 191–193

Neuroleptic drugs have been shown to block postsynaptic dopamine 2 (D_2) receptors. For each effect of neuroleptic drugs, select the dopaminergic tract thought to underlie the action.

(A) Tuberoinfundibular tract
(B) Nigrostriatal tract
(C) Mesolimbic tract
(D) Medullary periventricular tract
(E) Incertohypothalamic tract

191. Lactation

192. Parkinsonism

193. Antipsychotic effects

Questions 194–198

For each description of a bone of the skull below, choose the appropriate labelled area in the accompanying diagram.

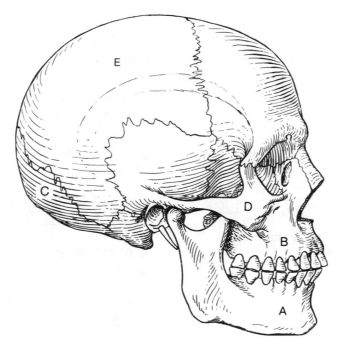

194. This bone is formed by intramembranous ossification and is part of the membranous viscerocranium; it contains no odontoblast derivatives

195. This bone is formed by endochondral ossification in its lower part and intramembranous ossification in its upper part

196. This bone is part of the membranous viscerocranium and is derived from the first maxillary component of the first pharyngeal arch; the lateral palatine processes form on its medial border

197. This bone is part of the membranous neurocranium, and the anterior fontanelle forms on its anterior border

198. This bone forms by intramembranous ossification around Meckel's cartilage

Questions 199–203

Match each description of muscles listed below with the appropriate rotator cuff component.

(A) Infraspinatus
(B) Subscapularis
(C) Supraspinatus
(D) Teres minor
(E) None of the above

199. A primary medial (internal) rotator of the arm

200. A muscle that forms the posterior wall of the axilla

201. A muscle that initiates humeral abduction (first 15°)

202. A muscle innervated by the axillary nerve

203. A muscle innervated by a branch of the musculocutaneous nerve

Questions 204–207

For each method of activating (fixing) complement listed, select the immunoglobulin most closely associated with that method.

(A) Immunoglobulin D (IgD)
(B) IgA
(C) IgE
(D) IgG
(E) IgM

204. Fixes complement efficiently via the C_H2 domain

205. Fixes complement via the C_H3 domain

206. Fixes complement via the alternative pathway only

207. Fixes complement most efficiently in lytic reactions

Questions 208–211

Match each description that follows with the anti-infective agent most likely to be associated with it.

(A) Clindamycin
(B) Gentamicin
(C) Nafcillin
(D) Tetracycline
(E) Rifampin

208. This agent is very effective in the treatment of *Chlamydia* infections

209. This agent is often administered along with isoniazid and ethambutol.

210. This agent is the drug of choice for *Bacteroides fragilis* infection.

211. This agent is poorly absorbed orally because it is polycationic.

ANSWER KEY

1-D	31-C	61-B	91-D	121-E
2-A	32-E	62-D	92-E	122-F
3-E	33-A	63-D	93-D	123-B
4-E	34-D	64-E	94-E	124-A
5-E	35-C	65-E	95-A	125-D
6-B	36-C	66-B	96-B	126-E
7-D	37-A	67-A	97-C	127-C
8-D	38-D	68-A	98-B	128-A
9-A	39-C	69-E	99-A	129-D
10-B	40-D	70-D	100-D	130-B
11-D	41-B	71-E	101-C	131-C
12-C	42-E	72-C	102-C	132-E
13-B	43-C	73-D	103-E	133-D
14-A	44-C	74-B	104-D	134-B
15-B	45-A	75-B	105-A	135-A
16-C	46-C	76-C	106-B	136-A
17-E	47-C	77-A	107-B	137-C
18-A	48-B	78-C	108-B	138-A
19-B	49-E	79-A	109-A	139-B
20-C	50-B	80-E	110-D	140-B
21-C	51-C	81-E	111-E	141-E
22-D	52-A	82-C	112-B	142-A
23-B	53-C	83-D	113-D	143-A
24-A	54-D	84-C	114-C	144-A
25-B	55-A	85-E	115-A	145-D
26-C	56-C	86-B	116-D	146-B
27-E	57-C	87-A	117-C	147-A
28-C	58-A	88-B	118-B	148-C
29-E	59-E	89-C	119-A	149-B
30-A	60-E	90-A	120-C	150-C

151-A	164-D	176-E	188-A	200-B
152-B	165-E	177-B	189-D	201-C
153-D	166-A	178-E	190-B	202-D
154-A	167-C	179-D	191-A	203-E
155-E	168-B	180-A	192-B	204-D
156-C	169-A	181-C	193-C	205-E
157-C	170-E	182-D	194-D	206-B
158-E	171-D	183-E	195-C	207-E
159-D	172-B	184-C	196-B	208-D
160-A	173-A	185-D	197-E	209-E
161-B	174-D	186-C	198-A	210-A
162-C	175-C	187-E	199-B	211-B
163-B				

ANSWERS AND EXPLANATIONS

1. The answer is D. *(Fetal hemoglobin)*
Fetal hemoglobin (Hb F) needs an increased affinity for oxygen because the Po_2 of the placenta is, like that of most other tissues, low. Decreased levels of 2,3-bisphosphoglycerate (2,3-BPG) cause the oxygen binding affinity of hemoglobin A_1 (Hb A_1) to increase. This does not happen in fetal red blood cells because, in the absence of 2,3-BPG, Hb F has a lower affinity for oxygen than Hb A_1. The 2,3-BPG levels of fetal red blood cells are similar to those of adult red blood cells. Hb F differs from Hb A_1 by having two γ subunits instead of two β subunits. The γ subunits do not bind 2,3-BPG well, and this gives Hb F a higher oxygen binding affinity than Hb A_1.

2. The answer is A. *(Relationship of nerve roots to somites)*
One of the most important principles of the development of the peripheral nervous system (PNS) is that somites retain axons from their original spinal cord levels when they migrate to different locations. The axons, which in the primitive state would run directly laterally from the spinal cord to the somite, rearrange their course as they go through the cervical, brachial, and lumbosacral plexuses to reach those somites that change their position as a result of migration.

3. The answer is E. *(lac operon)*
A gene that is expressed at a constant, unregulated, and often low rate is said to be constitutively expressed. A mutation in either the operator sequence or the *lac* I gene, so that it produces an inactive repressor, results in an operon that cannot be regulated by the presence or absence of lactose and is therefore inactive. With an inactive repressor, the *lac* operon can still be regulated by catabolite repression. With a mutated repressor and no glucose, the expression of the *lac* operon would be high because there would be no catabolite repression by glucose. In the presence of glucose, it would be expressed, but at a low level. A mutated promoter that prevents RNA polymerase from binding leads to a complete inhibition of expression under all growth conditions. A missense mutation in the β-galactosidase gene is likely to reduce the activity of the enzyme but is not likely to affect its cellular levels. A mutated β-galactosidase has no effect on either of the other two enzyme products of the operon. A mutation in the catabolite activator protein (CAP) affects the *lac* operon's ability to be regulated by catabolite repression. The *lac* operon is not regulated by attenuation.

4. The answer is E. *(Spinal tap)*
The physician can insert a needle into the subarachnoid space to withdraw cerebrospinal fluid (CSF) for diagnostic analysis. The needle tip passes successively through the epidural space, the dura mater, the subdural space, and the arachnoid membrane. The CSF is between the arachnoid membrane and the pia mater, the innermost of the three meningeal sheaths.

5. The answer is E. *(Exudate)*
An exudate is the fluid and cells that collect during acute inflammation; the fluid contains protein in excess of 3 g/dl and has a specific gravity exceeding 1.015. Exudates often have abundant neutrophils as their cellular element. In contrast, a transudate is a noninflammatory fluid that is characterized by few cellular elements, a protein content less than 3 g/dl, and a specific gravity less than 1.015. Edema is fluid collected in tissue as a result of various processes [e.g., congestive heart failure (CHF), liver failure, hypoalbuminemia, a blocked lymphatic vessel]; the fluid accumulates because of osmotic pressure, not as a result of acute inflammation, and it does not have a high protein content. An effusion is the accumulation of any type of fluid (exudate or transudate) into a body space, such as the pleural cavity. Serum is the cell-free portion of the blood that remains after the blood has clotted—and has nothing to do with inflammation.

6. The answer is B. *(Hair follicles)*
The epidermal appendages of the skin all form as epidermal invaginations under the inductive influence of the underlying mesenchyme. Only the papilla of a hair follicle forms from mesenchymal cells. Hair follicles are invariably associated with sebaceous glands. Lanugo hairs form before birth. Hair follicles per se do not contribute to the vernix caseosa, which is a mixture of sloughed dead cells and sebaceous gland secretions.

7–10. The answers are: 7-D, 8-D, 9-A, 10-B. *(Therapy for mild hypertension)*
Because this patient did not have severe hypertension and the physical examination was unremarkable, dietary restriction was indicated. However, the patient was told to return for a checkup in 1 month.

After 1 month, no perceptible difference was seen in the blood pressure reading. First-line therapy for black hypertensive men should include thiazide diuretics. In general, black individuals respond better to volume loss than to β blockers.

After 2 months of thiazide diuretics, the patient was switched to atenolol, which in low doses is the only cardioselective β blocker listed. All of the other agents are nonselective.

One month later, the blood pressure is 140/86; however, the patient reports feeling dizzy. The physician stops the atenolol and initiates captopril, which was initially well tolerated but ultimately caused cough and bronchospasm. Captopril is a competitive inhibitor of peptidyl dipeptidase, an angiotensin-converting enzyme, and is increasingly used for the treatment of mild to moderate hypertension.

11. The answer is D. *(Surgical lesions)*
Large parts of the nervous system can be removed or transected without abolishing consciousness. A cerebral hemisphere or the entire cerebellum can be removed. The spinal cord or the brain stem, from the caudal pontine levels downward, can be transected without abolishing consciousness if blood pressure and breathing are supported. Midbrain transection permanently abolishes consciousness.

12. The answer is C. *(Biopsy specimens)*
When in doubt, a clinician should send a fresh specimen to the pathology laboratory. This practice allows the pathologist to best deal with the tissue and aliquot portions, and use them in various ways for diagnostic tests.

13. The answer is B. *(Tubular loss of glucose)*
When the filtered load of a substance exceeds the Tm for that substance, the excess is not reabsorbed, and, thus, proportionately more of the substance is excreted. In this example, the Tm for glucose (*B* on the curve) is determined by extrapolation of the linear portion of the curve (from *C* to *D*) to the abscissa (filtered load). The splay of the curve (from *A* to *C*) indicates that all of the tubules are not uniform in length, number of glucose transporters, or renal threshold.

14. The answer is A. *(Reciprocal innervation)*
Reciprocal innervation is most accurately described as inhibition of the antagonist muscle when the agonist muscle is activated. For example, flexor muscles are inhibited during an extension. Reciprocal innervation allows extensor contraction to occur without interference from the flexor muscles that are being stretched during the movement. Under normal circumstances, stretching the flexors will elicit a stretch reflex leading to contraction of the flexor muscles. Inhibiting the alpha motoneurons that innervate the flexor muscles prevents the stretch reflex from interfering with the extension. Reciprocal innervation characterizes all movements, not just extension.

15. The answer is B. *(Areas of the brain)*
Although the pathology in many parts of the central nervous system (CNS) can impair problem solving, damage to the frontal lobes is the major cause of dysfunctional intellectual processes. The frontal lobe is the area of the brain that is most involved with the ability to solve problems.

16–21. The answers are: 16-C, 17-E, 18-A, 19-B, 20-C, 21-C. *(Diabetes)*
Metabolic acidosis is defined as a below normal level of serum bicarbonate. Respiratory alkalosis is defined as a below normal partial pressure of carbon dioxide (Pco_2). The respiratory alkalosis represents an attempt by the lungs to compensate for the metabolic acidosis. If the lungs do not compensate, the blood pH is even lower.

The primary cause of low blood pH in a patient with untreated diabetes is ketoacidosis caused by high levels of ketone bodies in the blood. The ketone bodies acetoacetate and β-hydroxybutyrate are acids that cannot be excreted by the lungs. Hyperventilation is a response by the lungs to compensate for the metabolic acidosis. Lactate is a product of glycolysis in the muscle and would not be expected to be present in a diabetic state, during which glucose is not taken up by tissues. Although the patient is experiencing loss of water and may eventually experience renal failure if the condition is not treated, these symptoms do not relate to the primary cause of acidosis in this patient.

The metabolic profile of the liver in people with untreated diabetes is very similar to what would be observed during starvation. Glucose-utilizing pathways such as glycolysis and glycogenesis are depressed. Biosynthetic pathways such as fatty acid synthesis are also inhibited. Gluconeogenesis, however, is stimulated in the liver so that it may continue to provide glucose for tissues, such as the brain, which have a strong preference for that fuel. In the diabetic state, the liver has not received a signal that adequate glucose is already present in the blood. Lipolysis also occurs until triacylglycerol stores are depleted, but this process occurs in the adipose tissue rather than in the liver.

The metabolic profile of skeletal muscle in a patient with untreated diabetes is very similar to what would be observed during starvation. Glucose is not taken from the blood, and the glycogen stores are quickly depleted so that no glucose is available for gluconeogenesis. As in starvation, proteolysis occurs to provide amino acids as a source of energy for the body. Gluconeogenesis, ketone body synthesis, and the urea cycle are active, but these pathways are located in the liver and not in the muscle.

In the diabetic state, as in postabsorptive and starved states, the liver exports whatever glucose it can generate from glycogenolysis and gluconeogenesis. The final step in the formation of glucose from these pathways is the dephosphorylation of glucose 6-phosphate (G6P). G6P is also an intermediate in glycolysis, the pentose phosphate pathway, and glycogenesis. These pathways are not active under these conditions. Fructose 6-phosphate is an intermediate in glycolysis, and pyruvate is the end product of glycolysis. Ribose 5-phosphate is a product of the pentose phosphate pathway. Glucose 1-phosphate is formed from G6P in glycogenesis.

Proper administration of insulin and correction of fluid and electrolyte imbalances should correct this patient's condition if he has insulin-dependent (type I) diabetes, which is caused by a destruction of the insulin-producing β-cells of the pancreatic islets. Diabetes that does not respond to insulin treatment is probably non–insulin-dependent (type II) diabetes, which is caused by a defect or deficiency of insulin receptors. The blood pH has no effect on the insulin therapy, and, if the patient were suffering from type I diabetes, the acid–base imbalance would return to normal once the metabolism returned to normal.

22. The answer is D. *(Renal allograft)*
Transplant recipients are at risk for a variety of opportunistic infections. Epstein-Barr virus (EBV) infection with posttransplant lymphoproliferative disorder (PTLD) is one such complication. In PTLD, the immunosuppressed host suffers from primary or reactivated infection. EBV exerts a proliferative pressure on the B cells. In the absence of regulatory T-cell control, B cells may expand and develop clonal populations (i.e., lymphoma).

23–24. The answers are: 23-B, 24-A. *(Ventricular and aortic pressure tracings)*
The gradient that occurs between the ventricular and aortic systolic pressures is diagnostic of aortic stenosis. The normal aortic valve provides a negligible resistance, and the aortic pressure is nearly identical to the

ventricular pressure during the phase of rapid ventricular ejection. A similar picture is seen if right ventricular and pulmonary pressures are measured in the presence of pulmonary valve stenosis, but the pressures are proportionately reduced because of the low resistance of the pulmonary circulation.

Semilunar valve stenosis represents an impediment to the ejection of blood from the ventricle and results in an ejection-type murmur during systole. An ejection murmur is diamond-shaped (i.e., it is a crescendo–decrescendo sound that has maximal intensity in midsystole, when the pressure gradient is largest).

25. The answer is B. *(Infection in immunocompromised patients)*
The pathologic description of the colonic biopsy is that of cytomegalovirus (CMV) colitis. Hemorrhagic necrosis related to cytomegalic change, with nuclear and cytoplasmic inclusions, is characteristic of CMV colitis. Superinfection with fungus, in particular, *Candida,* is common in CMV infection in immunocompromised patients.

26. The answer is C. *(AIDS screening)*
The current method of screening patients for evidence of infection by human immune deficiency virus (HIV) is to perform an immunoassay on their serum to detect the presence of antibodies to HIV. Immunoassay-positive sera are retested using a Western blot to confirm that the reactive antibodies are HIV specific. Currently, the direct detection of the HIV virus itself either by cultivation or by immunoassay is not reliable. The detection of viral RNA in blood looks promising in some cases but is still not enough to be anything more than a research tool.

27. The answer is E. *(Coronary arteries)*
The coronary arteries in cardiac allografts can show subintimal or mural accumulation of foam cells and lymphocytes. This inflammation combined with the accompanying fibrosis has been termed "accelerated atherosclerosis" because of its morphologic similarity to primary coronary atherosclerosis. Because this process may occur within months to years of engraftment, it is thought to be a manifestation of vascular rejection in the coronary arteries. Necrotizing, hemorrhagic, or granulomatous coronary artery disease in allografts is extremely uncommon.

28–30. The answers are: 28-C, 29-E, 30-A. *(Medical ethics)*
If the physician's sole concern is not to harm the patient with unnecessary worry, the guiding principle is nonmaleficence. If her sole concern is to be able to benefit the patient with urography (which is impossible if the patient refuses because of concerns about the risks), the guiding principle is beneficence. Both are possible. Justice is irrelevant, and gratitude (e.g., for the patient's patronage) is at most marginally relevant.

If the physician decides to do whatever others of her profession do in like circumstances, she is acting without appeal to the independent ethical principles of beneficence and nonmaleficence. Depending on what the professional practice standard dictates, the disclosure decision might prove to be respectful of autonomy or strongly paternalistic, but the decision would still be guided by professional practice. Weak paternalism is entirely irrelevant because the patient is competent.

If the physician is guided by respect for the patient's preferences, she is acting with respect for her patient's autonomy. If the patient would want disclosure, it is possible that such disclosure could fail to benefit him or could even harm him, so neither beneficence nor maleficence is guiding the physician's thinking. Clearly, the basis for her thinking is independent of the usual practice of her profession.

31. The answer is C. *(Renal allograft)*
Approximately 15% of donor kidneys show changes related to preexisting damage before harvest. Athero-emboli are pathologically recognized as needlelike spaces within the microvasculature. Atheroembolism is associated with severe atheromatous plaque in the donor vasculature and invasive procedures such as catheterization or vascular surgery. "Primary nonfunction" in a renal allograft may be secondary to a variety

of causes, however. Ischemic damage during harvest (i.e., "harvest injury") is most common. Preformed antibody directed against donor tissue can occasionally be missed during pretransplant cross-match testing and cause hyperacute rejection, but this situation is uncommon.

32–33. The answers are: 32-E, 33-A. *(Carcinoembryonic antigen)*
Carcinoembryonic antigen (CEA) is associated with carcinoma of the colon and pancreas; however, because CEA also occurs in nonmalignant conditions (e.g., as a result of cigarette smoking), it is not considered to be diagnostic of, but merely suggestive of, a cancerous condition. Assays for CEA show their greatest promise in monitoring for the recurrence of certain malignancies after surgery or chemotherapy.

The presence of CEA in the serum is correlated with the tumor burden of the host. The higher the level of CEA, the greater is the patient's tumor mass. Following surgical excision of the tumor, the CEA level should drop very low, perhaps even to indiscernible levels. If the CEA level rises again, it suggests that the tumor has metastasized and appropriate therapeutic or surgical intervention is indicated. The patient presented in the questions is gravely ill. Surgical removal of the tumor was incomplete, and metastases have developed, as indicated by the rise in CEA in months 10 to 12. The chemotherapeutic regimen should be reevaluated, and the patient should be thoroughly examined for possible radiologic and surgical treatment.

34–38. The answers are: 34-D, 35-C, 36-C, 37-A, 38-D. *(Statistics)*
The mean finishing time $(\overline{Y})$ for this group of eight subjects is the arithmetic average of their individual times:

$$\overline{Y} = \Sigma\, Y_i/n$$
$$= 36/8$$
$$= 4.5 \text{ minutes}$$

For an even number of observations, the median is the arithmetic average of the two middle values when the observations are arranged in order of ascending magnitude. Here, the eight running times, arranged in order of magnitude, are 2, 2, 4, 4, 5, 5, 5 and 9. Since n is even, the median is the average of the two middle values, 4 and 5: $(4 + 5)/2 = 4.5$ minutes.

The mode is the value in a set of observations that occurs most frequently. For these data, the modal running time is 5.0 minutes.

The range is the difference between the slowest and the fastest finishing time. Thus,

$$\text{range} = 9 - 2$$
$$= 7.0 \text{ minutes}$$

The standard deviation of the eight running times (s) is calculated from the formula

$$s = \frac{\Sigma Y_i^2 - \left(\Sigma\, Y_i\right)/n}{n - 1}$$

$$= \frac{196 - (36)^2/8}{8 - 1}$$

$$= \sqrt{34/7}, \text{ or } 2.2 \text{ minutes}$$

39. The answer is C. *(Corticosteroid therapy)*
Corticosteroids have a lympholytic effect and are good treatment for acute cellular rejection. Acute vascular rejection is less responsive to steroid therapy. Steroids have no effect on the renal toxicity of cyclosporine, the tubular damage of "harvest injury," or the fixed structural lesion of the recurrent glomerulosclerosis.

40–42. The answers are: 40-D, 41-B, 42-E. *(DNA typing for Huntington's disease)*
Evidently, the gene causing Huntington's disease (HD) in this family is inherited together with the A marker. However, II-1 has AB markers, and it is impossible to know whether she has inherited the A or the B marker from the affected father; therefore, her risk of having inherited the HD gene has not changed.

II-3 has inherited marker B from his affected father and marker B from his mother. In view of the fact that the gene for HD is inherited together with marker A, this man's risk of being affected with HD has significantly decreased.

II-4 has inherited an A marker from his mother. However, II-4 has a C marker. The supposed father (I-1) does not have a C marker. Therefore, it is highly unlikely that I-1 is the father of II-4. This being the case, II-4 has no risk of having inherited anything from I-1. The frequency of undisclosed illegitimacy is high in the population (3% to 5%) and can dramatically alter risk estimates.

43–44. The answers are: 43-C, 44-C. *(Coagulation abnormality)*
This patient's coagulation abnormality most likely is the result of vitamin K deficiency. A prolonged period of malnutrition with administration of broad-spectrum antibiotics is a common combination that frequently results in vitamin K deficiency. Correction of the prothrombin time (PT) and partial thromboplastin time (PTT) in the mixing test excludes the possibility of an acquired inhibitor. Coagulation factors would not have been diluted by the transfusion of 3 units of packed red cells; only massive transfusions might cause this effect. Folate deficiency is not associated with abnormalities of the coagulation cascade, and von Willebrand's disease does not affect the PT.

Replenishment of vitamin K is simple and without significant adverse effects, and it usually normalizes the PT within 12–24 hours. Although the patient is not bleeding, he is at increased risk for bleeding, and therefore treatment is justified. Fresh frozen plasma (FFP) and cryoprecipitate carry significant risks, and cryoprecipitation does not concentrate the necessary factors. A decision to discontinue the antibiotics must be based on the patient's infection; discontinuation would do little acutely to alter the established deficiency.

45. The answer is A. *(Immunohistochemical analysis)*
Immunohistochemical (IHC) analysis for tumor markers has revolutionized pathology because many antigens remain preserved in paraffin-embedded tissues—the routine way tissues are processed. The immunoperoxidase (IP) staining method provides a permanent slide (a major advantage of this method over immunofluorescence, which provides only temporary slides that may be difficult to read). Moreover, the IP method allows later review of the slide without loss of immunoreactivity. This method has greatly aided in tumor diagnosis by defining antigens in many tumor types. When comparing IP methods, the more enzyme molecules localized to the antigen site, the more substrate will be deposited there, making the method more sensitive. Because immune complexes are so small, they are better seen with the higher contrast of immunofluorescence—the one preferred use of this technique over IP methods. Polyclonal antibodies can be used, although they have some disadvantages.

46. The answer is C. *(Anamnestic response)*
The anamnestic response, or anamnesis, is also called the booster response, memory response, or secondary immune response. It is characterized by the prompt production of high levels of antibody (i.e., a rapid rise in antibody titers) following secondary exposure to antigen. Anamnesis is caused by the presence of B and T memory cells that were induced during the primary immune response. Immune paralysis is the inability to mount a response to a normally immunogenic substance.

47–48. The answers are: 47-C, 48-B. *(Lung compliance)*
Lung compliance is calculated as the change in volume per unit change in distending pressure. Because alveolar pressure is zero at the beginning and end of inspiration, the transmural (distending) pressure for the lung is zero minus the interpleural pressure. Only the change in interpleural pressure between the beginning

and end of inspiration is given. This difference divided into the tidal volume gives the lung compliance during dynamic conditions, or 150 and 60 ml/cm H_2O. Note that compliance is expressed as volume/pressure.

The change in this patient's lung compliance when she alters her respiratory rate is termed frequency-dependent compliance (FDC). FDC occurs in the presence of high airway resistance, which causes some acini not to fill completely at rapid rates of respiration, due to long time constants. Thus, FDC indicates the presence of high airway resistance, which is synonymous with obstructive lung disease.

49–51. The answers are: 49-E, 50-B, 51-C. *(Oxidation–reduction reactions)*
The equilibrium ratio of products to reactants is related to $\Delta G^{\circ\prime}$ by the equation:

$$\Delta G^{\circ\prime} = -RT \ln[\text{products}]/[\text{reactants}]$$

Under standard conditions, this becomes:

$$2.8 = -1.418 \log_{10}[\text{products}]/[\text{reactants}]$$
$$[\text{products}]/[\text{reactants}] = \text{antilog}(-2.0) = 0.01$$

An enzyme that catalyzes this reaction is an oxidase, which by definition uses O_2 only as an electron acceptor and does not incorporate the oxygen into the organic reactant as would an oxygenase. Peroxidases destroy H_2O_2 rather than generate them. Dehydrogenases can also convert alcohols to aldehydes but use a compound other than O_2 as an electron acceptor. Aldolases catalyze much different types of reactions.

Many oxidases possess tightly bound flavin adenine dinucleotide (FAD) as a cofactor. It is the only cofactor listed among the choices of pyridoxal phosphate, biotin, thiamine pyrophosphate, and coenzyme A that functions as an electron carrier in oxidation–reduction reactions.

52. The answer is A. *(Amanita muscaria poisoning)*
The mushroom *Amanita muscaria* causes muscarinic effects on the nervous system (i.e., sweating, narrow pupils, a slow heart rate, and low blood pressure); however, in contrast to poisoning with *Amanita phalloides*, patients usually recover without more severe problems. Methyl alcohol may cause blindness, and chloroform causes liver toxicity, which would not produce this patient's symptoms. Nasal bleeding secondary to perforation is a common presentation of cocaine sniffers. In heroin overdose, shortness of breath due to pulmonary edema is often seen.

53–55. The answers are: 53-C, 54-D, 55-A. *(Ethical theory)*
Any issue concerning the ethically correct way to allocate funds is essentially concerned with justice. Autonomy is only marginally involved (regarding the autonomy of the county in allocating its funds), and paternalism is irrelevant. Beneficence is somewhat relevant because either plan would benefit some persons, but the essential question is about which proposed allocation is ethically correct.

By arguing that spending the funds on a small number of persons would be wrong, and that it would be most productive to spend it on supplies for schoolchildren, the second council member is clearly thinking along the lines of maximizing benefits (good consequences)—the utilitarian approach. Libertarianism, rights theories, and virtue theories do not seem to play a role. The view obviously is not strict egalitarianism because the handicapped children, who have considerable needs, would not benefit from this arrangement.

The first council member's position is not libertarian, which states that one has no duty to benefit others, all charity being strictly optional. It might be a rights theory in that the children might be thought to have a right to better care. Her position might involve virtue theory, in that virtuous persons would want to correct the wrongs of the previous neglect she mentioned. And if she believes that justice requires egalitarian distributions of goods and services, her view could be either socialism or strict egalitarianism.

56–63. The answers are: 56-C, 57-C, 58-A, 59-E, 60-E, 61-B, 62-D, 63-D. *(Case–control study)*
This study uses a case–control study design; that is, it begins with the selection of cases of the disease in question (chronic otitis media) and disease-free controls. Both groups are then followed backward in time to determine exposure to the putative risk factor (parental history of ear infections).

Restriction is used in this study to equalize the comparison groups with respect to age (cases and controls are limited to children between the ages of 1 and 3. However, the comparison groups may differ with respect to other factors. If these extraneous systematic differences affect the response variable (parental history of chronic otitis media) as well as the outcome (chronic otitis media in children between 1 and 3 years of age), a biased comparison will occur. For example, low socioeconomic status (leading to a reduced access to health care, poor nutrition, etc.) may be the critical factor mediating the occurrence of chronic otitis media in both parents and their children. Case–control studies are particularly prone to recall bias. That is, the parents of children suffering from recurrent otitis media may be far more likely to remember their own history of this disorder.

The results of this study can be summarized in the following 2 × 2 table:

Parental History	Ear Infections; Cases (D+)		No Ear Infections; Controls (D−)	Totals
Childhood Ear Infections (E+)	30 a	b	20	50
No Childhood Ear Infections (E−)	20 c	d	30	50
Totals	50		50	100

The odds ratio (OR) can be calculated from the values in this table, using the formula

$$OR = (ad)/(bc)$$
$$= (30)(30)/(20)(20)$$
$$= 2.25$$

That is, the odds that children with chronic otitis media have at least one parent who also suffered from this disorder are 2.25 times greater than the odds of parental history of infection for controls.

Neither the absolute risk of chronic otitis media in children with a parental history of this disorder $[P(D+|E+)]$ nor the absolute risk for children with no such family history $[P(D+|E−)]$ can be calculated directly from the results of a case–control study. Thus, relative risk (RR), $P(D+|E+)/P(D+|E−)$, is also impossible to calculate directly. If the prevalence of otitis media in the general population were low, and if the control group is representative of the healthy population with respect to family history of chronic otitis media, then the OR would be an estimate of RR. Because otitis media is *common* rather than rare, no such estimate can be made.

The absolute risk of chronic otitis media, given a parental history of the disorder $[P(D+|E+)]$ cannot be directly calculated from the results of this case–control study. Estimates of absolute risk can be obtained only in a prospective cohort study, in which exposed and nonexposed subjects are followed forward in time to determine the incidence of the disease in question.

When an investigator wants to detect an association between two study variables (or differences among proportions) and the data are in the form of counts (such as number of children infected), the chi-square test is the appropriate statistical procedure. (For matched samples, McNemar's test, a variant of the basic chi-square test, is most appropriate.) The paired *t* test is used to detect differences between two means when study subjects have been matched and the data are continuous, whereas the independent sample (pooled) *t* test is selected for two independent samples. Correlation analysis allows the investigator to determine the magnitude of the association between two variables measured on an interval/ratio scale. Analysis of variance is used in studies involving interval/ratio data to compare the equality of several population means.

Statistical significance implies only that it is unlikely that an association at least as large as that observed would be obtained by random chance in two samples drawn from populations in which no such association actually exists. A statistically significant association is not necessarily either strong or clinically important; even a weak association may prove significant when the sample size is large. Furthermore, a statistically significant association is not proof of causality. Other confounding variables related to both exposure and the outcome may cause the two to "travel together." Statistical significance does not guarantee an absence of bias. Only careful attention to proper study design and the control of potential sources of bias can ensure internal validity.

The p value does not measure the strength of an association between two study variables, but is rather the actual probability of committing a type I error (concluding that an association exists, when, in fact, it does not). If $P \leq \alpha$, the preselected risk of a type I error the investigator is willing to tolerate, the null hypothesis is rejected.

64. The answer is E. *(Chronic renal allograft rejection)*
Active lymphocytic inflammation in tubules ("tubulitis") is a feature of acute cellular rejection. Chronic rejection of the kidney is represented by sclerosing pathology. In the vessels, chronic rejection shows vascular sclerosis; in the interstitium, fibrosis and tubular atrophy; and in the glomerular compartment, glomerulosclerosis.

65. The answer is E. *(Male external genitalia)*
The normal development of the male external genitalia requires at least one X and one Y chromosome although it also occurs in 47,XXY karyotypes as well. Testes and their steroid hormone, testosterone, are also required, but the testosterone receptor must be present as well as the hormone itself. In the male fetus, the labioscrotal swellings will ultimately form the scrotum. Paramesonephric duct derivatives form the female reproductive tract and form only vestigial structures in the male.

66. The answer is B. *(Signs of disease)*
The disease is the objective biologic phenomenon that is apprehended by a physician because of signs; disease signals a pathophysiologic alteration in normative functioning. Mood swings are not solely indicative of disease.

67. The answer is A. *(Ultrasound)*
Ultrasound provides images of fetal structure and the location of the placenta safely and noninvasively. Ultrasound by itself would not be useful for detection of Down syndrome, although ultrasound can be used to guide the sampling needle during amniocentesis, which can detect Down syndrome. Neural tube defects often show up on ultrasonography. The technique can also be used to measure skull size.

68. The answer is A. *(Lung allografts)*
Obliterative bronchiolitis (OB) refers to a progressive fibrosing lesion of the membranous and respiratory bronchioles. This chronic change may be seen in rejection, but it can also be seen in infection, ischemia, or graft-versus-host (GVH) disease. The features of acute cellular rejection in the lung depend on the severity of the rejection process. In early rejection, lymphocytic inflammation is confined to the perivascular space. With increasing severity, the inflammation spills into the interstitium and alveolar spaces, and more neutrophils are seen. Severe rejection may include hemorrhage and necrosis accompanied by hyaline membrane formation.

69. The answer is E. *(Teratogens)*
Teratogenic drugs are those known to cause structural defects in utero. Aminopterin inhibits cell division and is therefore a known teratogen. Alcohol in large doses is known to have deleterious effects on the fetus; the

effects of smaller doses are not certain. Synthetic progestins, including those in birth control pills, are known teratogens. Phenytoin is an anticonvulsant, and like certain other drugs active on the central nervous system, it is known to be teratogenic. Heroin crosses the placenta and causes addiction of the fetus, but it is not a well-established teratogenic agent.

70. The answer is D. *(Parietal lobe)*
The parietal lobe bounds the frontal lobe at the central sulcus and the temporal lobe at the sylvian fissure, and it is separated from the occipital lobe by an arbitrary line from the superior to the inferior preoccipital notches. Depending on definitions, the limbic lobe can be considered a lobe that borders the parietal lobe or as part of the parietal lobe. The calcarine sulcus splits the occipital lobe medially, and although it contacts the isthmus between the parietal and temporal lobes, it does not itself demarcate an extensive boundary of the parietal lobe.

71. The answer is E. *(Pericarditis)*
Hemochromatosis is not associated with pericarditis, although it may cause dilated or restrictive cardiomyopathy. Pericarditis is an inflammatory disorder of the visceral or parietal pericardium. Although of varied causes (infectious or noninfectious), pericarditis typically is the result of an extracardiac disorder rather than a primary cardiac disease. The varied causes of pericarditis are reflected by the different morphologic patterns of inflammation that are seen during the acute phase of pericarditis. This late sequela of pericarditis is characterized by dense fibrous thickening and, in some cases, calcification of the pericardium.

72. The answer is C. *(Role of prostaglandin in labor)*
Phosphatidyl ethanolamine (PE) contains a fatty acid called arachidonic acid. Lysosomal phospholipase would release arachidonic acid from PE. Arachidonic acid is a precursor of prostaglandin. The enzyme that converts arachidonic acid to prostaglandin is known as prostaglandin synthetase. When arachidonate levels in maternal blood increase, prostaglandin synthetase increases the prostaglandin levels. Subsequently, the prostaglandin stimulates uterine and cervical smooth muscle contraction, which is important during labor.

73. The answer is D. *(Malnutrition)*
Malnutrition has no known relationship to gastric carcinoma. The results of malnutrition obviously include emaciation. Because malnutrition depresses cellular and humoral immunity, numerous infections may occur. Malnutrition often results in fatty liver, which also may be associated with anorexia.

74. The answer is B. *(Electron microscopy)*
Electron microscopic (EM) study of tissues allows identification of a variety of disease processes. Ultrastructurally, it is easy to identify viruses, bacteria (e.g., as seen in Whipple's disease histiocytes), and immune deposits (e.g., as seen in the skin in pemphigus and in the renal glomeruli in glomerulonephritis). However, only immunohistochemistry (IHC) or DNA gene rearrangements can distinguish one type of lymphoma from another.

75. The answer is B. *(Turner syndrome)*
Turner syndrome is an example of gonadal dysgenesis. A patient with Turner syndrome has a 45, X karyotype. As a result of this genetic anomaly, normal ovaries fail to form. The abnormal ovaries that do form have no follicles in them. Therefore, secondary sexual characteristics, which are normally induced by follicular steroids, are also lacking. Sterility, lack of menses, and a webbed neck are all characteristics of patients with Turner syndrome.

76. The answer is C. *(Reticuloendothelial system)*
One of the major functions of the reticuloendothelial system (i.e., the body's storehouse of monocytes, histiocytes, and macrophages) is to clear the blood quickly of noxious matter such as bacteria, foreign particles, and cellular debris. For example, if particulate carbon were injected into the bloodstream, within minutes the carbon would be extracted from the blood by the reticuloendothelial system. The system consists of cells found in many organs, including the histiocytes in lymph node sinuses and splenic cords, the histiocytes lining hepatic sinuses (called Kupffer cells), and the histiocytes in glomeruli (called mesangial cells). Intestinal epithelial cells are not monocytes and are not directly related to the bloodstream; they can only absorb or engulf carbon from the gut lumen.

77. The answer is A. *(Renal agenesis)*
Normally, a reciprocal inductive interaction between the ureteric bud and the metanephric blastema leads to the development of the definitive adult kidney. Failure in this inductive system leads to renal agenesis. Failure of allantoic degeneration leads to urinary bladder fistula or to cysts in the umbilical region.

Renal agenesis can be unilateral or bilateral. Unilateral renal agenesis is often asymptomatic and is compatible with a normal life because of compensatory hypertrophy of the single normal kidney. Bilateral renal agenesis is associated with oligohydramnios (decreased volume of amniotic fluid) because of an absence of fetal urine production. A newborn infant with complete renal agenesis can be born normally at term because of the maternal elimination of fetal nitrogenous wastes by way of the placenta, but the infant will die soon after birth.

78–82. The answers are: 78-C, 79-A, 80-E, 81-E, 82-C. *(Nephrons)*
The solute concentration in the ascending limb of the loop of Henle (*C*) is less than that in any segment of the descending limb. The tubular fluid leaves the ascending limb at a lower concentration than it had when it entered the descending limb. Thus, the fluid presented to the distal tubule always is hyposmotic, regardless of the body's state of hydration.

Ultrafiltration separates water and nonprotein constituents (the "crystalloids") of plasma from the blood cells and protein macromolecules (the "colloids"). Except for proteins and lipids, the concentrations of crystalloids (e.g., Na^+, glucose) in the plasma and in Bowman's space (*A*) are nearly the same.

The wall of the ascending limb of the loop of Henle is relatively impermeable to water. Therefore, NaCl in this segment is reabsorbed to the virtual exclusion of water, a process that renders the medullary and papillary interstitium hyperosmotic to plasma. The medullary interstitial osmolality is higher in antidiuresis than diuresis, due largely to urea. Thus, the highest osmolality exists in the papillary interstitium. With continued reabsorption of water, urea becomes even more concentrated at the terminals of the collecting ducts (*E*).

During dehydration with maximal ADH secretion, the U_{osm}/P_{osm} approaches 4 to 1 (at *E*) because of the increased free-water reabsorption.

The macula densa is located at the junction of the thick segment of the ascending limb of the loop of Henle and the distal convoluted tubule (*C*).

83–87. The answers are: 83-D, 84-C, 85-E, 86-B, 87-A. *(Characteristics of protozoa)*
Domestic cats and other felines are the primary definitive hosts of *Toxoplasma gondii*. Infectious oocysts are excreted in the feces of these animals, and humans become infected by the fecal–oral route.

Naegleria fowleri is the etiologic agent of primary amoebic meningoencephalitis. This fulminant disease typically causes death in 3–5 days. The free-living amoeba appears to be acquired from water and dust by the respiratory route.

Trichomonas vaginalis is the etiologic agent of a sexually transmitted disease frequently seen in women. It is estimated that 3 million women acquire the disease annually in the United States. Men who acquire the infection tend to be asymptomatic.

Entamoeba histolytica is the etiologic agent of amoebic dysentery; the disease usually occurs in debilitated people and during pregnancy. It is characterized by abdominal pain, fever, and profuse bloody stools. Hepatic abscess is seen in approximately 5% of patients with clinically overt amoebiasis caused by *E. histolytica*.

Pneumocystis carinii is the etiologic agent of pneumonia in immunosuppressed people. The disease generally is rare, but it has become an important cause of fatalities in AIDS patients.

88–92. The answers are: 88-B, 89-C, 90-A, 91-D, 92-E. *(Characteristics of complement components)*
The binding of C1 and C4 by a virus–antibody complex can neutralize virus activity; it is probable that the C4 prevents viral attachment to target cells. In the alternative pathway, the $\overline{C3bBb}$ complex is cleaved by factor $\overline{D}$. The Ba fragment is released, and the $\overline{C3bBb}$ complex, stabilized by properdin, becomes a C3 convertase. C2 is thought to be involved in the symptoms of hereditary angioedema, a disease caused by uncontrolled C1s activity. C2 cleavage has been reported to be linked to the production of a kinin-like molecule that increases vascular permeability and contracts smooth muscle. C3e provokes a release of neutrophils from the bone marrow, causing prompt leukocytosis. C3e is derived, by proteolytic cleavage, from C3c, which, in turn, is derived from C3b. C3b plays an important role in opsonization.

93–97. The answers are: 93-D, 94-E, 95-A, 96-B, 97-C. *(Organelles)*
The GERL produces lysosomes that are called primary lysosomes until they participate in another metabolic event. Primary lysosomes that fuse with phagosomes form phagolysosomes, one type of heterolysosome. Primary lysosomes that fuse with cytosegresomes form autolysosomes. Partially degraded autolysosomes and phagolysosomes may be reabsorbed by the cytoplasm, expelled from the cell as cytostools, or stored in the cell as residual bodies.

98–101. The answers are: 98-B, 99-A, 100-D, 101-C. *(Testing for hematologic disorders)*
In the Ham test, the presence of paroxysmal nocturnal hemoglobinuria (PNH) is determined by incubating the patient's red cells in acidified normal serum. A positive result indicates the presence of sensitive, abnormal PNH II and PNH III cells; their hemolysis is the result of the activation of complement. Because some normal serum is inactive in this test and may give a false-negative result, the sugar water test is performed to check if the negative Ham test result is a true- or false-negative.

Although the indirect Coombs' test may give positive results in two thirds of patients with autoimmune hemolytic anemia, the direct Coombs' test will demonstrate the presence of autoantibodies, complement, or both on the red cell surface. The indirect Coombs' test demonstrates antibodies in the serum, and they are specific to antigens in the donor red cells, causing a delayed hemolytic transfusion reaction.

The formation of Heinz bodies (unstable hemoglobin precipitates) can be seen on crystal violet stain in glucose-6-phosphate dehydrogenase (G6PD) deficiency during episodes of hemolysis. Although the test is nonspecific, diagnosis is made by transiently assaying enzyme levels in red cells during the stable phase.

The test for hereditary spherocytosis (HS) is the osmotic fragility test, in which the patient's red cells are exposed to a series of sodium chloride solutions that vary from isotonic concentration (0.9%) to much lower concentrations. HS is demonstrated when hemolysis occurs at concentrations of 0.6% to 0.8%; normal cells do not demonstrate hemolysis until concentrations of 0.4% to 0.5% are reached. HS red cells are already in the form of spherocytes and do not have much leeway for expansion in response to the low sodium concentration of their test environment. Normal cells are able to withstand much lower sodium concentrations.

102–106. The answers are: 102-C, 103-E, 104-D, 105-A, 106-B. *(Inherited disorders)*
A disorder is said to be nonpenetrant when there is no clinical evidence of a mutant allele in an individual known to have inherited the gene. When the gene is expressed, the form of expression may be highly variable, with some family members being severely affected and others having few signs of the disorder. This is common with autosomal disorders and is called variable expression. Different mutations of either the same

gene (i.e., at the same locus) or different genes may give a similar clinical picture. Consanguineous individuals have a proportion of their genes in common by inheritance from a common ancestor. In some villages originated by a few settlers, disease alleles may be in higher frequencies, and a particular recessive disorder may be more common in that community.

107–111. The answers are: 107-B, 108-B, 109-A, 110-D, 111-E. *(Afferent fibers of the cerebellar cortex)* The afferent tracts to the cerebellum generally terminate in specific regions. The vermis receives the bulk of the spinocerebellar tracts and the trigeminocerebellar tract.

The hemispheres receive projections from the principal olivary nuclei and from the basis pontis.

The flocculonodular lobe is the oldest part of the cerebellum phylogenetically and the part from which the whole cerebellum originates. It originally received the vestibular connections, both through direct connections to the vestibular nerve and through the vestibular nuclei, and it retains these connections although the phylogenetically newer parts of the cerebellum are much larger in higher animals. From its original role as an integrating center for the vestibular system in controlling the axial muscles, the cerebellum now has the role of coordinating the appendicular or limb muscles. The parts of the cerebellum that perform this function have increased in size in accordance with the size of the cerebral motor cortex and the cortical efferent system through the pyramidal and corticopontocerebellar tracts.

The rostral vermis also receives projections from the visual and auditory systems, although the functional role of these projections is not well understood. Many of the afferent pathways to the cerebellum also send collaterals to the deep cerebellar nuclei as they pass through the deep cerebellar white matter on their way to the cerebellar cortex. The nucleus locus ceruleus projects diffusely to the cerebellum just as it projects diffusely to most other parts of the central nervous system (CNS).

112–115. The answers are: 112-B, 113-D, 114-C, 115-A. *(Glucose 6-phosphate metabolites)* Glucose 1-phosphate, which is formed from glucose 6-phosphate (G6P), is the precursor for glycogen formation. Conversion of G6P to fructose 6-phosphate occurs in the glycolytic pathway. Subsequent reactions yield pyruvate, which is the end product of glycolysis. Conversion of G6P to 6-phosphogluconate is the first step in the pentose phosphate pathway, which yields ribose 5-phosphate as a product. In gluconeogenic tissues, such as the liver, G6P may be dephosphorylated to directly form glucose.

116–119. The answers are: 116-D, 117-C, 118-B, 119-A. *(Embryonic structures)* The site where the liver diverticulum (A) and the pancreatic buds (C) arise is the boundary between the foregut and the midgut. The liver diverticulum (A) forms the epithelial parenchymal cells, which have both an endocrine and an exocrine function. The pancreatic buds (C) form part of the pancreas, including the islets of Langerhans. The midgut (B) forms the distal small intestine, including most of the duodenum, all of the jejunum, and all of the ileum, as well as the ascending and proximal transverse colon. The cloaca (D) is a hindgut derivative that receives the excurrent ducts of the urinary and reproductive systems. The vitelline duct (E) is a midgut diverticulum that projects into the umbilicus and serves as the axis of rotation of the midgut loop along with the superior mesenteric artery.

120–125. The answers are: 120-C, 121-E, 122-F, 123-B, 124-A, 125-D. *(Stages of neutrophil maturation)* Neutrophil maturation progresses through several morphologic stages, beginning with the myeloblast. The myeloblast (C) is characterized by immature nuclear chromatin but no cytoplasmic differentiation; the promyelocyte (A) has cytoplasmic azurophilic granules; the myelocyte (F) demonstrates progressive chromatin condensation and emergence of secondary granules; the metamyelocyte (D) has additional secondary granules and nuclear indentation; the band neutrophil (E) demonstrates further nuclear constriction; and the mature neutrophil (B) exhibits nuclear segmentation.

Most peripheral blood or bone marrow cells are easily classified according to this scheme, but cells with morphologic features intermediate between different stages can always be found. Some hematologists prefer to place such cells in the more mature group. In disorders characterized by significant disturbance of myeloid maturation with asynchrony of cytoplasmic and nuclear development (e.g., myelodysplastic syndromes), classification according to normal differentiation schemes may be difficult for many cells.

126–130. The answers are: 126-E, 127-C, 128-A, 129-D, 130-B. *(Brain lesions)*

The topographic representation of the visual fields is very strict. For this reason, lesions affecting particular sites along the optic pathway cause very characteristic and reproducible field defects. Lesions of the parts of the geniculocalcarine pathway as it courses through the hemispheric wall cause different field defects, depending on the location. Because the geniculocalcarine fibers course deep in the white matter, in the external sagittal stratum (which is a few millimeters lateral to the ventricular wall), the cerebral lesions that cause field defects must be deep within the white matter rather than limited to the cortex or immediately subjacent white matter. A lesion of the most anterior fibers of the geniculocalcarine tract as it loops around the temporal horn causes a contralateral superior quadrantanopia, which is more or less complete, depending on the number of fibers affected.

As the geniculocalcarine tract proceeds backward, the fibers that represent the inferior visual fields course through the inferior part of the parietal lobe. Hence, lesions of the inferior parietal region that interrupt these fibers give rise to a contralateral inferior homonymous field defect.

Lesions of one occipital lobe likewise cause contralateral defects, which may vary from partial quadrantanopia to a complete contralateral hemianopia. Bilateral occipital lobe destruction causes double hemianopia or, in essence, complete blindness.

Lesions of the superior or inferior banks of the calcarine fissure, either unilateral or bilateral, cause quadrantanopias or hemianopias, depending on the extent of the tissue destroyed. Destruction of either the superior banks or the inferior banks on both sides causes an altitudinal hemianopia. Destruction of the superior banks causes an inferior altitudinal hemianopia in both eyes; destruction of the inferior banks causes a superior altitudinal hemianopia.

Lesions of the cerebral white matter beyond the actual course of the geniculocalcarine tracts do not cause field defects, nor do lesions of the corpus callosum. The latter lesions interfere with transfer of visual information from one hemisphere to the other but do not cause field defects.

131–135. The answers are: 131-C, 132-E, 133-D, 134-B, 135-A. *(Pathologic responses)*

Caseating granulomas are found in tuberculosis, whereas noncaseating granulomas are seen in berylliosis as well as many other diseases. Simple emphysema has a variety of causes, such as smoking, but the emphysematous changes seen in the pneumoconioses are not simple. Pleural calcifications are typical of asbestosis, and nodules with polarizable silica are seen in silicosis.

136–144. The answers are: 136-A, 137-C, 138-A, 139-B, 140-B, 141-E, 142-A, 143-A, 144-A. *(Pathophysiological mechanisms of sickle cell disease)*

The normal deformation of red cells as they move through the microcirculation to release oxygen is not possible for sickle cells, which become trapped and block the vessels. As adjacent cells attempt to compensate for the resultant tissue anoxia, they also become plugged, which starts a cycle of vaso-occlusion and tissue anoxia. Tissue necrosis results and is the source of the chronic and acute pain of sickle cell anemia. Sickle cells also become trapped in the cords of the spleen when their inclusions grow in response to the relatively anoxic environment, preventing them from squeezing through into the sinuses. These patients lose their splenic function by late infancy because of infarction and anemia, resulting in predisposition to infection by encapsulated organisms. Gallstones result in precipitation of excess bile from the metabolism of heme, which is increased because of hemolysis.

145–149. The answers are: 145-D, 146-B, 147-A, 148-C, 149-B. *(Distal lung components)*

Alveoli (*C*) in the lungs are lined by an epithelium that contains type I cells and type II cells. Type I cells (*A*) are extremely attenuated squamous cells specialized for gas exchange. Type II cells (*B*) are rounded cells containing phospholipid-rich multilamellar bodies of secretion product (surfactant). Alveoli are adjacent to capillaries, which are filled with erythrocytes (*D*). Macrophages are abundant in alveoli, where they phagocytose and destroy inspired debris such as bacteria.

150–152. The answers are: 150-C, 151-A, 152-B. *(Acid–base disturbance)*

Hyperventilation is defined as alveolar ventilation in excess of the body's need for CO_2 elimination, which results in decreased arterial P_{CO_2}—the underlying factor in respiratory alkalosis. Although P_{CO_2} is not given, it can be calculated using the mathematical relationship: $[HCO_3^-]/S \times P_{CO_2} = 20/1$. Applying this equation, it is clear that the values in *set C* indicate a decrease in P_{CO_2}, as

$$\frac{15}{S \times P_{CO_2}} = \frac{20}{1} \text{ , or S} \times P_{CO_2} = 0.75 \text{ mmol/L}$$

Since

$$S \times P_{CO_2} = 0.75 \text{ mmol/L}$$

and

$$S = 0.03 \text{ mmol/L/mm Hg,}$$

then

$$P_{CO_2} = \frac{0.75 \text{ mmol/L}}{0.03 \text{ mmol/L/mm Hg}} = 25 \text{ mm Hg}$$

A P_{CO_2} of 25 mm Hg is significantly lower than normal (40 mm Hg). In acute respiratory alkalosis, there is a decrease in urinary H^+ excretion and an increase in urinary HCO_3^- excretion. In this case, there has been complete renal compensation, as evidenced by the return of the $[HCO_3^-]/S \times P_{CO_2}$ ratio to normal (20:1).

In chronic respiratory tract obstruction (e.g., due to tracheal stenosis, foreign body, or tumor), alveolar ventilation is insufficient to excrete CO_2 at a rate required by the body, which leads to increased arterial P_{CO_2}—the underlying factor in respiratory acidosis. When P_{CO_2} is increased, the kidney is unable to reabsorb HCO_3^-. The kidney increases H^+ secretion, resulting in the addition of HCO_3^- to the ECF. The values in *set A* coincide with these changes. In this case, there is partial compensation of the respiratory acidosis as evidenced by the lesser increase in $[HCO_3^-]$. In chronic respiratory acidosis, the respiratory centers become less sensitive to hypercapnia and acidosis and rely on the associated hypoxemia as the primary drive to ventilation. Correction of the low P_{O_2} by the administration of O_2 will diminish respiratory drive, resulting in hypoventilation, a further increase in P_{CO_2}, and possibly CO_2 narcosis. For this reason, O_2 must be given with extreme caution to patients with chronic hypercapnia.

Metabolic acidosis exhibits the characteristics of increased $[H^+]$ (decreased pH), a reduced $[HCO_3^-]$, and a compensatory hyperventilation resulting in hypocapnia. The kidney responds to the increased H^+ load by increasing the secretion and excretion of NH_4^+ and the excretion of titratable acid ($H_2PO_4^-$). The values in *set B* coincide with these changes.

153–156. The answers are: 153-D, 154-A, 155-E, 156-C. *(Presynaptic inhibition)*

In presynaptic inhibition, an inhibitory neuron forms an axo-axonic synapse with the neuron that is excitatory to the alpha motoneuron. The inhibitory neuron releases γ-aminobutyric acid [GABA] (*A*), which opens Cl^- channels on the postsynaptic membrane (*C*). The action potential invading the nerve terminal is reduced in size. As a result, less Ca^{2+} enters the nerve terminal (*D*), less transmitter is released, and the magnitude of the excitatory postsynaptic potential on the motoneuron is reduced (*E*). (*B*) is the portion of the axon that is not affected by presynaptic inhibition.

157–161. The answers are: 157-C, 158-E, 159-D, 160-A, 161-B. *(Gametogenic cells)*
The primordial germ cells are diploid proliferative cells derived from the wall of the yolk sac. They differentiate into diploid spermatogonia and oogonia. Primary spermatocytes are tetraploid cells that are produced in vast quantities by mitosis of spermatogonia in the male after puberty. The proliferation of spermatogonia and production of primary spermatocytes continue until death. Primary oocytes are tetraploid cells that are arrested in meiosis I from their time of formation (before birth) until ovulation at some time later, up to menopause. Secondary oocytes are diploid cells that undergo unequal cytoplasmic divisions to produce small polar bodies and ova. Secondary spermatocytes are diploid cells that undergo equal cytoplasmic divisions to form spermatids, which subsequently differentiate into spermatozoa during spermiogenesis.

162–166. The answers are: 162-C, 163-B, 164-D, 165-E, 166-A. *(Factors and proteins)*
Catabolite activator protein (CAP), also called cyclic adenosine monophosphate (cAMP) receptor protein (CRP) is a positive transcription regulatory factor in prokaryotes. In the presence of cAMP (caused by low levels of glucose), CAP greatly enhances the initiation of transcription at CAP-responsive promoters.

The dnaA protein is required for proper initiation of replication in *Escherichia coli*. It binds to specific sequences within the origin of replication, and, in the presence of adenosine triphosphate (ATP) and other components of replication, dnaA protein facilitates initiation of replication.

Although the exact mechanism is unknown, rho (ρ) protein binds as a hexamer to rho-dependent termination sequences, and, upon cleavage of ATP by rho, termination of transcription takes place.

The eukaryotic transcription factor IID (TFIID) is needed to initiate transcription from TATA box promoters by RNA polymerase II. TFIID recognizes and binds to the TATA box sequences independently of RNA polymerase II.

Sigma (σ) factor is required for proper initiation of transcription in prokaryotes. It enables the RNA polymerase holoenzyme to recognize and bind to the promoter sequences and accurately initiate transcription.

167–171. The answers are: 167-C, 168-B, 169-A, 170-E, 171-D. *(Organs and tissues in the postabsorptive state)*
The flow of metabolites shown in the figure occurs during the postabsorptive state, several hours after a meal. The adipose tissue releases fatty acids, which are used by the heart, skeletal muscle, and liver for fuel. Glycerol, which is taken up by the liver and converted to glucose, is also released by adipose tissue. The liver releases glucose into the blood. The glucose, which is derived from glycogenolysis and gluconeogenesis, is taken up and used for fuel by the brain and skeletal muscle. The skeletal muscle releases lactate, formed from glucose via pyruvate, which is taken up by the liver and used as a substrate for gluconeogenesis.

172–176. The answers are: 172-B, 173-A, 174-D, 175-C, 176-E. *(Inflammatory heart disease)*
Chronic rheumatic heart disease refers to the long-term cardiac complications (especially valvular) of acute rheumatic fever. Typically, the mitral and aortic valve leaflets become thickened and deformed by fibrosis, with commissural fusion. The damaged valves represent a fertile ground for the development of infective endocarditis (subacute type).

Chronic rheumatic heart disease is a complication of rheumatic fever, which is a nonsuppurative systemic disorder related to an untreated pharyngitis caused by group A β-hemolytic streptococci. Although the precise mechanism of acute rheumatic fever is unknown, the presence of antistreptococcal antibodies that cross-react with heart antigens in these patients suggests an autoimmune basis for this disorder.

Subacute bacterial endocarditis most commonly is caused by α-hemolytic (viridans) streptococci, an organism that is a normal component of the oral flora. Typically, the organism gains entry to the circulation with minor oral trauma, and a transient bacteremia ensues. The bacteria then colonize a platelet–fibrin thrombus that has formed on a valve previously damaged by chronic rheumatic heart disease, mitral valve prolapse, previous cardiac surgery, or some other cause.

The acute form of bacterial endocarditis, in contrast to the subacute form, typically involves a normal heart valve in the setting of a well-defined bacteremia. In this case, the infectious agent usually is a virulent organism (e.g., *Staphylococcus aureus*) that causes the initial damage to the valves by way of a toxin.

Libman-Sacks endocarditis (also known as nonbacterial verrucous endocarditis) may occur as a complication of systemic lupus erythematosus. This disorder is characterized by the presence of warty endocardial vegetations along the valve margins and, most distinctively, on the undersurface of the valves.

177–182. The answers are: 177-B, 178-E, 179-D, 180-A, 181-C, 182-D. *(Adenohypophysial cells)*

Corticotropes are basophils that secrete adrenocorticotropic hormone (ACTH). ACTH regulates adrenal cortical steroid production and, thus, regulates blood and urine ionic composition. Corticotropes have large granules and abundant cytoplasmic filaments.

Gonadotropes are basophils with medium-sized granules. Their granules are larger than the small granules of thyrotropes and smaller than the large granules of corticotropes. Gonadotropes secrete luteinizing hormone (LH) and follicle-stimulating hormone (FSH), which are hormones that help control spermatogenesis and ovulation.

Somatotropes are acidophils that secrete growth hormone (GH). GH secretion is decreased in pituitary dwarfs.

Thyrotropes are basophils with small granules. Thyrotropes secrete thyroid-stimulating hormone (TSH), a hormone that regulates basal metabolic rate.

Lactotropes are acidophils that secrete prolactin, a hormone that stimulates mammary gland development and lactation.

183–185. The answers are: 183-E, 184-C, 185-D. *(Drug action)*

Mitomycin is both a natural product and an alkylating agent. Isolated from a *Streptomyces* species, mitomycin C is reduced by a reduced nicotinamide adenine dinucleotide phosphate (NADPH)–dependent reductase and alkylates DNA.

Cytarabine inhibits DNA polymerase and, thus, kills cells in S phase. Cytarabine nucleotides can be incorporated into DNA and RNA, but the significance of this is not known.

Vincristine, a natural product, is an M-phase–specific agent, blocking proliferating cells as they enter metaphase.

186–190. The answers are: 186-C, 187-E, 188-A, 189-D, 190-B. *(Measurements of renal function)*

The use of inulin clearance (C_{in}) to measure glomerular filtration rate (GFR) is valid because all of the filtered inulin is excreted in the urine without being reabsorbed or secreted by the renal tubules. Thus, GFR is equal to C_{in} as

$$GFR = C_{in} = \frac{U_{in} \times \dot{V}}{P_{in}}$$

where U_{in} and P_{in} = the urinary and plasma inulin concentrations, respectively, and $\dot{V}$ = the urinary volume/minute. Substituting,

$$GFR = C_{in} = \frac{150 \text{ mg/ml} \times 1.2 \text{ ml/min}}{1.5 \text{ mg/ml}}$$

$$= \frac{180 \text{ mg/min}}{1.5 \text{ mg/ml}}$$

$$= 120 \text{ ml/min}$$

Note that with a unit analysis, both mg/ml terms cancel out.

Renal plasma flow (RPF) is calculated from the clearance of para-aminohippuric acid (PAH); however, there are no PAH data provided for this patient. Therefore, it is necessary to determine RPF from the filtration fraction (FF), defined as the ratio of GFR to RPF, or

$$FF = \frac{GFR}{RPF}$$

FF can be calculated from the arterial and venous inulin concentrations as

$$\text{fraction of inulin filtered} = \frac{A_{in} - V_{in}}{A_{in}}$$

where A_{in} and V_{in} are the arterial and venous inulin concentrations, respectively. Substituting,

$$FF = \frac{1.50 \text{ mg/ml} - 1.20 \text{ mg/ml}}{1.50 \text{ mg/ml}}$$

$$= \frac{0.3}{1.50} = 0.20$$

With FF and GFR determined, the RPF is easily determined as

$$FF = \frac{GFR}{RPF}; RPF = \frac{GFR}{FF} = \frac{120}{0.2} \text{ ml/min} = 600 \text{ ml/min}$$

Because FF = the ratio of GFR to RPF, FF also can be calculated using the extraction of a substance such as inulin to determine RPF. If the urinary concentration of inulin is 150 mg/ml and the urine flow rate is 1.2 ml/min, the urinary excretion rate of inulin is 180 mg/min. If, when the excretion rate was measured, the inulin concentration was 1.50 mg/ml in renal arterial plasma and 1.20 mg/ml in renal venous plasma, each milliliter of plasma traversing the kidneys must have contributed 0.30 mg to the 180 mg that was excreted. Therefore, the RPF must have been

$$\frac{180 \text{ mg/min}}{0.3 \text{ mg/ml}} = 600 \text{ ml/min}$$

Thus, with the RPF determined, FF can be calculated as

$$FF = \frac{GFR}{RPF} = \frac{120 \text{ ml/min}}{600 \text{ ml/min}} = 0.2$$

Once RPF is determined, renal blood flow (RBF) can also be discerned. RBF is calculated by dividing RPF by the term (1 − hematocrit), or

$$RBF = \frac{RPF}{1 - \text{hematocrit}} = \frac{600 \text{ ml/min}}{1 - 0.40} = \frac{600 \text{ ml/min}}{0.60} = 1000 \text{ ml/min}$$

The quantity (or amount) of the substance filtered per unit time is termed the filtered load (FL), or amount filtered. It is equal to the product of the GFR (or C_{in}) and the plasma concentration of that substance, or

$$FL = GFR \times P_G$$
$$= 120 \text{ ml/min} \times 0.9 \text{ mg/ml}$$
$$= 108 \text{ mg/min}$$

Note that the ml terms cancel out with a unit analysis and that it is necessary to express the plasma glucose concentration (P_G) in mg/ml and not in the unit of mg/dl given in the original data.

191–193. The answers are: 191-A, 192-B, 193-C. *(Effects of neuroleptic drugs)*
Lactation (via the tuberoinfundibular tract) and parkinsonism (via the nigrostriatal tract) both are associated with the effects of neuroleptic drugs on postsynaptic dopamine 2 (D_2) receptors. Some of the antipsychotic effects are also thought to be mediated by dopaminergic blockade, but the brain tracts involved are believed to be the mesolimbic and possibly the mesocortical pathways. There is little evidence that the nigrostriatal and tuberoinfundibular tracts are important in the direct antipsychotic effects of neuroleptics. However, other neurotransmitter systems probably are involved in the neuroleptic effects.

194–198. The answers are: 194-D, 195-C, 196-B, 197-E, 198-A. *(Skull bones)*
The mandible (*A*) and maxilla (*B*) are both parts of the membranous viscerocranium, as is the zygomatic arch (*D*). The mandible forms around Meckel's cartilage. The maxilla has lateral palatine processes on its medial borders, and these form the secondary palate. Both the mandible and the maxilla have teeth with dentin (an odontoblast derivative) but the zygomatic arch does not. The parietal bone (*E*) is part of the membranous neurocranium and is on the posterior border of the anterior fontanelle. The lower portion of the occipital bone (*C*) is part of the cartilaginous neurocranium, and the upper portion is part of the membranous neurocranium.

199–203. The answers are: 199-B, 200-B, 201-C, 202-D, 203-E. *(Muscles)*
The supraspinatus, infraspinatus, teres minor, and subscapularis comprise the rotator cuff that acts across the glenohumeral joint and dynamically stabilizes the shoulder. The subscapularis, forming the posterior wall of the axilla, is a strong medial rotator of the arm. It is innervated by the upper and lower subscapular branches of the posterior cord of the branchial plexus. The supraspinatus, innervated by the suprascapular nerve, initiates abduction of the arm through the first 15°, at which point the deltoid muscle assumes this function. The infraspinatus and teres minor are both lateral rotators, the former of which is innervated by the suprascapular nerve, and the latter by the axillary nerve. The musculocutaneous nerve innervates the coracobrachialis, biceps, and brachialis muscles.

204–207. The answers are: 204-D, 205-E, 206-B, 207-E. *(Immunoglobulins)*
The complement system, which plays a major role in host defense and the inflammatory process, can be activated (fixed) via the classic or alternative pathways. Activation of the pathways may occur via antigen–antibody complexes or by aggregated immunoglobulins. IgG molecules (mainly the IgG1 and IgG3 subclasses) are capable of fixing complement. Activation of the classic pathway follows binding of complement to the C_H2 domain on the Fc fragment of IgG. Serum IgA fixes complement via the alternative pathway only. Activation of this pathway can be triggered immunologically primarily by IgA (and to a lesser degree by some IgG). IgM is the most efficient immunoglobulin at activating complement via the classic pathway. Only one molecule of IgM is required to react with complement. Activation of the classic pathway follows binding of complement to the C_H3 domain on the Fc fragment of IgM.

208–211. The answers are: 208-D, 209-E, 210-A, 211-B. *(Anti-infective agents)*
Tetracyclines (e.g., demeclocycline) are effective in the treatment of *Chlamydia* infections. Agents such as demeclocycline can produce a severe phototoxic skin reaction.

Rifampin, which is used in combination with isoniazid and ethambutol for the treatment of tuberculosis, may cause urine, sweat, tears, and contact lenses to have a harmless orange color.

Clindamycin is the drug of first choice for *Bacteroides fragilis* infections. It can produce pseudomembranous colitis as an untoward effect.

The aminoglycosides (e.g., gentamicin) are polycations, which accounts for their pharmacokinetic properties, including poor oral absorption. These agents have a predilection for causing both ototoxicity and nephrotoxicity.

Dr. Patel
Dermatology slides

810 - 548 - 6767

step 2
- Geriatrics
- Emergency care

pg 226

24 - D
25 - C
26 - C
27 - B - A
28 - C
29 - C
30 - C
31 - B
31 - D
32 - D
33 - C